MILADY'S AESTHETICIAN SERIES

Advanced
Hair Removal

MILADY'S AESTHETICIAN SERIES

Advanced
Hair Removal

PAMELA HILL, R.N.
HELEN R. BICKMORE

THOMSON

DELMAR LEARNING

Australia Canada Mexico Singapore Spain United Kingdom United States

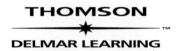

Milady's Aesthetician Series: Advanced Hair Removal
Pamela Hill and Helen R. Bickmore

President, Milady:
Dawn Gerrain

Managing Editor:
Robert L. Serenka

Acquisitions Editor:
Martine Edwards

Product Manager:
Jennifer Anderson

Editorial Assistant:
Falon Ferraro

Director of Content and Media Production:
Wendy A. Troeger

Content Project Manager:
Nina Tucciarelli

Composition:
Pre-PressPMG

Director of Marketing:
Wendy Mapstone

Director Beauty Industry Relations:
Sandra Bruce

Marketing Coordinator:
Nicole Riggi

Text Design:
Essence of Seven

Library of Congress Cataloging-in-Publication Data
Hill, Pamela, RN.
   Advanced hair removal / Pamela Hill, Helen Bickmore.
      p. ; cm. -- (Milady's aesthetician series)
   Includes bibliographical references and index.
      ISBN-13: 978-1-4018-8174-0
      ISBN-10: 1-4018-8174-2
   1. Hair--Removal. I. Bickmore, Helen R. II. Title. III. Series: Hill, Pamela, RN. Milady's aesthetician series.
      [DNLM: 1. Hair Removal. 2. Hair--physiology. WR 450 H647a 2008]
      RL92.A3885 2008
      617.4'779--dc22
                          2007014857

NOTICE TO THE READER

Contents

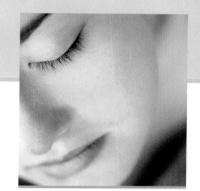

■ CHAPTER 4

■ CHAPTER 5

■ CHAPTER 10

225 | THREADING AND SUGARING

■ CHAPTER 11

243 | ELECTROLYSIS

Preface

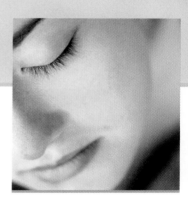

In mainstream U.S. culture we aspire to smooth, silky, hair-free skin, whether it be a man's back or a lady's legs. Superfluous hair on a woman's face is considered undesirable. For these reasons and many others, hair removal is among the more popular treatments in the United States. The treatments range from temporary methods like waxing to permanent reduction by laser hair removal to permanent removal by electrolysis with many other options in between. A technician who understands the anatomy and physiology of hair growth, skin typing, and options in hair removal can develop a very nice business of repeat clients. In many cases hair removal is an art as well as a science. Understanding which procedure is right for the client and having an aesthetic eye to create a pleasing result (such as the correct eyebrow shape) are keys to success. This book will guide the reader through procedures such as waxing to the high-tech treatments of electrolysis and laser hair removal. Specific chapters are dedicated to particular methods of hair removal. Within the chapter, the reader will learn the most important aspects of the treatment methods, how to apply them to a specific situation, and the problems that can occur from incorrect applications or not following protocol.

Because hair removal is so popular, it is important to understand all of the options that are available and be able to perform the treatments correctly. This book will help you to improve and refine your skills, answer questions, and become successful in these very popular techniques.

About the Authors

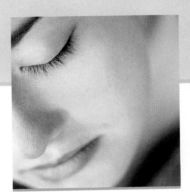

Pamela Hill received her nursing diploma from Presbyterian Hospital and Colorado Women's College, Denver, Colorado, and has practiced as a registered nurse for more than 20 years. Her background includes 15 years of operational and leadership experience in the medical spa, medical skin care, and educational sector. Ms. Hill has been instrumental in the growth and development of Facial Aesthetics, Inc. ("FAI"), a successful Colorado-based medical spa. An astute results-oriented leader with a proven track record of building and growing companies in the medical appearance sector, she has been actively involved in the evolution of the medical spa model as well as the research and development of the Pamela Hill Skin Care product line. Ms. Hill has been active with patient care, the development of policy and procedure, and clinician education. Passionate about the education of aestheticians in the medical spa setting, Ms. Hill began a relationship with Milady, an imprint of Thomson Delmar Learning, in 2003. This relationship launched Ms. Hill's authoring of the Aesthetician Series, a 12-book series dedicated to the education of medical aestheticians and the must-have information for on-the-job success. Currently six of the books are in print.

Helen R. Bickmore received her diplomas for Beauty Therapy (aesthetics), Body Treatments, Massage, and Electrolysis in 1979 through both the London College of Fashion and the City and Guilds of London Institute (CGLI).

She is a New York State Licensed Esthetician and Massage Therapist (LMT), is a Certified Professional Electrologist (CPE) with the American Electrology Association (AEA), and a Certified Medical Electrologist (CME) with the Society for Clinical and Medical Hair Removal, Inc. (SCMHR).

Ms. Bickmore has taught aesthetics at (the former) Scarborough Technical College, now called the Yorkshire Coast College, in Yorkshire, England, and over the years has worked in salons and had her own business in the United Kingdom and the United States. She has worked as a Spa Director and continues to provide services to a large clientele.

Ms. Bickmore is the author of *Milady's Hair Removal Techniques, A Comprehensive Manual* (Thomson Delmar Learning, 2004). In addition, she has reviewed manuscripts, written articles, appeared on television news programs, given workshops, and served on a number of panels. She currently serves on the board of the New York Electrology Association.

She resides in Albany, NY, with her husband of 20 years and three children.

Acknowledgments

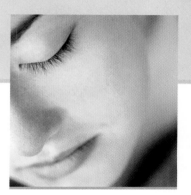

Books that require the knowledge of techniques and technology are typically not written by a single person. Such is the case in this situation. Contributing authors, reviewers, and the editors at Milady have helped to bring this book to print.

Milady and the authors would like to thank the following for contributing to this text:

Christine Gordon, President of International Education Group, Graham Webb Academy, for hosting our photo shoot at her school in Arlington, VA

Elena L. Reichel, PR and Partners

All location photographs were provided by Larry Hamill Photography, Columbus, OH

Models who participated in the photo shoot:

Anastasia Arnold
Julianne Baddock
Robin Carlson
Randi Engel
Swaroopa Giangapathy
Isabella Gomez
Michaela Hulgaard
Courtney Hungerford
Jenna McDonald
Tram Nguyen
Lisa Nyden
Janice Ricketts
Barry Smithers
Sarah Tope
Jenny Vo
Kim Williams
Tania Williams

Photo credits

Chapter 1: Figure 1–4: Courtesy of Leon Prete, LMT, and Barbara Prete, CE, SafeLase Institute for Cosmetic Laser Training. Figure 1–5: Photograph courtesy of Facial Aesthetics.

Chapter 5: Figure 5–4: LightSheer® diode hair removal laser, courtesy of Lumenis®. Figure 5–5: Courtesy of Syneron. Figure 5–6: Courtesy of Dectro International.

Chapter 6: Figure 6–11: Courtesy of Leon Prete, LMT, and Barbara Prete, CE, SafeLase Institute for Cosmetic Laser Training.

Chapter 7: Figures 7–5, 7–8, 7–10, 7–12, 7–13, 7–14, 7–15: Courtesy of Leon Prete, LMT, and Barbara Prete, CE, SafeLase Institute for Cosmetic Laser Training. Figure 7–11: LightSheer® diode hair removal laser, courtesy of Lumenis®.

Chapter 8: Figure 8–3: Courtesy of CDC/ Dr. Herrmann. Figure 8–5: Courtesy of Thom Cammer, Albany, NY.

Chapter 11: Figures 11–5, 11–6: Courtesy of Thom Cammer, Albany, NY.

Reviewers

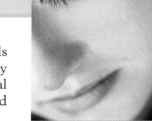

The authors and publisher would like to thank the following individuals who have reviewed this text and offered invaluable feedback. This very important task, although time consuming for each reviewer, is a critical component to the success of a book. We are grateful for your time and honest comments.

Elizabeth Myron,
General Manager, Hive Beauty USA

Kathy Phelps,
Moore Norman Technology Center, Norman, OK

Michael A. Herion, MD,
Institute for Medical Aesthetics, Scottsdale, AZ

Kathy Hernandez, L.Ac. Dipl. Ac.,
San Bernardino, CA

Maggie McNerney,
Holyoke, MA

Sandra Peoples,
Counselor, Instructor,
Pickens Technical Center, CO

Leon Prete, LMT,
SafeLase Institute for Cosmetic Laser Training, Milford, CT

Nancy Tomaselli,
Instructor,
Cerritos Community College, Norwalk, CA

Natasha Amber Ogorodnitsky, LE, LMBT, NCTMB,
Florida College of Natural Health, Ft. Lauderdale, FL

Introduction to Hair Removal

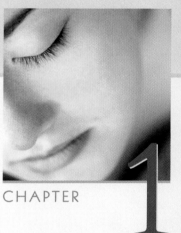

CHAPTER 1

KEY TERMS

Achard-Thiers syndrome

adrenogenital syndrome

bloodborne pathogens

career plan

clinic protocols

contaminated

Continuing Education Units (CEU)

Cushing's syndrome

hirsutism

hypertrichosis

mission statement

Occupational Safety and Health Administration (OSHA)

polycystic ovary syndrome

professional ethics

progressive improvement plan

pseudofolliculitis barbae

reflexology

Safety Bill of Rights

safety manual

technique sensitive

thioglycolate

Universal Precautions

LEARNING OBJECTIVES

After completing this chapter, you should be able to:

1. Identify the different types of hair removal.
2. Develop a plan for marketing yourself.
3. Know the basics about licensure.

INTRODUCTION

Beginning in adolescence, boys and girls experience a sequence of body changes that carry into adulthood. Although these changes are often difficult for teenagers to appreciate, the changes signify signs of normal development and growth. Changes that involve unwanted hair growth can be especially difficult to accept, especially for women. As a result, some individuals may try one or more methods to reduce, permanently remove, or temporarily remove unwanted hair. Finding the best treatment for hair removal usually depends on the characteristics of hair (i.e., quantity, quality, color), the location of hair, and the cost of removal techniques.

While general statements can be made about skin type and ethnicity, hair quality (thinness and thickness) and quantity (amount of hair) can vary significantly. The hair on one person may be thicker, longer, or curlier than on another person, and this is true for related or unrelated individuals. Coloration can also vary from one person to the next and from one strand of hair to another. All these factors can contribute to an individual's decision to consider removal as well as the type of hair removal process an individual may select.

Location is another consideration for hair removal. Hair removal is a personal choice that can be influenced by convenience, societal norms, appearance, and self-esteem. Common areas for hair removal for women include face, legs, face/eyebrows, arms, pubic region, and underarms, and for men, the back and shoulders.

Cost is another consideration when it comes to hair removal. Costs vary significantly with hair removal. A razor and shaving cream might cost $5 to $10, while laser hair removal might cost $50 to $1,000 per area. Because of the wide range in cost, many individuals might not be able to afford the removal technique they would prefer.

■ INTRODUCTION TO HAIR REMOVAL METHODS

Hair removal can be divided into four main categories: permanent hair removal, permanent *reduction,* temporary hair removal, and camouflaging. The FDA (Food and Drug Administration) and AMA (American Medical Association) only allow the term permanent *reduction* for laser hair removal. Permanent hair removal is long term (at least one year) and is accomplished by destroying or injuring the dermal papilla of the hair. Because individuals have varying degrees of follicular density, many treatments may be necessary to accomplish complete hair removal in a given area.

The second removal procedure is temporary hair removal, which is accomplished by eliminating the hair at the root and causes little or no damage to the hair follicle. Some types of temporary hair removal include eradicating the hair root from the follicle (i.e., waxing, tweezing, sugaring), while others leave the root intact by clipping or removing the hair at the surface (i.e., shaving, depilatory remedies). The treatments that remove the hair from the root will have longer lasting results. Shaving and depilatory treatments have to be done more often but, obviously, are less expensive.

The final type of hair removal is camouflage. This method is accomplished by bleaching or coloring the hair so the natural color is less noticeable. While this treatment is not hair removal per se, it is a viable option for sparse, fine hairs. It is also a good treatment modality for persons with low pain thresholds.

Now that we have identified the categories of hair removal, we can discuss in more detail the techniques that can be performed at home or by a qualified technician.

Shaving

Shaving is the most widely performed means of hair removal and is the most temporary, inexpensive, and least effective means of hair removal. Shaving involves cutting the hair shaft at the skin's surface. The remainder of the hair shaft remains below the skin's surface for a short time, but will eventually penetrate the surface, which creates what we commonly refer to as "stubble."

Technique is a very important component of shaving. Aside from the obvious risks of dragging a razor sharp edge along your skin, there are other harmful consequences of inappropriate technique. One consequence is pseudofolliculitis barbae (PFB), which is a condition common to individuals with curly or wiry hair types. It is the result of shaven hairs that have become trapped beneath the skin, resulting in inflammation and infection. Another consequence of shaving is "razor burn," which is the result of repeated passes with the razor over one section. After several passes, the razor eliminates any lubrication and strips the outer layers of skin. The resulting redness and pruritus is painful and irritating. Individuals who routinely suffer from PFB will benefit from using an electric razor rather than a wet shave. Wet shaving produces a very close shave, causing sharp edged hairs to drop back below the epidermis causing PFB. Hair shaved with an electric razor is not as close, and the level can even be adjusted so it is even less close, reducing or preventing PFB from developing.

pseudofolliculitis barbae
form of folliculitis, commonly seen as a result of shaving or waxing

> ## Proper Shaving Techniques
>
> - Do not shave immediately after waking. Wait 15 or 20 minutes.
> - Wash the skin with a mild cleanser prior to shaving.
> - Splash warm water on area immediately before shaving, even if you just showered or washed.
> - Make sure razor is sharp. Disposables can be used only 2 or 3 times.
> - Use shaving cream, lotion, or oil.
> - Shave in the direction of the hair growth.
> - Rinse your razor in warm water often while shaving.
> - Avoid repeated passes.
> - Rinse the shaved area(s) with cold water.
> - Consider using a toner or aftershave balm. Do not use alcohol-based aftershave lotions.

Because shaving is most often done at home rather than at a spa by an aesthetician, further discussion is outside the scope of this text.

Depilatories

Depilatory creams are chemical-based remedies that use substances that essentially melt away the hair at the skin's surface. The main chemical ingredient, thioglycolate, breaks down the hair by dissolving the hair's protein and cystine, which is a main component of the bond that holds hair together. By dissolving the cystine, the individual hairs are reduced to a substance that resembles a pile of jelly. This residual hair matter can be easily wiped away.

> **thioglycolate**
> a salt used in the solutions for hair permanents

Although depilatories are inexpensive, easy to use, and easy to purchase in drug stores, they have several disadvantages. First, depilatories are effective for a relatively brief period of time. Second, they cause the appearance of a residual shadow of the former hair, especially for those with darker hairs. Third, depilatories cause skin irritation, especially for those with sensitive skin. Depilatories also cause problems for those who do not follow the manufacturers' instructions and leave the product on the skin longer than the recommended time to dissolve coarser hair. Topical application of hydrocortisone may reduce irritation for these individuals.

Because depilatories are mostly done at home rather than at a spa by an aesthetician, further discussion of depilatories is outside the scope of this text. However, as part of a comprehensive discussion of hair removal, it is important to know how they work.

Bleaching

Bleaching is a method of hair camouflage that involves lightening hair to reduce the noticeable appearance. This method is most often done for fine sparse hairs, often on the upper lip and the underside of the jaw. Bleaching is done by applying hydrogen peroxide to the hair for a brief period of time until the hair lightens to the desired shade. This treatment should not be done around the eyes or in the bikini area. If the recipient experiences irritation following an application, the peroxide should be removed immediately. To avoid irritation, testing should be done a couple of days prior to treatment.

The advantage of this treatment is that it reduces the appearance of the hair in the privacy and convenience of home. As a result, the cost is minimal. However, the disadvantage of this treatment is that it is not an actual removal.

Because bleaching is mostly done at home rather than at a spa by an aesthetician, further discussion is outside the scope of this text.

Tweezing

Tweezing of individual hairs is a form of temporary hair removal in which the hair and root are removed from the hair follicle. Although tweezing is a very effective means of removal, it can be time consuming and painful. For areas with a few rogue hairs that require removal (such as the eyebrows after waxing), it is very effective. Conversely, it is not the best means of removal for larger areas of unwanted hair growth. Disadvantages of tweezing include these requirements: a steady hand, dexterity, patience, and a high pain threshold. The hair must be long enough to grasp with tweezers. For those especially concerned with unwanted hair, the period of letting hair become long enough to tweeze can be uncomfortable and embarrassing.

Tweezing is often used by technicians to clean up areas following a hair removal procedure treatment. Whether tweezing follows waxing, electrolysis, or laser hair removal, it is a common process used to improve the overall appearance of the area that may have been treated by other modalities. While tweezing may seem simple, it requires the proper tools and a good hand to yield a professional result.

Waxing

Waxing is an effective method of temporary hair removal, especially for large areas of hair that require removal at one time. For this reason, it is more easily tolerated than tweezing in areas of similar size. To begin, a warmed wax is applied in the direction of hair growth. A strip is placed onto the area and rubbed. This process achieves a firm grasp on the hair. The strip is then quickly removed against the hair growth, thus removing the hair from the follicle. Waxing is traditionally used on the eyebrow, chin, upper lip, legs, and bikini line. While effective, it takes an experienced individual to master the detailed aspects of this treatment. Subtle nuances to effectiveness include the types of wax, wax temperature, speed, and the clean-up process. Clean-up or removing the wax from the skin can be particularly tricky, but efficiency increases with experience.

Waxing is a common treatment that salons and spas provide. It is the preferred treatment modality for areas such as the legs, back, and bikini area. It is an effective, relatively inexpensive, and easily performed treatment. There are many types of waxing, with many different properties associated with each, which will be discussed in greater depth later in the text.

Sugar Waxing

Hair removal with sugar paste is a derivative of waxing that is thousands of years old, but has been gaining popularity in more recent times. It uses a melted sugar substance that resembles caramel and is applied to the skin in the same manner as traditional waxing.

The major distinction between traditional waxing and sugar waxing is the clean-up process. Because sugar is water soluble (unlike wax), it can be easily cleaned. *However, manufacturers of sugar paste are now adding other ingredients, like resins, changing how it is traditionally used.* We will discuss sugaring in greater detail later in the text.

Electrolysis

Electrolysis is a form of permanent hair removal in which a thin needle is inserted into the hair follicle and treatment energy of high frequency or galvanic current *is applied in sufficient quantity to destroy the papilla* of the hair follicle. The process injures the hair follicle and renders it useless. Ideally, the follicle will be damaged enough to prevent new hair growth. This method requires that each hair be treated individually, which makes for an expensive, time-consuming, and painful method of hair removal.

Electrolysis does have a few disadvantages worth mention. First, guidelines for licensure can vary from state to state. Consequently, the educational processes may be different, and, as such, the technician knowledge base may differ. Another disadvantage is that the procedure can be performed only while the hair is at certain stages of growth, so some appointments may yield better results than others. Unfortunately, cases of poor results are common. However, this is true with most hair removal processes. Finally, *for more than just a few hairs* this method is very time consuming and expensive, and requires repeated treatments over an extended period of time.

The technical aspects of this treatment will be discussed at greater length later in the book.

Laser

Lasers are used for a variety of aesthetic treatments including skin resurfacing, treating spider veins and varicose veins, repairing solar damage, and removing hair. Laser hair removal is by far the most popular use of laser light. There are three ways the laser can affect the hair: thermal, mechanical, and photochemical.[1] Laser hair removal is not for everyone. The best candidate has light skin and dark hair. Because of the fact that lasers target pigment in the hair, individuals with blonde, light red, gray, and white hair will have poor results. Because hair is of varying color and texture, laser hair removal is challenging and the skin can be susceptible to injury. Further, because laser hair removal is a technique-sensitive treatment, extensive training is necessary for optimal outcomes.

Because laser hair removal is one of the most popular treatments in the aesthetic environment, this topic will be discussed in more detail later in the text.

■ HISTORY AND ORIGINS OF HAIR REMOVAL

People have desired a hairless appearance for centuries, and, in fact, the history of hair removal is as old as civilization itself. (See Figure 1–1.)

Timeline

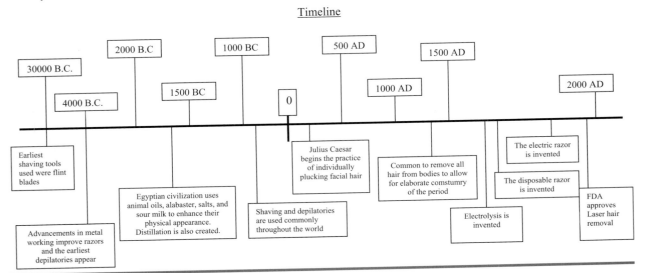

Figure 1–1 A timeline of the history of hair removal

Archeologists have unearthed flint blades that date back to 30,000 B.C. These flint blades dulled rather quickly, and actually could be considered the world's first disposable razors. Aside from flint, clamshells were used as tweezers to pluck individual hairs. Few advancements were made until 4,000 B.C. when depilatory remedies began to surface. Early depilatories included bizarre and often dangerous materials including arsenic. Around the same time, advancements in metalworking ushered the dawn of the razor. It is thought that the invention of the razor occurred concurrently in India and Egypt. Also around this time, the hair removal technique known as threading became common in Arabia. In the Middle East, shaving and hair removal are common practices intended to promote hygiene. Middle Eastern women do not remove hair until they marry. At that point, every hair on the bodies (except the scalp) is tweezed, and the women continue the practice as a sign of respect toward their grooms.

By 500 B.C., hair removal was a common practice throughout the world. In India, Greece, and the Roman Empire, men shaved their faces, chests, and pubic regions, while women used tweezers and crude depilatory creams to remove leg hair. By 50 B.C., Julius Caesar began the trend of having every facial hair individually tweezed from men's faces.

In Europe during the Middle Ages, it was a common practice for women to remove all the hair from their bodies, including the scalp, eyebrows, and eyelashes. This was done to accommodate the lavish costume wigs and makeup that were in vogue at the time.

By colonial times, men and women alike shaved anywhere and everywhere that hair grew. This practice continued until the Victorian era when beards came back into fashion.

In 1875, an ophthalmologist named Charles E. Michel discovered electrolysis. He used the treatment to correct ingrown eyelashes. It was not long before the aesthetic community became apprised of this technology and perfected the technique for removing unwanted body hair, particularly facial hair.

In 1901, the first disposable razor was patented by King Camp Gillette. It was also the first double-edged razor cut from a template rather than forged individually. In 1935, the first dry electric shaver was introduced. In the 1920s X-rays were implemented to treat superfluous hair with disastrous consequences of ulcerations, cancer, and bone deterioration. It was eventually banned in 1946.

In the early part of the twentieth century, Gillette launched a marketing campaign in *Harper's Bazaar* that proclaimed that underarm hair on women was unfeminine. Thus the tradition of shaving the underarms was prompted, a practice common only to American women.

"Shaving makes hair grow back thicker or faster."
This old wives' tale is still told between mothers and daughters. Hormones affect the hair growth, regardless of what your mother said. The reason this myth still exists is likely due to the fact that stubble forms after hair is shaved. It may feel thicker and coarser, but it is not.

In the late twentieth century, the laser hair removal era began. Lasers were first used on skin in the late 1960s, and the FDA approved a laser device in the mid-1990s.

■ DISEASES THAT INCREASE HAIR GROWTH

For the most part, hair growth varies a great deal from one individual to the next. While one person may have excessive hair growth, another may have virtually none. The difference in hair growth may be hormonal or impacted by a disease process. The conditions that cause sudden hair growth can be quite distressing to the affected individual. Among the conditions that affect hair growth are hypertrichosis, hirsutism, adrenogenital syndrome, polycystic ovary syndrome (PCOS), Achard-Thiers syndrome, and Cushing's syndrome.

Hypertrichosis is a condition in which excessive hair growth appears on the posterior and lateral sides of the body. This abnormal hair growth is caused by a number of different reasons. For some, hypertrichosis is hereditary or a side effect of hormonal fluctuations (as with cases of menopause or pregnancy). Hypertrichosis could also be caused by a drug reaction or a side effect to certain cancer treatment modalities.

Hirsutism is a common condition caused by an imbalance of male hormones, which results in male pattern hair growth on the chest and/or face. For women, this can be a particularly distressing condition. The reasons for the hormonal imbalances vary. Like hypertrichosis, hirsutism could have a genetic component or could be a side effect of medication.

Rare conditions that affect hair growth include adrenogenital syndrome, PCOS, Achard-Thiers syndrome, and Cushing's syndrome. The increased hair growth and other symptoms from these diseases usually are a result of hormonal irregularities, such as an abundance of androgens.

Hair growth patterns also change as we age. This can result in either a net loss of hair density (as with male patterned baldness) or a net gain of

hypertrichosis
condition characterized by excessive hair

hirsutism
condition characterized by abnormal hair growth

adrenogenital syndrome
condition characterized by excessive androgen production

polycystic ovary syndrome
a disease that may constitute the following symptoms typically in childbearing women: high levels of androgens, an irregular or no menstrual cycle, possible small ovarian cysts

Achard-Thiers syndrome
a disorder mainly affecting postmenopausal women, marked by diabetes mellitus and hirsutism, deep masculine voice, facial hypertrichosis, and obesity

Cushing's syndrome
condition characterized by excessive pituitary gland secretions

hair. Excessive hair growth that occurs with age is hormonal in nature. Many women who experience menopause will notice an increase in facial hair growth, which is caused by a decrease in estrogen that "buffered" the percentage of androgens that women also have, present in their blood, stimulating the beard area, which is a secondary sexual characteristic of hair growth occurring in boys at puberty.

■ TRAINING TECHNICIANS ON HAIR REMOVAL PROCEDURES

Technicians must be trained before they can perform hair removal techniques. (See Figure 1–2.) Because hair removal techniques and processes can be technique sensitive, technicians must understand the different methods, indications, and contraindications, as well as proper precare and postcare management, all of which are important factors for success.

The training process for hair removal should be specific to the treatment type [e.g., waxing (see Figure 1–3), laser, or electrolysis]. State licensure is fairly specific as to who can provide which types of hair removal. For example, in New Jersey, only physicians are authorized to operate laser hair removal devices while other states are not as strict. Nevertheless, training is key. Because certain types of hair removal are risky, it is imperative that spas and clinics ensure that technicians have

technique sensitive
a procedure that is performed differently from aesthetician to aesthetician based on his or her experience and knowledge

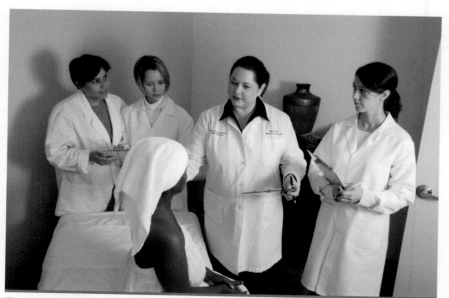

Figure 1–2 Training is the first and most important step in beginning a career in hair removal

the necessary training. Requiring technicians to be adequately trained will give the spa the confidence to allow technicians to provide effective care to clients. If technicians are not previously trained, it is incumbent on the spa to have a trainer available to teach and mentor new technicians in the different types of hair removal and in what it takes to be successful when providing these treatments.

Hair removal training should take place in a dedicated class using a combination of theory and hands-on application. Classroom work should include a review of the anatomy and physiology of skin, the basics of wound healing, as well as the indications and contraindications of procedures.

The course should include information about clinic protocols for hair removal and the variety of treatments and programs available. Once students complete classroom work and have passed the recommended examinations, they can move on to hands-on, clinical training.

The review of anatomy and physiology should be specific to the layers of the skin and the response of the skin to waxing, electrolysis, and hair removal laser. Also, the trainer should be able to tie those responses into wound healing and the anticipated results of treatments. All conditions that reflect indications and contraindications should be covered. The information may vary by facility, and classroom agendas are usually based on established policy and procedures.

The ability to reproduce a treatment comes with practice; therefore, extra time should be built into the training process. Technicians should not provide treatments to clients until they have completed a comprehensive clinical training program. However, completion of a training program does not always reflect competency. Skill testing and observation of technicians in training are critical for the safety of clients.

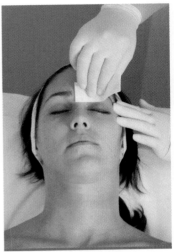

Figure 1–3 Waxing is one of many hair removal techniques

clinic protocols
any set of rules or guidelines established by a clinic for safe practice. These guidelines will vary by location, yet are expected to be observed by clinicians working within the individual clinic.

Training Protocols

Training protocols are documents that describe the processes deemed acceptable for training. Protocols address subjects such as who can be trained, how training takes place, and what test scores are required to be considered a skilled technician. Each clinic should have protocols to guide training processes.

In a medical spa, directors and physicians should develop protocols that outline who can be trained. In a day spa, those in charge of operations should be in charge of training protocols. The qualifications of the personnel category (aesthetician versus nurse) should be used to differentiate among whether laser, electrolysis, or waxing procedures can be used and why. The training environment is also important to differentiate in training protocols, which protects facilities from potential litigation. The

Company Name Training and Certification as a Hair Removal Specialist

Date of Origination: June 1992

Creator: Pamela Hill, R.N.

Date of Review: June 1997

Revisions by: S. Smith, M.E.

Date of Revisions: June '98, June '99, June '00, June '01, June '02, June '03, June '04, June '05

Policy #: 05-005

Attachments: Policy and Procedure document for Hair Removal, Certificates of Completion, Written Test, Clinical Test

Title of Policy: Training and Certification for Hair Removal

Policy: All clinical staff will be licensed and insured in the state of employment. Certification through the company training program is required prior to client care.

Purpose: To ensure that all employed clinical staff are properly trained and certified in hair removal techniques, policies, and procedures through the company training programs

Scope: All clinical personnel

Definition: Clinical Aesthetic Personnel

Procedure Indications: Supervisors will recommend that all technicians seeking certification complete the training program.

Procedure Contraindications: Not applicable

Required Paperwork: "Recommendation for Training # PER- 42" signed by the technician supervisor.

Testing if Necessary: Score of 80% or greater on written examination is required before proceeding to clinical training. A score of 90% or greater on the clinical examination is required to treat clients.

Required Reading: Articles and technical information provided by the instructor.

Classroom Training: Training consists of two classroom days. The curriculum includes a review of anatomy and physiology of the skin, wound healing, principles and techniques of hair removal (i.e., waxing and laser hair removal). A written test will be administered at the conclusion of the two-day classroom course. A score of at least 80% is required to move to the clinical training.

Clinical Training: The technician will be responsible for finding 25 models on whom to practice laser hair removal and 25 models on whom to practice waxing. These models should have different skin types and different indications. A full consultation will be done, followed by a treatment. Technicians need to prove competency in consultation skills, the development of home programs, and the techniques of hair removal described in the policy and procedure document. A passing score of 90% is required on the clinical training to be released to treat clients.

Technician Requirements: Licensed professional

training outline should be complete and available for others to review. Additionally, training protocols should be updated yearly. Finally, evaluating the training process is important since meaningful feedback can improve the training protocols.

Clinical Training Process

In the clinical segment of training, technicians should work one-on-one with the clinic educator or instructor to master the use of the hair removal laser (see Figure 1–4), wax, or electrology unit. The clinical training should be directed at three specific processes: the consultative process, the hair removal techniques, and the appropriate home care programs. When learning about the consultative process, technicians should take the specifics learned in the classroom, such as indications and contraindications, and apply them appropriately to specific skin types and clients' complaints. When focusing on laser hair removal, technicians will learn the issues of skin quality, the types of lasers available, recovery time, and potential complications. Finally, home adjunct therapy for the client is a critical component of the long-term success of clinical hair removal programs.

The clinic must require at least 25 "model" clients with varying skin types and clinical concerns to be treated prior to treatment of "client" clients. A clinical examination is also required to ensure technicians understand the application of different hair removal processes.

Evaluating Technician Skills

While written testing is a great tool to evaluate students through the treatment-related educational process, it is not always an accurate indicator of clinical abilities. For example, a technician may be adept at performing waxing treatments, but he or she will also need to be reviewed on the nonclinical aspects of performing in the clinic. (See Table 1–1.) A simple

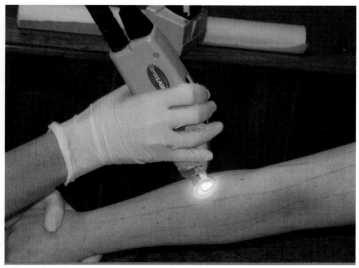

Figure 1–4 Hair removal laser is a common hair removal technique

Table 1–1   Additional Technician Skills

Clinical Skills	Score 1–10	Recommended Improvements
Communications Skills		
Clarity		
Education		
Sales		
Safety Skills		
Wears protective gear		
Understands waxes		
Understands lasers and electrolysis		
Charting		
Understands the record		
Makes appropriate notes		
Takes pictures		
Products		
Understands product lines		
Professionalism		
Appropriate to client		
Appropriate to peers		

checklist for technician and clinical instructors might be useful, which can include tasks such as draping the client, client communication skills, home program evaluation, and the ability to orient to the physical space. These skills and those identified in Table 1–1 will help technicians expand their knowledge.

Continuing Education

Continuing education is a privilege as well as a professional obligation. Educational updates can take place by three methods: an annual recertification process through the clinic, **Continuing Education Units (CEU)** obtained at professional meetings, or online study and education. Annual recertification processes within a clinic or spa usually have two phases.

Continuing Education Units (CEU)
any certified training or event which is intended to build or add skills

The first phase is through self-managed workbook reading and quizzes. These workbooks can be printed or put on your intranet (an efficient way of managing the process) in the spa. The second phase is the clinical recertification, which includes having the clinic educator or physician observe technicians treating clients. The educator uses a score sheet to evaluate the technician in all areas of the treatment and the treatment room, including the actual treatment, cleanliness of the room, professionalism with the client, etc. The score on this evaluation must be at least 90 percent. If technicians do not achieve a passing score, then a problem solving document called a progressive improvement plan should be implemented to help technicians improve their skills.

Although it is difficult to find continuing education classes on hair removal (other than electrolysis and hair removal lasers), technicians should keep their eyes open for courses that interest them and advance their knowledge.

Many associations like the Society of Clinical and Medical Hair Removal (SCMHR) and the American Electrology Association (AEA) require CEUs for continued membership, available by attending classes at conferences or trade shows and online.

Requirements for Training

Hair removal training should be comprehensive and include laser treatments, waxing, tweezing, electrolysis, and other types of hair removal used in the clinic or spa. Technicians dedicated to the process of hair removal will often render better results than those who provide hair removal intermittently. Each procedure should be taught in the clinic and followed with clinic experience. Technicians should provide at least 25 treatments and be able to pass the written test.

There should be a specific document within the clinic protocols called "Requirements for Training" that outline the specific actions that must take place *for technicians to be placed* in a training program as well as for after they complete the training, before they can be authorized to treat clients. Within this document should be an outline of requirements for previous experience, additional education (e.g., college courses), written recommendations by physicians, or number of years that the technician must be employed with the company prior to training. Once the qualifications have been met, the criteria to treat clients must be addressed (e.g., a passing score on the written examination, treatment of 25 models, written permission of the physician). Several additional training requirements include having a valid license in the state in which the technician is practicing and receiving a recommendation from the physician or clinic manager for training.

progressive improvement plan
administrative document that is intended to record a problem and the actions that will be taken to improve the problem in order to prevent its reoccurrence

Ongoing education is one of the most important activities you can pursue to advance your career. It is your annuity for increasing wages, improving treatment results, and realizing self-improvement.

Ongoing training can be part of a yearly "self-improvement" plan. After graduating from school, it is helpful to take at least one course a year about a new subject to add depth and power to your resume.

Safety Bill of Rights
original name for OSHA manual

Occupational Safety and Health Administration (OSHA)
federal agency responsible for defining and regulating safety in the workplace

bloodborne pathogens
infectious substances present in the blood that can cause infection or disease. HIV and HCV are bloodborne pathogens.

Universal Precautions
preventative actions taken to prevent the transmission of infectious diseases; involves the use of protective procedures and equipment, such as gloves and masks

safety manual
OSHA document that outlines the hazardous materials and equipment specific to each location and the safety protocols for each

contaminated
the act of making an item or compound nonsterile or impure

▪ OSHA AND SAFETY

It is hard to separate the notion of safe practices and sanitation because the concepts are really intertwined. For example, leaving dirty instruments on the counter is not only unsanitary but can also be dangerous to clients and technicians. Having electrical cords strung across a room collecting dust is unsanitary, but walking across the room and tripping over the cord is dangerous. Keeping the environment clean and safe should be the priority of everyone in the facility. Sometimes safety and sanitary issues are points of contention between employers and technicians for various reasons. Nevertheless, spas are required to observe Occupational Safety and Health Administration (OSHA) rules to protect employees and clients.

OSHA has many rules and regulations—far too many to cover in this text. However, we must discuss OSHA rules that apply to laser hair removal, waxing, and electrolysis, such as bloodborne pathogens, the use of Universal Precautions, and the management of used wax (waste disposal). The protocol we will highlight should be outlined in your spa's safety manual.

Universal Precautions

The subject of bloodborne pathogens, in and of itself, is an extensive topic that includes a variety of issues mostly related to needle safe handling of sharps and exposure to body fluids, usually blood. While it is possible that technicians will be exposed to blood or bodily fluids during laser hair removal, waxing, or electrolysis, the amounts will be miniscule. Nevertheless, it is important for technicians to *always* follow "Universal Precautions," which includes assuming that all body fluids technicians come into contact with are contaminated. For protection during a laser hair removal procedure, technicians must always wear protective eye goggles, lab coats, and gloves. Also, clients must wear protective goggles. These rules are for your safety and protection.

Gloves

Gloves are an important component of self-protection and should be worn during *all* treatments. There are two types of gloves: latex and nonlatex. (See Table 1–2.) Latex allergies have become more common and can be significant. If a client states that he or she might have a latex allergy, be sure to use a nonlatex glove. Latex allergies are also common in technicians who wear gloves everyday, but can be resolved by wearing

Table 1–2 Protective Glove Materials[2]

Material Type	Tensile Strength	Softness	Elasticity	Tear Strength	Cost
Natural Rubber	Good	Very Good	Very Good	Good	Low
Polyisoprene	Good	Very Good	Very Good	Moderate	High
Nitrile	Good	Good	Good	Poor	Moderate
Neoprene	Good	Good/Very Good	Good/Very Good	Poor	Moderate/High
Block copolymers	Good	Good	Very Good	Fair	Moderate/High
PVC	Fair	Good	Poor	Poor	Low
Polyurethane	Very Good	Good	Good	Good	High

gloves without latex. For certain treatments, such as waxing, nonlatex gloves are preferred, due to the tackiness of the wax.

Eye Wear

Using protective eyewear is simple. Eyewear is used to protect technicians from dangers of the laser beam. Likewise, clients' eyes must be protected. The type of eyewear will be dictated by the laser being used. Some technicians like to place a gauze pad under the goggles to make them more comfortable or use metal eye shields.

■ EMPLOYMENT OPTIONS

Career opportunities abound for the hair removal specialist. (See Table 1–3.) Creating a career plan is the first step to becoming a successful technician. Many professionals recommend identifying the goal and working backward to achieve that goal.

Using this technique, identify where you want to be in five years and what you want to be doing. Then create a list of objectives to achieve the goal. For example, if you are currently an aesthetician without medical experience and you would like to be in a medical spa as a hair removal specialist, identify objectives that will allow you to meet the goal. Find out where to gain the training, expertise, and experience that will allow you to be a valued employee in this setting. Identify internships or learning situations that will help you to hone your skills. Take communication courses to help learn how to communicate with clients, peers,

Within the facility there should be a "safety coordinator" who is responsible for maintenance of the OSHA manual. The manual includes guidelines for communicating safety practices for the business, maintains all required documents, and contains the safety training protocol for the facility.

career plan
action taken on by an aesthetician to set goals and actions taken to ensure their realization

Table 1–3	Career Opportunities	
Location	**Specialist**	**Types of Hair Removal**
Medical Office	• Plastic Surgery • Dermatology • Family Practice • Gynecology • Otolaryngology (ENT) • Opthamology	• Laser Hair Removal • Waxing • Electrolysis
Spas	• Salon Spas • Fitness Club Spa • Country Club Spas • Holistic Spas • Day Spas	• Waxing • Electrolysis • Sugaring • Threading
Resorts	• Destination Spas • Resort/ Hotel Spas • Cruise Ship Spas	• Waxing • Electrolysis • Sugaring • Threading

and superiors. Take sales courses to help make contributions to your employer and to yourself. Learn the basics of building a business. Create a professional resume. Practice interviewing skills to help you get a desirable job.

Marketing yourself to a business will become an important skill in acquiring the right job. Whether you want to land a job in a medical spa, a destination spa, or a holistic spa, the tactics you use to get there will be the same. Remember, just as you are looking for the perfect job, the employer is looking for the perfect employee. Not every opportunity will be a good match for you or the employer, and that is okay. Understanding the components of a good match will be the key to long-term success. By marketing yourself, you will have a sound understanding of what positions will be a good match for you personally.

There are several components of marketing yourself that should be addressed, including your values, integrity, skills, and needs. Before looking for a job, it would be worthwhile to write out each category. This exercise will help you to ask potential employers the right questions, which will assist in your own determination. Then practice with a friend. Remember, you are interviewing the employer as much as the employer is interviewing you.

Values are defined as "the abstract concepts of what is right, worthwhile or desirable; principles or standards."[3] Ask questions about the business's philosophies and goals (businesses should have both financial and nonfinancial goals). Specifically ask about client care philosophies. Then discuss those values with which you can identify. Important values may include: being on time, following company protocol, providing quality care of clients, and volunteering services. Think twice about taking a position where your values differ from those of the clinic or employer.

You may want to consider factors such as the location and reputation of your educational institution. Include a list of your advanced education, including college (name, location, and degree) and advanced aesthetic education classes (with whom and where). And, finally, include experience in the field in which you are looking to be employed.

Integrity is different from values. Integrity is defined as "uncompromising adherence to moral and ethical principles; *honesty*."[4] In this category you may want to ask questions about client care, such as how complications are handled, how unhappy clients are handled, and how fee disputes are managed. Also, ask direct questions about the ethical principles of the company. There should be a written philosophy, which is usually reflected in an organization's mission statement. Then consider if these ethical principles are similar to your own.

mission statement
written statement of a business's individual philosophy

Your skills are important to an employer, but sometimes the position does not fit the position you are seeking. You may be underqualified or overqualified. You need to assess this with the employer. Ask questions about specific skills needed, and respond with information about your skills. If you are underqualified but there is otherwise a match, what training will be available to help you become qualified? How quickly will training occur, and who will do the training? Will there be a pay increase after the training is complete? These are important questions to ask prior to committing to an employment position. What you hear at the interview and what comes to pass in a job are not always the same thing. It is in your best interest to put into writing some of what would otherwise be a "handshake" deal. This approach eliminates any future misunderstandings or hard feelings. If the employer is unwilling to do this, maybe it is not a match.

Although your needs are especially important, they are not exclusive of the employer's needs. The best situation is when you find a "need match." List your needs, such as salary or pay rate, benefits, vacation time, sick day policies, hours to be worked, desired job description, and any other important needs you may have. In advance, decide which needs you can compromise on, and which needs are deal breakers. Making this decision in advance prevents you from feeling resentful if you give in and regret it later.

> Technicians must be properly licensed by the states in which they plan on working.

Once you have your credentials, resume, and marketing plan, you are ready to get the job for which you are uniquely qualified.

License and Insurance

Whether an aesthetician, nurse, physician's assistant, or medical assistant, you must be licensed in the state in which you work. Confirmation of licensure should be provided to the employer and kept in the employee record. Many technicians like to keep their license hanging in their treatment rooms, and, in some states, this is a requirement.

Some states are very particular about who can operate a laser and where the laser is stored. Before accepting a position to perform laser hair removal, be sure to check the state requirements. Do not put yourself in the position of doing procedures that may jeopardize your license.

There are several types of insurance necessary for a spa business. The most important insurance policy for technicians to carry is malpractice insurance. This is true whether you provide facials, waxing, or hair removal laser. The insurance policy covers your actions when treating clients. If something goes wrong, the malpractice policy will protect you. In medical offices, sometimes physicians have a broad policy under which technicians are covered. This is also true in luxury spas.

For individual technicians, getting proper coverage is a fact-finding mission. First, speak with your employer to find out the status of any provided coverage. Second, find a reputable insurance company and consult with an agent. Take his or her counsel and then consider a discussion with an attorney to ensure your best interests are evaluated.

> Before you begin employment, be sure to call the state board that recognizes your license and find out what specific implications should be noted when you are providing hair removal services. Once you have completed this phone call, the next call is to your insurance agent to make sure you have the proper coverage for the procedures you will be doing.

Medical Offices

Busy aesthetic medical offices (see Figure 1–5) are always looking for proficient aestheticians. Often a physician looks for employees who can multitask and take on increasing job responsibilities. Depending on the scope of the practice, you may have an opportunity to learn more than just hair removal techniques.

Working in medical offices has many rewards, among them prestige, advanced knowledge, complex treatments, and working with other medical professionals. Medical professionals, physicians, nurses, physician assistants, residents, and interns are unlike any other professionals. Their training has spanned life and death, and their commitment to clients is unlike any other commitment to a customer. Physicians, nurses, and clients do not tolerate unnecessary mistakes, which can make for an intense and intimating work environment, but the payoffs are usually worth the effort.

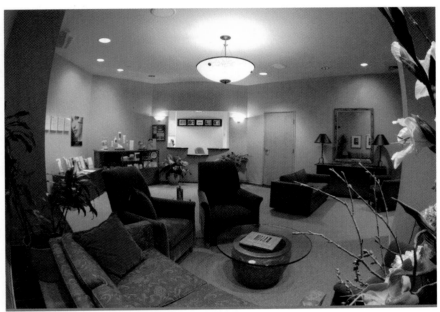

Figure 1–5 A medical spa may have all varieties of hair removal treatments available to patients

The ability to make a difference in the lives of clients is among the most meaningful rewards. To learn and become more skilled, to participate, and to bring visible results to clients in need—these are some of the benefits of working in a medical office. Working in a medical office requires expert skills, a willingness to learn, true compassion and empathy, as well as expert professionalism.

Salons and Spas

Salons and spas offer a sense of well-being and luxury to clients. (See Figure 1–6.) As treatments become more sophisticated and tools become more advanced, technicians have the opportunity to provide clients with treatments that may supplement hair removal services (e.g., iontophoresis) or help to reduce stress (e.g., reflexology).

Many different types of spas exist, including (but not limited to) salon spas, resort spas, cruise ship spas, day spas, club spas, destination spas, and holistic or mineral bath spas. Each type of spa has a different focus and requires the aesthetician to develop a hair removal program that will complement other spa treatments. No matter what type of spa in which you are seeking employment, hair removal services will be an integral component of the services offered. Regardless of the spa specialty, the spa director will expect employees to be professional, educated, and willing to work diligently to build clientele.

reflexology
system of massage in which certain body parts are massaged in specific areas in order to favorably influence other body functions

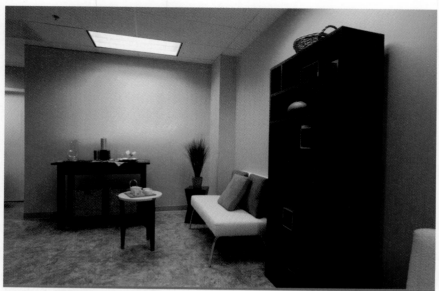

Figure 1-6 A salon spa is a common location for hair removal therapies to be found

Liability Issues for the Technician

Liability issues for technicians are an important factor in planning a career. Our U.S. society is far more litigious than ever before. If something goes wrong, the client is always looking for someone to blame. Whether a case comes to settlement or trial, the stress of being blamed will be unbelievable, and the situation should be avoided if at all possible.

Many potential liability risks exist for technicians. The most common injuries at risk related to hair removal include scarring, burns, hyperpigmentation, hypopigmentation, infections, and failure to keep information confidential.

Burns caused by hair removal lasers can develop into deep wounds and scars if left untreated. These burns are usually due to a failure to understand the skin and the potential injury the machine can cause. It is important to understand wound healing and wound care so that technicians can quickly recognize problems and seek immediate help.

Scarring is an obvious concern. No one is exempt from possible scarring; for instance, improper extraction techniques during a facial are susceptible to scarring. With laser hair removal, each technician must follow protocol carefully to ensure that he or she is skilled in laser procedures. It is important for technicians to be qualified and to know when to ask for help from physicians, which is an important skill in and of itself, a skill that is often directed by protocol and experience.

Infection is most commonly the result of a technician's failure to provide an adequate standard of care. While other treatments such as peels or microdermabrasions are more likely to result in an infection, it is still important for technicians to understand the signs of infection. Lifting skin when waxing or causing a blister when treating with electrolysis or laser hair removal can allow bacteria to enter the broken skin and an infection to ensue. Not using sterilized probes or forceps on a client when performing electrolysis can also result in an infection.

Regulatory Agencies

The agencies that regulate the spas are not federalized, but are implemented on a state-by-state basis. Therefore, it is important to check with the licensing agency in your state to determine if there are specific requirements related to your job, aside from general licensure. For example, you might need a certificate indicating you have completed a course on laser hair removal in order to perform the treatment.

Professional Organizations

Many organizations are trying to accomplish lofty goals for industry, only to be in conflict with another organization with the same goals. It will be important over the coming years for us to support organizations that have our best interests in mind as we work toward goals to create uniform educational requirements. The most progressive organization is the National Coalition of Esthetic and Related Associations, which is a catch-all organization. Check with NCEA to find out if there is a professional organization that meets your individual needs. Meanwhile, if you work for a plastic surgeon, check into the Society of Plastic Surgical Skin Care Specialists, and if you work for a dermatologist, check into The Society of Dermatology Skin Care Specialists. Also for electrologists, there is the American Electrology Association, and for electrologists and laser practitioners, the Society of Clinical and Medical Hair Removal.

> Belonging to a professional organization can be educational as well as a great place to network. However, finding a good fit is important. Usually the physician with whom you are working belongs to a professional organization. If there are associations for ancillary staff, consider these organizations first.

Professional Code of Ethics

There are two types of ethical codes: personal ethics and professional ethics. (See Table 1–4.) While they may overlap, each individual document is important. Individually, the code of ethics is a very personal document that discusses how you will live your life and what your priorities will be in daily decision making.

A professional code of ethics should be very public and well known to all in our profession, as well as to our clients. If we are to be considered

professional ethics
set of guidelines that should set a framework for professional behavior and responsibilities

Table 1–4   Writing a Professional Code of Ethics

Component	Considerations
Preamble	• What is the purpose of the organization?
Statement of Intent	• What is the purpose of the code?
Fundamental Principles	• What population is affected by the organization? • What is the organization's area of expertise?
Fundamental Rules	• What unethical situations does your organization want to prevent? • What are the likely problem situations in which unethical solutions might arise?
Guidelines for the Fundamental Principles and Fundamental Rules	• How can these unethical situations be prevented? • How can employees prevent conflicting principles?

members of the trained service professionals (sometimes referred to as allied health professionals) as our counterparts in nursing, social work, nutrition, or others are, we should extend ourselves to the highest level, and this includes professional ethics. So, exactly what does a code of ethics need to include? It should discuss appropriate and inappropriate behavior, promote high standards of client care, be used for self-evaluation, establish a framework for professional behavior and responsibilities, identify professionals, and create an image of occupational maturity.[5]

Given all these criteria, we recognize that creating a code of ethics is not an easy task. Although the National Coalition of Esthetic and Related Associations does publish a code of ethics, creating one in your place of work is a good idea. In order for codes of ethics to be meaningful, the group that is going to *use* the document should develop the code. Creating a code may feel like an overwhelming task because the subject matter can be broad and diverse, especially if the group writing the code of ethics is large.

The focus of a code is based on moral principles. The process should begin by asking certain questions such as: Why establish a code of ethics? What is the purpose of our organization? What will the code be used for? In order for the code to be useful, it must reflect the qualities of the group, which can often be difficult because each person within the group has different qualities and moral viewpoints. However, finding a compromise will create a useful document.

The code of ethics must be broad enough to take into consideration the number of people using it, but specific enough to direct behavior. Therefore, if the code fails to provide substantive guidance for the organization, it creates confusion. As for the skin care industry at large and your business specifically, a few tips are offered in Table 1–4.

National Code of Estheticians, Manufacturers/ Distributors & Associations (NCEA) *ESTHETICIAN CODE OF ETHICS*

Client Relationships

Estheticians* will serve the best interests of their clients at all times and will provide the highest quality service possible.

Estheticians will maintain client confidentiality and provide clear, honest communication.

Estheticians will provide clients with clear and realistic goals and outcomes and will not make false claims regarding the potential benefits of the techniques rendered or products recommended.

Estheticians will adhere to the scope of practice of their profession and refer clients to the appropriate qualified health practitioner when indicated.

Scope of Practice

Estheticians will offer services only within the scope of practice as defined by the state within which they operate, if required, and in adherence with appropriate federal laws and regulations.

Estheticians will not utilize any technique/procedure for which they have not had adequate training and shall represent their education, training, qualifications and abilities honestly.

Estheticians will strictly adhere to all usage instructions and guidelines provided by product and equipment manufacturers, provided those guidelines and instructions are within the scope of practice as defined by the state, if required.

Professionalism

Estheticians will commit themselves to ongoing education and to provide clients and the public with the most accurate information possible.

Estheticians will dress in attire consistent with professional practice and adhere to the Code of Conduct of their governing board.

*For the purpose of the NCEA Code of Ethics, the use of the term Esthetician applies to all licensed skin care professionals as defined by their state law.

Reprinted with permission from the NCEA

A Code of Ethics is a means of uniquely expressing a group's collective commitment to a specific set of standards of conduct while offering guidance in how to best follow those codes.[6]

A Higher Standard of Professionalism

When we work in the profession of aesthetics, more is expected of us. We are expected to adhere to a higher level of professionalism and customer service than in other settings. Technicians must display professional conduct at all times to maintain a client's confidence. Also, informal atmospheres do not reflect positively on the image of technicians or on the profession. In fact, improper behavior could negatively reflect on the technician or the organization in the eyes of the client. Professional conduct must be present when interacting with clients, perusing their medical records, and communicating with colleagues about clients. In medical offices, the information technicians share about the client to colleagues should comply with HIPAA regulations (see below). To this effect, any client information belongs to the physician and, according to HIPAA regulations, cannot leave the medical office.

Conclusion

Before making a choice to pursue a career as a hair removal specialist, you should be aware of the importance of being properly trained to provide safe and effective treatments. The training should include a working knowledge in hair removal lasers, as well as other methods of hair removal. Once training is completed, technicians have a host of employment options ranging from the day spa to the medical spa, and finally as an entrepreneur. A career in hair removal is becoming a specialty within the aesthetic field and can be a lucrative and rewarding career choice.

▷ ▷ ▷ TOP 10 TIPS TO TAKE TO THE CLINIC

1. Know the different types of hair removal processes.
2. Be aware that there are diseases or physical conditions that can cause increased hair growth.
3. Professional training allows the greatest opportunity for success.
4. Join professional organizations.
5. Decide where you want to work and devise a plan to reach these goals.
6. Be ethical.
7. Be professional; the areas you could be treating might be embarrassing to the client.
8. Know your state laws and how they impact the ability to effectively develop skills.
9. Obtain insurance before you begin to practice.
10. Use protective equipment such as eye protection or gloves.

CHAPTER QUESTIONS

1. What are the different types of hair removal?
2. Why is insurance important to technicians providing hair removal services?
3. What are some injuries that can occur from hair removal treatments?
4. How would you define "professionalism"?
5. What makes hair removal an interesting career choice?

CHAPTER REFERENCES

1. Dierick, C. C., & Grossman, M. C. (2005). Laser and Lights. In D. Goldberg (Ed.), *Laser Hair Removal*. Philadelphia, PA: Elsevier Saunders.
2. Health and Safety Executive. (2004, April 11). *Non-latex Glove Alternatives*. Available at http://www.hse.gov.uk
3. *Webster's College Dictionary*. (1992). New York: Random House (p. 1473).
4. *Webster's College Dictionary*. (1992). New York: Random House (p. 700).
5. MacDonald, C. (2004, March 9). *Why Have a Code of Ethics?* Available at http://www.ethicsweb.ca
6. Olson, A. (2004, March 11). *Authoring a Code: Observations on Process and Organization*. Available at http://www.iit.edu

BIBLIOGRAPHY

Bickmore, H. (2003). *2004 Milady's Hair Removal Techniques*. Clifton Park, NY: Milady, an imprint of Thomson Delmar Learning.

Dierick, C. C., & Grossman, M. C. (2005). Laser and Lights. In D. Goldberg (Ed.), *Laser Hair Removal*. Philadelphia, PA: Elsevier Saunders.

Health and Safety Executive. (2004, April 11). *Non-latex Glove Alternatives*. Available at http://www.hse.gov.uk

MacDonald, C. (2004, March 9). *Why Have a Code of Ethics?* Available at http://www.ethicsweb.ca

Olson, A. (2004, March 11). *Authoring a Code: Observations on Process and Organization*. Available at http://www.iit.edu

Webster's College Dictionary. (1992). New York: Random House.

Anatomy and Physiology of the Hair and Skin

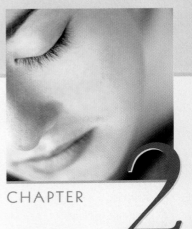

CHAPTER

2

29

After completing this chapter, you should be able to:

1. Name the layers of the epidermis.
2. Name appendages within the dermis.
3. List the major functions of the skin.
4. Name components of the pilosebaceous unit.
5. Name the three stages of hair growth.

INTRODUCTION

"The beauty of a face is a frail ornament, a passing flower, a moment's brightness belonging only to the skin."[1]

The skin is the largest human organ. It is our protection from outside elements, it identifies us, and it defines our beauty.

integumentary system
the skin and its accessory organs, such as the sebaceous and sweat glands, sensory receptors, hair, and nails

The skin and its appendages—nails, hair, nerve endings, sweat and oil glands—compose the integumentary system, sometimes referred to as "integument." (See Figure 2–1.) Skin not only keeps our bodies and their various components intact, but, and equally important, it is also our most immediate contact with our environment. Our skin senses vital information about the world in which we live; therefore, it ensures our survival.

While seemingly uniform and simple in its presentation and purpose, skin is far more complex and variant than meets the eye. It varies in thickness and in sensitivity. (See Table 2–1.) Parts of it develop from brain tissues and remain attached to the brain through nerves, which conduct signals we feel as pleasure or pain.[2] These signals are vital to our success as a species. While not all of the sensations we feel are pleasurable, they are all purposeful. If we could not sense cold air, we would all freeze to death. If we could not feel a cut, we could bleed to death or die from infection. These sensations are sensed by nerves, which in turn send the information to our brains for processing and translation. Overall, the skin possesses most of the nerve endings that transmit vital information about our environment to the brain. There are relatively few on our posterior sides; however, in lips, fingers, and genitals they are abundant.

Similarly, because the skin is our outermost organ, it also serves as a unique identifier, which we see and use to associate with one person and differentiate from the next. Being the psychosocial creatures we are, we have put great emphasis on how others perceive our appearance. The

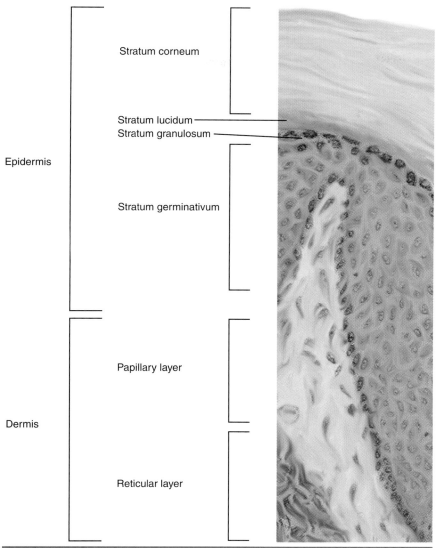

Epidermis

Stratum corneum

Stratum lucidum
Stratum granulosum

Stratum germinativum

Dermis

Papillary layer

Reticular layer

As clinicians in the field of dermal and, in this instance, hair removal techniques, we must be familiar with the skin, its layers, and the cells within them. Your deeper understanding of skin structure and function will help you to be a better clinician. In turn, this will provide your client with improved results and safer care.

Figure 2–1 The layers of the skin are important for the hair removal technician to understand

way we dress, beautify, and posture ourselves conveys gender, age, strength, and, most noticeably, attractiveness.

The appearance of the skin has become a synonym for beauty in our society, and we strive to optimize it. New scientific developments allow for the promise of creams that act longer, stronger, or faster to turn back

Table 2–1   Fun Facts About the Skin[3]
Fun Facts About the Skin
Humans shed millions of dead skin flakes every minute.
In adults, the skin usually covers about two square meters (about the size of a shower curtain) and weighs about 7 pounds. It also has 300 million skin cells.
The skin is between 1.5 mm and 4 mm thick, about as thick as a few sheets of paper.
The thickest areas of the skin (plantar and palmar regions) contain no hair follicles or sweat glands.
Millions of coiled sweat glands discharge sweat and salts to the surface where evaporation begins to cool the body in seconds.
Just below the surface, the dermis feeds miles of blood vessels with nutrients.
The brain and skin become connected very early in fetal development. Even in the womb, a baby's hand can feel its way to the mouth.
Touch is the first sense to develop.
The skin's array of nerves is sensitive enough to feel the weight of a mosquito as it lands.
On average, each square inch of skin contains 10 hairs, 15 sebaceous glands, 100 sweat glands, and 3.2 feet of blood vessels.

the clock. Some consumers are extraordinarily sophisticated in finding the newest treatments and the latest products to counteract the aging process. Others are overwhelmed by the options available to them. Either way, there are things we can do to maintain and even regain beautiful skin. In order to do so we must ask ourselves how we can determine what works best and why. How much change is even possible? Even the savviest of consumers need help answering these questions. Most of them will turn to you for advice. It is here our quest begins.

▪ SKIN ANATOMY

If one of the skin's main functions is to act as a barrier against intruding substances, how, then, do lotions that we apply "soak in"? The primary answer is through the appendages.

Appendages are defined as smaller parts to a greater part. For the skin, they include the pilosebaceous unit (hair follicle and accompany-

appendages
any anatomical structures associated with a larger structure; for the skin, its appendages include hair, glands, and pores

pilosebaceous unit
hair follicle and accompanying sebaceous glands and arrector pili muscle

ing sebaceous glands and arrector pili muscle), sweat glands, and nails.[4] Appendages originate in the dermis but extend into the epidermis.

External substances, such as skin creams, ointments, and salves, can enter the skin through the appendages of the hair and sweat ducts, and also through the intercellular spaces between the cornified cells. Smaller molecules can pass through cells at the surface of the skin.

■ THE LAYERS OF THE SKIN

The skin comprises three main layers. (See Figure 2–2.) The epidermis is the outer layer and is constantly being worn down and replaced.[5] It shields us from the environment, bacteria, pollution, and the sun's rays. It contains no blood vessels or nerves and is vital in preventing loss of moisture from the body. The next layer of skin is the dermis, which lies below the epidermis. Finally, the subcutaneous (meaning "sub"— beneath "cutaneous"—the skin) fat layer lies beneath the dermis. The subcutaneous layer, also known as the hypodermis, acts as a thermal barrier and mechanical cushion varying in thickness from person to person and at different places on the body. Sturdy collagen within the hypodermis prevents tearing and sustains the main dermal strength. Within these three layers of skin are sublayers with cells that perform specific functions.

sebaceous glands
oil glands of the skin connected to hair follicles

arrector pili
an appendage that is attached to the dermal papilla and to the hair shaft

cornified
hardening or thickening of the skin

dermis
underlying or inner layer of the skin

hypodermis
layer of subcutaneous fat and connective tissue lying beneath the epidermis

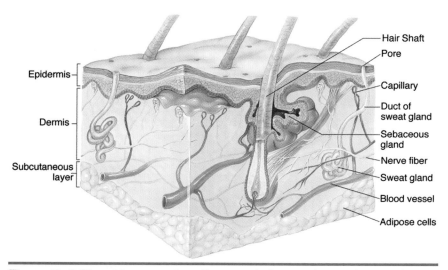

Figure 2–2 The skin comprises three main layers, the epidermis, the dermis, and the hypodermis

The Epidermis

epidermis
the thin, outermost layer of the skin

stratified epithelium
layers of tissue that lack blood vessels;
acts as a surface barrier

avascular
lacking in blood vessels and, thus,
having a poor blood supply

keratin
a protein found in the skin that helps
guard against invasion

keratinization
the process of living cells moving
upward and changing to dead cells

The epidermis consists of layers made of stratified epithelium. (See Figure 2–3.) Compared to the dermis, the epidermis is often very thin, approximately 0.12 millimeter, but its thickness also varies dramatically over the body.[6]

It is thickest on the palms of the hands and soles of the feet and thinnest on the eyelids. The epidermis is avascular (without blood vessels), impermeable to water, physically tough, and dry at the surface to impede the growth of microorganisms.

Skin cells divide in the lowest layer and migrate upward to replace the dead skin cells that have been shed. When the epidermis is injured or diseased, its replacement speeds up in response, and this is important to us as clinicians. As the cells, called keratinocytes, move upward, they become filled with a protein substance called keratin that helps protect the skin against invasion. The process of living cells moving upward and changing to dead cells is known as keratinization.

The many epidermal layers are divided into two main zones: 1. horny zone, and 2. germinal zone. The horny zone, the outer portion of the epidermis, is divided into three layers of differing cells:

1. stratum corneum
2. stratum lucidum
3. stratum granulosum

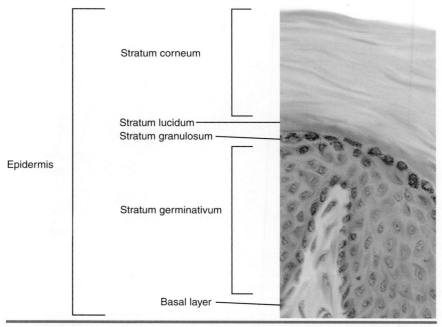

Stratum corneum

Stratum lucidum
Stratum granulosum

Epidermis

Stratum germinativum

Basal layer

Figure 2–3 The epidermis consists of layers made of stratified epithelium

The Stratum Corneum

The outermost layer of the skin is the stratum corneum. It is this outermost layer of dead, cornified skin cells that is constantly shed, even through the gentle friction of changing clothes. These cells are flat and without nuclei, and are predominantly bound by sebum, the skin's natural lubricant. However, this is not enough to prevent the regular shedding of dead skin cells. The stratum corneum varies in thickness: thin on the upper arm, and thicker on the palms and soles of the feet and in areas of chronic friction. Its thickness can be affected by simple dry skin as well as by disease processes such as psoriasis.

The Stratum Lucidum

Below the stratum corneum lies the stratum lucidum. This layer gets its name from the transparent nature of the cells that contain eleidin, a clear substance derived from keratohyalin, which allow light to pass through

> Psoriasis is a malfunction of the epidermal cellular reproduction rate. The accelerated process creates a phenomenon known as psoriasis plaques. Psoriasis can also be environmentally precipitated, but usually people are genetically predisposed.

stratum corneum
superficial sublayer of the epidermis; varies in thickness over the body

psoriasis
skin disease marked by red scaly patches

stratum lucidum
the layer between the stratum corneum and the stratum granulosum in the palms of the hands and the soles of the feet

eleidin
a substance in the stratum lucidum

transepidermal water loss (TEWL)
the process by which our bodies constantly lose water via evaporation

natural moisturizing factor (NMF)
compound found only in the top layer of skin that gives cells their ability to bind with water

As long as we are not submerged, our bodies constantly lose water via evaporation through our skin. This process is called **transepidermal water loss (TEWL)**.[7]

In normal epidermis the water content decreases the closer we get to the surface. Water makes up to 70 to 75 percent of the weight of layers beneath, but only 10 to 15 percent of the weight of the stratum corneum. When too much water evaporates, our skin and also our bodies suffer ill effects. Preventing excessive water loss is important both to the skin and to the body as a whole.

The stratum corneum contains **natural moisturizing factor (NMF)**. NMF helps to keep the skin soft and moisturized even in dry climates.[8] NMF is composed of amino acids and filaggrin, water-soluble chemicals capable of absorbing large quantities of water. The presence of NMF in the stratum corneum is critical for soft and flexible skin. Although NMF is contained only in the uppermost layer of the skin, its existence is made possible by ingredients provided by deeper structures.[9]

It is worth noting that NMF and TEWL have nothing to do with water loss associated with sweating. It is a common misconception that drinking water will improve hydration levels of the skin. This is simply not true. Drinking water improves water level inside the body, but is used up there. The best way to rehydrate the skin is by applying a topical moisturizer. NMF is diminished by age and excessive exposure to soap. This is key to understanding the phenomenon of dry skin.

stratum granulosum
the granular layer of skin found at the bottom of the horny zone

keratohyalin granules
substance in cytoplasm cells of the stratum granulosum

filaggrin
synthesizes lipids (fats) that are thought to serve as "intercellular cement"; mportant component of NMF

stratum spinosum
the superior layer of the stratum germinativum; named for its shape and spiny, thorn-like protrusions; also known as the "prickle cell layer"

desmosomes
small hair-like structures in the spiny layer of the epidermis

lamellar granules
control lipids that produce NMF

lipids
fat or fat-like substances, descriptive not chemical

cholesterol
an alcohol distributed in animal tissues and synthesized in the liver. A precursor to certain hormones and, in some individuals, coronary artery disease.

fatty acids
one of many molecules that are long chains of lipid-carboxylic acid found in fats and oils

ceramides
a class of lipids that do not contain glycerol

them. The cells in this layer also lack nuclei, and they lose their shape. The stratum lucidum is present only in the palms of the hands and the soles of the feet where the epidermis is thickest. It is not found in thin skin.

The Stratum Granulosum

At the bottom of the horny zone lies the stratum granulosum, also known as the granular layer, because of the granules that appear in the cells here. Unlike the flatter stratum corneum, the stratum granulosum cells have a distinct shape. The lower cells have nuclei and are still living. As these cells are pushed upward by new cells, they lose their nuclei and organelles and die. This layer gives the skin its opaque appearance due to the presence of keratohyalin granules in the cytoplasm. The stratum granulosum also contains a compound called filaggrin, which assists keratinocytes in creating the natural moisturizing factor found in the stratum corneum. Filaggrin also combines with other cells found within the granular layer to provide strength and stability for the epidermis. The stratum granulosum varies in thickness. It is at its thickest on the soles of the feet, followed by the palms of the hands, and it is at its thinnest on the eyelids. Persistent friction and pressure cause areas to thicken for protection and form calluses, as found on the soles of the feet, elbows, and knees.

The Stratum Spinosum

The stratum spinosum is also known as the "spiny layer" or prickle cell layer because of the cells' prickly shape. They are living cells, each containing a nucleus. Each cell is attached to the cells around it by prickly shaped fibers called desmosomes. The hair-like desmosomes permit materials to move around them in the intercellular space (the spaces between cells). Lamellar granules are also found here. These granules control lipids that migrate to the stratum corneum and become another component of natural moisturizing factor, along with cholesterol, fatty acids, and ceramides. It is in the stratum spinosum that keratinocytes depart the basal layer and show the first signs of keratinization. Many books refer to the stratum basale and the stratum spinosum together as forming the stratum germinativum.

The Stratum Basale

The stratum basale is appropriately named as it is located in the basement of the epidermis, also known as the stratum germinativum or germinating layer. As the lowest layer of the epidermis, it is in contact with the dermis. It is the layer in which cell division called mitosis takes place and where new epidermal tissue is formed and begins migrating to the surface of the skin, replacing the dead skin cells that have been shed. Basal cells remain in the basal layer, creating a solid skin foundation, and keratinocytes begin their upward migration to the stratum corneum. This desquamation process takes approximately 28 days—much less in babies and younger children and longer in mature adults, particularly people in their late twenties and older.

In the stratum basale are melanocytes. Ultraviolet rays from sunlight react with the amino acid tyrosine found in the melanocytes and produce melanin, a dark pigment that gives skin its color and protects the dermis from ultraviolet radiation and sun damage. Approximately one in every ten cells in this layer is a melanocyte. The color of the skin depends on the melanin produced. Generally, people of different races have approximately the same number of melanocytes. People with dark skin have melanocytes that are more active and produce more melanin.

Stratum Mucosum

The stratum mucosum, combined with the stratum basale, is known as the malpighian layer. The stratum mucosum is only a single cell layer above the stratum basale, and there is a difference of opinion as to whether it should be considered a separate layer or part of the stratum basale.

Specialized Epidermal Cells

Within the epidermis there are four specialized cells: keratinocytes, melanocytes, Langerhans', and Merkel cells. (See Table 2–2.)

---

stratum basale
single cell layer that is the deepest layer of the epidermis

stratum germinativum
the lower level of the epidermis where cell division occurs

mitosis
the process by which a cell divides into two daughter cells

desquamation
the act of exfoliating dead skin cells

melanocytes
melanin-forming cells

tyrosine
an amino acid present in melanocytes

melanin
grains of pigment that give hair and skin its color

stratum mucosum
single-cell layer of the epidermis; found above the stratum germinativum

---

Table 2–2	Specialized Epidermal Cells	
Specialized Epidermal Cells	**Location**	**Function**
Keratinocytes	Generated in the strata basale, and half begin to migrate upward, eventually to be sloughed off	Basic skin cells that collectively make up the skin; undergo desquamation
Melanocytes	Between epidermis and the dermis	Secrete pigments that give skin, hair, and eyes their color
Langerhans' cells	Strata spinosum and strata basale	Patrol the epidermis for foreign invaders, ingest them, for removal by the lymphatic system
Merkel cells	By nerve endings throughout epidermis	Exact function unclear; likely involved in sensation

Keratinocytes

The majority of cells in the epidermis are keratinocytes. These cells are generated in the lower basal layer or stratum germinativum and then move upward to replace the dead skin cells that have been shed. Keratinocytes are filled with a protein substance called keratin that helps protect the skin against invasion. Fifty percent of the keratinocytes produced remain in the basal sublayer of the epidermis; the others, retaining their keratinocyte identity, begin the process of keratinization.

During differentiation, keratinocytes go through critical changes. The shape flattens, then organelles are "lost" and fibrous proteins are shaped, and, finally, as the cell becomes dehydrated, the cell membrane thickens. Keratinization takes approximately 28 to 35 days in younger people and up to 45 days as people age. When it takes longer, it shows. Delays in the migration process as well as extrinsic factors, such as smoking, solar damage, and pollution, cause our skin to turn sallow and gray. It causes the complaint so often heard from our clients that "my skin just looks dull and dirty."

Melanocytes

Located in or near the basal layer are melanocytes. (See Figure 2–4.) These are the melanin producing cells that give the skin and hair its color. Melanin is a form of pigment that lends color to skin, eyes, and hair. The pigment provides the skin with protection from the sun's ultraviolet rays. The UV rays from sunlight react with the amino acid tyrosine found in the melanocytes and produce the melanin.

Keratinocytes carry the melanin as they migrate upwards.[10] In this cellular relationship *melanocytes* are the melanin-*making* cells and keratinocytes are the melanin-*taking* cells, and thus it is that, although melanocytes produce melanin, in the end keratinocytes contain it. The proportion of melanocytes to keratinocytes varies from 1:4 to 1:10, depending on age, with the melanocyte proportion decreasing with age. As we age, therefore, our ability to protect our skin with melanin decreases.

Langerhans' Cells

Langerhans' cells are found in the epidermis and warn against the invasion of microorganisms, responding to that invasion. These cells are smaller in breadth than keratinocytes, and stretch finger-like processes between keratinocytes to the surface, where they scan like periscopes. Upon encountering "bad bacteria" they "acquire" them and transport the offenders to specialized white blood cells called T lymphocytes in the regional lymph nodes for disposal.

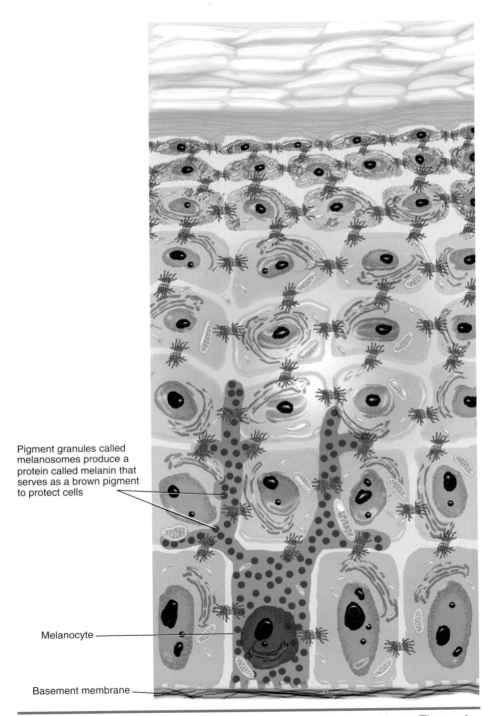

Pigment granules called melanosomes produce a protein called melanin that serves as a brown pigment to protect cells

Melanocyte

Basement membrane

Figure 2–4 The melanocytes are located in or near the basal layer. The melanocytes lend color to the skin.

Merkel cell
usually close to nerve endings and may
be involved in sensory perception

hyperpigmentation
overproduction and overdeposits of
melanin

hypopigmentation
a lack of melanin product

Merkel Cells

The Merkel cell is found in the basal layer of the epidermis and around the hair follicle. These cells are believed to work as receptors that mediate the sense of touch as well as hair movement. They are numerous about the lip, hard palate, palms, finger and foot pads, and proximal nail folds. The Merkel cell is known in the dermatology field as the source of a rare but aggressive form of skin cancer called Merkel cell carcinoma that begins in the germinating layer and the hair follicle, most commonly on the face and neck.

THE SKIN'S PIGMENTATION

Pigmentation of the skin is caused by the production of melanin in the stratum basale. Pigmentation is the result of both intrinsic and extrinsic factors. An excessive production of melanin is called hyperpigmentation, while an underproduction of melanin is called hypopigmentation.

Hyperpigmentation

Hyperpigmentation can be caused by intrinsic and extrinsic factors. Intrinsically, an individual can be genetically predisposed to melasma gravidarum, the mask of pregnancy. Extrinsically, sun damage can manifest itself during the aging process as chloasma or liver spots. Compromised skin that has areas of inflammation or erythema from unprotected exposure to UV rays can become hyperpigmented. (See Figure 2–5.) Intrinsically, pregnancy, the birth control pill, and other medications can also overstimulate the melanocytes in a haphazard fashion. (See Table 2–3.)

Unfortunately, hyperpigmentation can also result from aggressive or mismanaged peeling, lifting of the skin during a waxing service, overtreatment or incorrect application of electrolysis or laser hair removal, and intense pulsed-light therapy (FotoFacial™)—from any procedure in which the skin is overstimulated or injured. Hyperpigmentation is especially common in type IV, V, and VI skin types. These skin types should be treated with care both in the clinic and at home to avoid hyperpigmentation.

Hypopigmentation

Hypopigmentation occurs when melanocytes no longer produce melanin, leaving areas of the skin without pigment. Scarring caused by excoriation or a blistering burn are extrinsic causes, while diseases such as

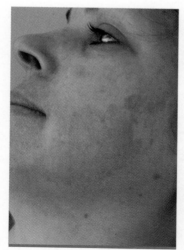

Figure 2–5 The skin can become hyperpigmented from the sun, pregnancy, the birth control pill, and other medications

Table 2–3   Diseases of Pigmentation

Actinic lentigines: caused by sun damage to the skin presenting as freckling

Merkel cell carcinoma: a rare but aggressive cancer that occurs in the germinating layer where melanin is produced, causing discoloration

Kaposi's sarcoma: a skin cancer that presents as brown and purple lesions, symptomatic in people with advanced stage AIDS

Melasma: the general term used for disorders and diseases that cause hyperpigmentation, the most common usage of which is the mask of pregnancy

Chloasma: liver spots appearing in mature skin due to previous sun damage

Tinea versicolor: also called pityriasis versicolor is a yeast infection that compromises the skin's ability to produce melanin, resulting in hypopigmentation

Vitiligo: possibly caused by an autoimmune disorder that destroys the melanocytes. The resulting hypopigmentation can present in an area as small as a macule or over much larger portions of the body.

Basal cell carcinoma: cancer that forms in the germinal layer of the epidermis where pigment is produced, and as a result it presents with hyperpigmented and multiple colored lesions

Melanoma: cancer that gets its name from the melanocytes that produce this cancer; may present like that of the basal cell, but it is far more deadly as it spreads (metastasizes) more aggressively

> Vitiligo affects approximately 4 percent of the world's population.[11] Affecting the melanocytes of the skin, vitiligo causes hypopigmentation that is irreversible. Those afflicted with vitiligo are often physiologically impacted and self-conscious of their appearance.

vitiligo and leukoderma (in association with inflammatory diseases such as atopic dermatitis) are two intrinsic and relatively common disorders that create hypopigmentation.

Just as with hyperpigmentation, hypopigmentation can also occur when skin has been damaged through aggressive treatment. Any treatment that affects melanocytes may result in hypopigmentation. (See Figure 2–6.) "White spots" are indicative that melanocytes have been damaged and will no longer produce pigment. This can be seen, following an incorrectly applied laser hair removal treatment, scabbing from electrolysis (see Table 2–4), deep dermabrasion, chemical peels, and laser resurfacing. Microdermabrasion is a less common cause.

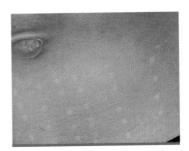

Figure 2–6 Hypopigmentation is caused when the melanocytes cease to function from either injury or disease

connective tissue
fibrous tissue that binds, protects, cushions, and supports the various parts of the body

reticula
a protein fiber

collagen
fiber made of protein that gives the skin its form and strength

■ THE DERMIS

The dermis, often called the *living layer* or "true skin," is made of dense connective tissue. This tissue is crisscrossed with three types of fibers that lend strength and elasticity. These fibers—reticula, collagen, and

Table 2–4   Pigment Changes with Hair Removal

Waxing: Lifting of the skin during waxing exposes the basal layer and damages melanocyte production causing hyperpigmentation and hypopigmentation. UV exposure to a scabbed or inflamed area can cause hyperpigmentation.

Electrolysis: Incorrect probing or excessive treatment energy applied too close to the surface of the hair follicle can cause eschars, which can lead to hypopigmentation. Overtreatment of an area with electrolysis can cause inflammation. If the area is inflamed, UV exposure can cause hyperpigmentation.

Laser hair removal: Hairs not adequately trimmed may cause blistering during a treatment, which may lead to hyperpigmentation. Incorrect wavelengths and fluences for the skin/hair type can result in extreme erythema causing both hyper- and hypopigmentation.

elastin
connective tissue proteins

dermal-epidermal junction
where the dermis and the epidermis meet

papillary dermis
the most superficial layer of the dermis

dermal papilla
small, cone-shaped indentation at the base of the hair follicle that fits into the hair bulb; also called the hair papilla

collagenous
of collagen fibers

papillae
cone-shaped, finger-like projections that protrude into the epidermis

glycosaminoglycans (GAGs)
polysaccharide chains, most prominent in the dermis, that bind with water, smoothing and softening the surface from below

elastin—form a network that creates stability for the skin. On its superficial side the dermis holds the epidermis at the dermal-epidermal junction (DEJ). On its distal side it attaches to subcutaneous tissue. It is about 2 millimeters thick.

The dermis is divided into layers called the papillary layer and the reticular layer (see Figure 2–7). Differing collagenous fibers subdivide these layers.

The Papillary Dermis

The papillary dermis or papillary layer, not to be confused with the dermal papilla at the base of the hair, lies directly below the epidermis and is made of elastic collagenous and reticular fibers. Reticular fibers are cone-shaped, finger-like projections called papillae or rete-pegs, which protrude upward into the epidermis and downwards into the reticular dermis, locking the layers together. Intertwined in this layer are superficial capillaries looped around the papillae.

Papillary dermis, the most superficial layer of the dermis, is the first skin layer to contain capillary blood vessels, small nerves, and lymphatic vessels. Blood vessels provide temperature changes when they constrict or dilate; thus, it is papillary dermis that is specifically responsible for thermoregulation of the body. It is widened vessels in the rete-pegs that cause "broken capillaries." People with transparent or very light skin may flush or blush, which is caused by a dilation of the capillaries in the rete-pegs.

The papillary dermis also contains glycosaminoglycans (GAGs), a variety of "chains" made of polysaccharide, a type of complex carbohydrate. GAGs are attracted to water and are thought capable of binding up

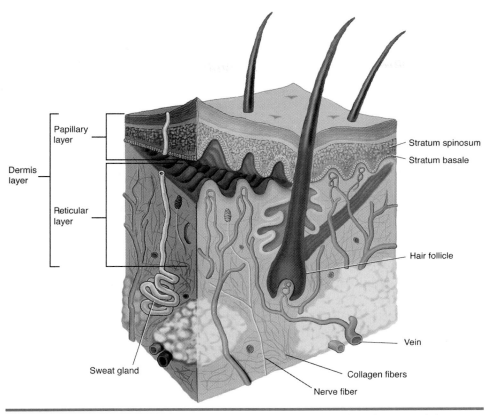

Figure 2–7 The dermis is divided into two layers: the papillary layer and the reticular layer

to 1,000 times their weight in water. An understanding of this and moisture content in general is important to electrologists and is further discussed.

The papillary layer also forms the connective tissue sheath around hair follicles. Meissner's corpuscles, which are the tactile nerve endings sensitive to touch, are in this layer.

The Reticular Dermis

The thickest layer of the skin, making up the greatest portion of it, is the reticular dermis. It is located beneath papillary dermis and rests on the thick pad of fat known as subcutaneous tissue. Here lies the real anchor of the skin.

The reticular layer is composed of dense bundles of collagen fibers. These fibers run in parallel layers and are denser closer to the papillary layer; they thin as they incorporate into the fatty subcutaneous tissue. In the reticular layer are numerous appendages: arrector pili muscles, blood

Meissner's corpuscles
nerve endings in the skin that are sensitive to touch

reticular dermis
a deep layer of the dermis; composed of dense bundles of collagen fibers; contains vessels, glands, nerve endings, and follicles

vessels, fat cells, hair follicles, lymph vessels, nerve endings, sebaceous glands, and sudoriferous glands.

Specialized Dermal Cells

Specialized dermal cells have multiple functions ranging from providing nutrition, eliminating waste and building collagen. (See Table 2–5.)

Fibroblast Cells

Fibroblasts are the "command" cells for the dermis. They direct the production of collagen, elastin, *reticulin,* and the ground substance for the dermis. In response to injury, fibroblasts proliferate to manufacture new collagen, from which scarring occurs.[12]

Mast Cells

Along with lymphocytes and macrophages, mast cells reside in connective tissue of the dermis, usually in the neighborhood of blood vessels. These cells protect against injury and invasion. Release of histamine by mast cells produces the inflammation that ousts intruders and begins wound healing.[13] In allergic reactions manifested in the skin, such as hives, there are large numbers of mast cells. Large numbers of mast cells are seen in conditions such as urticaria pigmentosa.

Ground Substance

Through diffusion, ground substance provides nutrients to and removes wastes from other tissue components.[14] It is integral to the healing process. As a wound heals, the available ground substance creates a moister wound that will heal more quickly. It is constantly undergoing synthesis and degradation. The ground substance of the dermis consists largely of glycosaminoglycans. Age probably brings a decrease in the ground substance.

ground substance
consists mainly of glycosaminoglycans (hyaluronic acid, chondroitin sulfate, and dermatan sulfate); involved in maintenance and repair of dermis

urticaria pigmentosa
hives that pigment; Dariers sign

Table 2–5   Specialized Dermal Cells

Specialized Dermal Cells	Location	Function
Fibroblasts	Reticular dermis, papillary dermis	Direct the production of collagen, reticulin, and ground substance
Mast cells	Papillary dermis	Protect skin against invasion and infection
Ground substance	Reticular dermis, papillary dermis	Provide nutrients and remove waste

■ HYPODERMIS OR SUBCUTANEOUS TISSUE

Subcutaneous tissue is the fatty layer beneath the dermis that gives the body smoothness and contour. (See Figure 2–8.) It contains fats as an energy source and acts as a protective cushion for the outer skin. Subcutaneous tissue is also called subcutis tissue or adipose tissue. This layer separates the dermis from the underlying musculature of the body. It also helps the skin to move over it as the attachment of subcutaneous tissue to reticular dermis is not tight or rigid. The subcutaneous tissue is crisscrossed with connective tissue, fibers, and layers interspersed with fat to hold it together. When pockets of fat accumulate between the connective tissue bands beyond the ability of the connective tissue to hold it smooth, the appearance is called "cellulite" or "orange-peel"

adipose tissue
connective tissue in animal bodies that contains fat

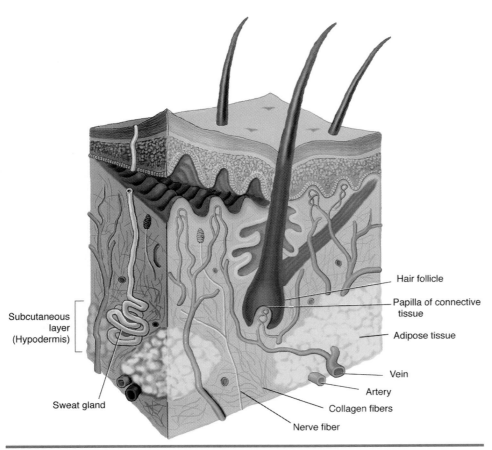

Subcutaneous layer (Hypodermis)

Sweat gland

Hair follicle

Papilla of connective tissue

Adipose tissue

Vein

Artery

Collagen fibers

Nerve fiber

Figure 2–8 The hypodermis or subcutaneous tissue is the fatty layer beneath the dermis that gives the body smoothness and contour

skin. Cellulite is generally more apparent in women. It is also more likely to appear in certain areas of the body as well, such as the hips, thighs, and buttocks.

This layer also varies in thickness depending on the individual's sex, age, and overall health. Many of the arteries, veins, and lymphatics circulate through this area, as do nerve endings and an abundance of fat cells.

Blood and Lymph Supply

A vascular network of arteries and veins circulate their way into the dermis, where they branch off into smaller capillaries at the hair follicles, the hair papillae, and the skin's various glands. As the blood supply circulates through the skin via tiny capillaries, it transports the oxygen-rich blood and nutrients essential for growth, reproduction, and tissue repair of the skin, hair, and nails.

Lymph glands produce lymph, which is made of white blood corpuscles and plasma. Vessels carrying the lymph, which contains waste products, salts, and nitrogenous wastes, run parallel to the blood supply and return to the deeper lymph nodes, where the lymphatic fluid is filtered for excretion. (See Figure 2–9.)

Sudoriferous Glands

The sudoriferous glands, the sweat glands, are under the control of the sympathetic nervous system. They are found deep in the dermis and have tubular ducts extending all the way up to the pores in the epidermis. There are two kinds of sweat glands: (1) apocrine and (2) eccrine.

The Apocrine Glands

The apocrine glands, found in the genital area and in the axillae, or underarm, usually open into hair follicles. During perspiration, water, salts, cellular waste, and fatty substances emit from these glands and combine with bacteria at the skin's surface to create body odor. Apocrine glands are also believed to excrete pheromones, which are thought to play a role in sexual attraction.

The Eccrine Glands

The eccrine glands are found all over the body but in increased numbers on the forehead, the palms of the hands, and the soles of the feet. They excrete mainly water with a little salt, urea, and other water-soluble substances.

arteries
carry oxygenated blood away from the heart

veins
carry unoxygenated blood to the lungs

lymph
a fluid found in the lymphatic vessels

sudoriferous glands
the skin's sweat glands

apocrine
glands in the axillae and groin that secrete sweat and substances that, when contaminated with bacteria, produce body odor

axillae
underarm

pheromones
chemicals produced by humans and other animals that, when secreted, influence other members of the same species

eccrine
glands throughout the skin that excrete mainly water and salt

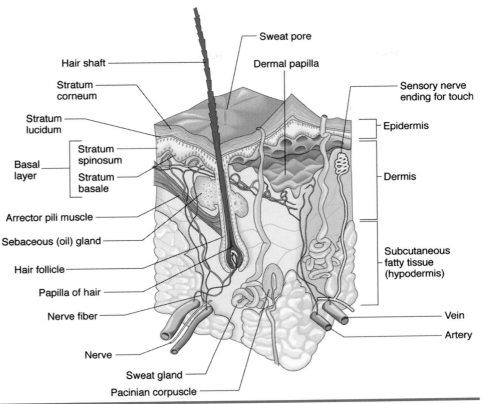

Figure 2–9 The skin has many structures that are relevant to the body's survival

Sebaceous Glands

The *sebaceous glands* are found all over the skin. They are mainly, though not always, appendages to the hair follicles and open into the shafts of hair follicles. These glands are found in greater numbers on the scalp, the T-zone (forehead, nose, and chin), and the cheeks. The sebaceous glands vary in size and shape and in their production of a waxy, oily substance called sebum, which lubricates the skin.

The endocrine system influences these glands, which are most active during puberty.

Nerve Endings

Nerve endings carry impulses to the brain. They are found at various levels of the skin and have different shapes, depending on the jobs they must do. As mentioned previously, Meissner's corpuscles are the most superficial and are responsible for touch, as opposed to **Pacinian's corpuscles**, which are round and lie much deeper in the dermis so that more pressure

Pacinian's corpuscles
found in the subcutaneous tissue; sensory nerve endings

is required to register sensation. Also closer to the surface is the pain receptor. Below the pain nerve endings are the receptors for heat, which are thread-like, and those for cold, which are round.

Hair

The hair, also called the pilosebaceous unit, is discussed in greater depth later in the chapter.

Suffice it to say that the hair and its follicle, including the sebaceous gland and arrector pili, are major appendages to the structure of the skin. Hair is found all over the body, with the exception of the soles of the feet and the palms of the hands. A great deal of hair on the body is invisible to the naked eye. Hair is denser on the head and limbs, and, after puberty, in the groin area and in the axillae. Hormones and genetic inheritance influence hair growth at different ages in males and females. The root or papilla of the mature terminal hair is found in the lower part of the dermis, and the hair shaft reaches up to its follicular opening in the epidermis. The arrector pili muscle is an appendage that is attached to the underside of the papillary layer and to the hair shaft between the bulb and the sebaceous gland. This is responsible for lifting the hair to trap a layer of air on the skin's surface.

■ SKIN PHYSIOLOGY

Not much thicker than a sheet of paper, skin is quite complex. In general terms, it protects, senses, and aids temperature regulation, excretion, immunologic responses, and metabolism.

The Functions of the Skin

As the body's largest sensory organ, the skin has multiple functions, including protection, heat regulation, excretion, secretion, absorption, sensation, and the synthesis of vitamin D. (See Table 2–6.) Hair

terminal hair
hair found on the scalp, arms, legs, axillae, and pubic area (postpuberty)

excretion
the act of discharging waste matter from tissues or organs

secretion
the process of producing and discharging substances from glands

absorption
the uptake of one substance into another

Table 2–6　The Six Functions of the Skin
Protection and Immunologic Response
Thermoregulation
Excretion
Secretion
Absorption/Penetration
Sensation

plays an important role in many of these functions. Healthy skin should have hair.

Protection and Immunologic Response

Skin covers the body and protects it against the environment and the invasion of bacteria.

Normal skin is usually not sterile and is often covered by legions of bacteria. These bacteria are generally noninvading and nonpathogenic. The skin has a built-in protective aid known as the acid mantle, which has a pH of 5 to 5.6 (7 is neutral). The acid mantle is caused by the combined activity of the sweat and sebaceous glands. Perspiration is acidic. As it lies on the skin's surface, it can act as a bactericide by inhibiting the growth of bacteria. (However, this is not true of areas of higher perspiration, like the axillae and groin area, where the skin is softer and where there is less acidity in excessive perspiration, allowing bacterial growth.)

Reactions, often inflammation, swelling, and welts, occur when an unwanted organism invades the skin. Unwanted organisms are recognized by the mast cells and the Langerhans' cells in the epidermis that warn against invading microorganisms. Leukocytes are released to engulf and destroy the invading organism. The reaction may seem extreme, but it is the skin's natural way of preventing the spread of infection to the surrounding tissue.

Starting with the outermost layer of the epidermis, the horny layer acts as a barrier against bacterial invasion and water absorption. The skin is waterproof, in part due to the aid of sebum secreted from sebaceous glands that lubricates and waterproofs the epidermal layers and makes the skin soft and supple. Sebum also prevents drying and cracking and thereby prevents bacteria and germs from entering the skin and, in turn, the body.

Adult sebum is also believed to be fungicidal and may play a role in preventing some types of ringworm. When intact, the skin also prevents harmful fluids from entering the body. It not only prevents water from entering the body, it prevents water (transepidermal water loss), blood, and lymph from leaving the body.

The germinal layer, particularly the stratum germinativum, contains melanin-producing melanocytes that protect the body from harmful ultraviolet radiation. People with dark skin get better protection from ultraviolet radiation and generally have fewer incidences of skin cancer.

The adipose tissue in the subcutis cushions the body from falls, protects against minor trauma, and provides a source of energy.

The lymphatic system acts as a second line of defense against bacterial invasion. Lymphatic fluid and lymphocytes are produced in the lymph nodes. Lymphocytes are the only cells in the fluid and are

acid mantle
the bacteria-killing layer made of sweat and lipids

mast cells
large tissue cells present in the skin that produce histamine and other acute symptoms of allergic reactions

Langerhans' cells
cells found in the epidermis that warn against the invasion of microorganisms and respond to that invasion

leukocytes
white blood cells or corpuscles

subcutis
a layer of subcutaneous tissue

lymphocytes
cells produced in the lymph nodes, spleen, and thymus gland that produce antibodies capable of attacking infection

transported through lymph vessels, where they engulf bacteria and are carried to the lymph nodes for filtration and draining of waste products.

Thermoregulation

A healthy body temperature is usually around 98° Fahrenheit (37° Celsius) although the skin's surface temperature is slightly cooler at around 91° Fahrenheit (33° Celsius) depending on the temperature of the air it is exposed to. As changes occur in the environment, the body adjusts with various mechanisms to counteract those changes and to maintain a safe and appropriate internal body temperature. The skin plays a vital role in maintaining the body's temperature and homeostasis. It does so in numerous ways that all work together to help keep the body at a safe and healthy temperature. These ways include evaporation, perspiration, radiation, and insulation.

Evaporation of perspiration on the skin's surface produces cooling, also known as thermoregulation. Radiation from constriction and dilation of tiny blood vessels, called capillaries, affects body temperature. The dilation or expansion of capillaries causes the surface heat of the body to be reduced through radiation, visible in some skin types as a flushed pink appearance (e.g., in the face). Conversely, the constriction or contraction of capillaries slows blood flow, preserving heat and giving the skin a bluish tint.

The arrector pili muscle fiber is stimulated by the body when the body feels cold or experiences fear, contracting and lifting the hair, which then traps a layer of insulating air on the skin's surface. Even sebum, which is produced in the sebaceous gland, plays a role in heat regulation, lubricating the hair, keeping it supple, and preventing the hair from becoming brittle and breaking. The adipose tissue of the subcutis also acts as an effective insulator, keeping the body warm.

Excretion and Secretion

The sebaceous glands, as mentioned earlier, secrete sebum, the skin's natural lubricant.

During perspiration, salts, urea, and other waste materials are excreted through the sudoriferous glands and rise to the surface of the skin.

Absorption and Penetration

The skin can absorb oil- and fat-based substances to differing levels, but it cannot absorb water. Pharmaceutical topical creams and lotions, which can effect dramatic changes in the skin, can penetrate the dermis and absorb into the blood supply. For this reason, these creams and lotions

dilation
the process of widening or expanding

constriction
the process of narrowing

require medical guidance and physicians' prescriptions to be obtained and used.

Cosmeceuticals, which contain no drugs or medications that could cause drug interactions or carry warnings against usage if pregnant or nursing, may have deeper absorption qualities than standard over-the-counter cosmetics. They are believed to be able to effect greater change in the skin than drugstore brands. Cosmeceuticals are obtained from, and require the professional guidance of, a dermatologist, plastic surgeon, or skin care professional.

Another important factor in the skin's ability to absorb is the way it absorbs ultraviolet rays that are synthesized in the form of ergosterol and converted to vitamin D, a deficiency of which can cause soft bones as well as poor bone and teeth structure.

cosmeceuticals
those products that do more than decorate or camouflage but less than a drug would do

Sensation and Communication

Skin is capable of receiving a diverse amount of tactile information from a variety of receptors. (See Figure 2–10.) Neural receptors, some of them quite elaborate, mediate touch, position, pressure, temperature, and pain. The communication goes two ways and occurs instinctively. The skin releases signals such as blushing, pheromones (unique chemical signals), and body odor.

Through the skin's ability to register sensation we are aware of heat, cold, pain, pressure, and even an annoying itch. Nerves that receive and send these sensory signals to the brain show a variety of sensory endings, including expanded tips (Merkel's disks and Ruffini's endings), encapsulated endings (Pacinian's corpuscles, Meissner's corpuscles), and free

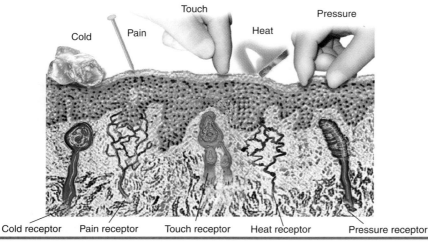

Cold   Pain   Touch   Heat   Pressure

Cold receptor   Pain receptor   Touch receptor   Heat receptor   Pressure receptor

Figure 2–10 The sensory nerve endings sense temperature, pain, and pressure

nerve endings. Pacinian's, Meissner's, and Merkel's corpuscles are all mechanoreceptors, responding to various types of touch. Pacinian's corpuscle registers deep pressure and vibration, Meissner's corpuscle registers fine tactile sensations like stroking and fluttering, Merkel's corpuscles register the pressure of a finger gliding across a surface, and Ruffini's corpuscle registers the tension and stretch of the skin.

Thermoreceptors register the sensations of hot and cold. If the body cannot react to escape the sensation of increased heat and damage results causing pain, the pain is perceived through nociceptors. Whereas a minor burn can be very painful, a third degree burn that causes nerve damage can leave the skin numb and without sensation once the tissue has healed over.

Metabolism

Blood vessels within the lower layer of the skin provide nutrition for the skin. Blood carries some of the minerals and vitamins important to skin's health and appearance, such as oxygen. Oxygen requirements for skin are *greater* than that for connective tissue, and if not enough oxygen is supplied, the health of the skin may suffer. This is why smoking cigarettes may cause problems with healing. Skin health not only affects how we look but also how quickly and smoothly injuries such as cat scratches and paper cuts heal.

■ THE PILOSEBACEOUS UNIT

Healthy hair is continually growing, shedding, and being replaced. To understand the physiology of the hair and its follicle, it is best to study it initially as one unit in its active stage. The hair sits in a pocket in the skin. The epidermis goes down around the base of the hair and back up to the surface. The space the hair occupies is known as the follicular canal. The outer sheath of the canal is formed from the basal cell layer. The inner side of the follicular canal that is made up of horny epidermal tissue is called the external root sheath. (See Figure 2–11.)

The Hair Follicle

The hair shaft is lined with epidermal tissue and in full-grown, active-hair stage extends downward, through the dermis to the subcutaneous tissue. The epidermal cells are responsible for producing the hair follicle and the hair matrix. The base of the follicular canal widens to the

follicular canal
the depression in the skin that houses the entire pilosebaceous unit

external root sheath
the inner side of the follicular canal, which is made of horny epidermal tissue

hair matrix
the germinating center of the hair follicle where mitotic activity occurs

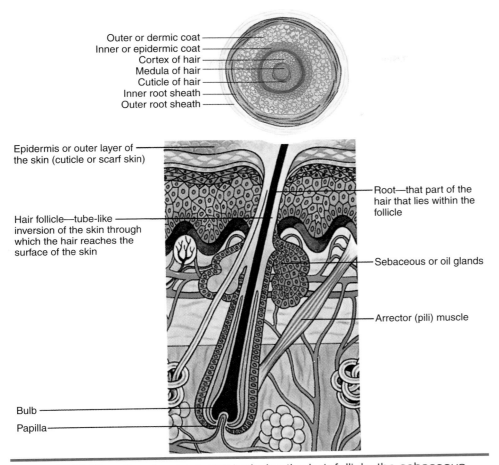

Outer or dermic coat
Inner or epidermic coat
Cortex of hair
Medula of hair
Cuticle of hair
Inner root sheath
Outer root sheath

Epidermis or outer layer of
the skin (cuticle or scarf skin)

Root—that part of the
hair that lies within the
follicle

Hair follicle—tube-like
inversion of the skin through
which the hair reaches the
surface of the skin

Sebaceous or oil glands

Arrector (pili) muscle

Bulb

Papilla

Figure 2–11 The pilosebaceous unit includes the hair follicle, the sebaceous glands, and the arrector pili muscle

hair follicle bulb. (See Figure 2–12.) The bulb, the area where the hair grows, contains the dividing cells of the hair matrix that produce the hair and the protective external and internal root sheath. The internal root sheath is sometimes visible on a tweezed hair, looking to the naked eye like a clump of petroleum jelly around the base of the hair. It protects the hair up as far as the sebaceous gland, where it disappears.

The Dermal Papilla and Papillae

The dermal papilla at the base of the hair bulb is an indentation that, as mentioned previously, is the layer of dermal tissue that attaches itself to the epidermis with protrusions called papillae. These papillae contain the

hair follicle bulb
the bulbous base of the hair follicle that houses the dermal papilla

internal root sheath
the innermost layer of the hair follicle, closest to the hair

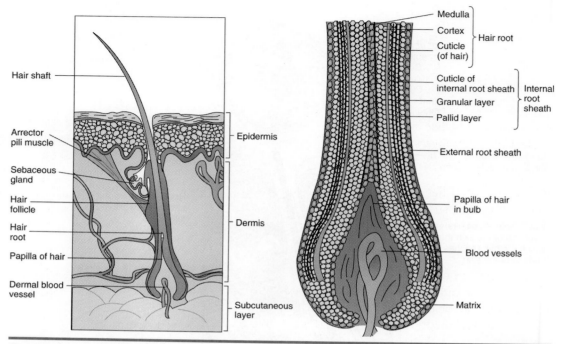

Figure 2–12 The hair follicle is made of many important structures

blood supply needed for providing nutrients for growth as well as the hormones that stimulate hair growth. This indentation is also called the papilla.

The Arrector Pili Muscle

The arrector pili muscle is an appendage that attaches to the underside of the papillary layer and to the hair shaft midway between the bulb and the sebaceous gland. This tiny muscle fiber is responsible for lifting the hair, thus trapping a layer of air on the skin's surface, making it partially responsible for heat regulation. Both fear and cold stimuli cause the arrector pili muscle fiber to contract, lifting the hair straight up. This action can be seen as "goose bumps" or "goose flesh."

The Sebaceous Gland

The sebaceous gland is attached to the hair follicle and opens into the follicular shaft. It secretes sebum, a protective fatty substance that lubricates the hair, preventing it from becoming dry and brittle and breaking. It also prevents the epidermis from drying and cracking and prevents bacteria and germs from entering the skin.

Layers of the Hair

The structure of a strand of hair is composed of three distinct layers: the cuticle, the cortex, and the medulla.

The Cuticle

The outermost of the hair layers is the cuticle. The cuticle is composed of transparent cells that overlap like scales. The purpose of the cuticle is to protect the inner layers of the hair.

The Cortex

Below the cuticle lies the cortex. This middle layer is made of elongated cells of fibrous tissue and the pigment that gives hair its color. The cortex is also the layer that gives hair its strength and elasticity.

The Medulla

The innermost layer of the hair is the medulla. Made of round cells, the medulla is also called the pith or marrow. Fine hair lacks the medulla, but the medulla can be found in all wavy hair. In general, the curlier the hair, the stronger the medulla.

The Pilosebaceous Unit and Superficial Healing

Because the outer sheath of the canal is formed from the basal cell layer and the external root sheath is made up of horny epidermal tissue, cells can reproduce and move upwards to form new epidermal tissue, replacing epidermal tissue that has been removed through trauma or laser resurfacing. This process is called epithelialization.

The Pilosebaceous Unit and Topical Product Absorption

External substances such as skin creams, ointments, and salves can enter the skin through the hair follicle openings at the surface of the epidermis.

Different Types of Hair

The three main types of hair that are found on the human body at one time or another are lanugo, vellus, and terminal hair.

Lanugo

Lanugo, soft, downy hair, is also called fetal hair because it is on fetuses in utero and on infants at birth, covering their bodies and scalps. It may

cuticle
the outermost layer of hair consisting of one overlapping layer of transparent, scale-like cells

cortex
the middle layer of the hair; a fibrous protein core formed by elongated cells containing melanin

medulla
the innermost layer of hair; composed of round cells; often absent in fine hair

lanugo
soft, downy hair present on fetuses in utero, and infants at birth

contain pigment and be light or dark. Lanugo often sheds a few weeks after birth. The part of the scalp that rests on the crib mattress often loses lanugo first due to friction. Eventually, the permanent hair begins to grow in.

Vellus

This is often confused with lanugo, but vellus is present through adulthood. It is fine, short, and often called "peach fuzz." Vellus often has no pigment or medulla. Women are believed to have 55 percent more vellus than men, and it can be found on women's faces where men produce beard and mustache hair at puberty onward. Vellus hair follicles that are overstimulated on women's faces, often due to tweezing or waxing and shaving against the direction of hair growth, can produce terminal hairs.

Terminal

Terminal hair is the longer, coarser, pigmented hair that covers the scalp and is found on the arms and legs of both males and females. At puberty, it is also found in the groin area and axillae of both males and females, as well as on the face of men and occasionally the chest and back.

Hair follicles are capable of producing vellus or terminal hair, which can be affected by age, genetics, and the hormonal changes of puberty, pregnancy, menopause, and hair removal procedures.

The Stages of Hair Growth

A clear understanding of the different stages of hair growth is of the uttermost importance to all clinicians offering any hair removal treatment, and especially laser hair removal and electrolysis. Determining a hair's particular stage can determine the success of a hair removal treatment. There are three main stages of hair growth: growing, transitional, and resting. Recent research, however, alludes to a fourth stage, the exogen stage. The percentage of hair in each stage and the length of time hair may be in a stage vary for different parts of the face and body. The three most common phases, anagen, catagen, and telogen, can be easily remembered in their growth sequence by using the acronym ACT. (See Figure 2–13.)

Anagen: The Growing Phase

Anagen is the hair's active growing phase, when the hair follicle is at its deepest. At this stage, the hair matrix is active, encapsulating the dermal

vellus
fine, short hair with no pigment, found mainly on women's faces; also referred to as "peach fuzz"

exogen
fourth stage of hair, currently being studied

anagen
the growth phase in the hair cycle in which a new hair is synthesized

catagen
the transition stage of the hair's growth cycle; the period between the growth and resting phases

telogen
the resting phase of the hair follicle in its growth cycle

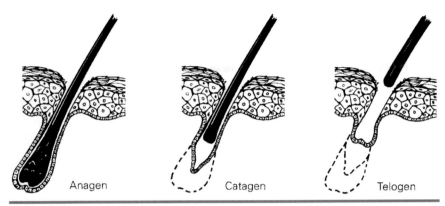

Figure 2–13 The three phases of hair growth are anagen, catagen, and telogen. They can be easily remembered in their growth sequence by using the acronym ACT.

papilla, and the bulb of the hair is visibly darker. Anagen can be affected and altered by the health of the individual, by the use of certain drugs and medications, and by pregnancy. Once a growing anagen hair has reached its full length, it can remain there, depending on location, for varying amounts of time—a few weeks on the fingers to eight years on the scalp.

Catagen: The Transitional Phase

Catagen occurs when the hair follicle separates from the dermal papilla. The follicle shrinks to about a third of its anagen size. A thin cord of epidermal tissue attaching the follicle to the dermal papilla retracts upward, with the dermal papilla. Catagen is the shortest hair-growth phase, lasting for only a few days up to a few weeks. Only a very small percentage of hairs are at this stage at any given time.

It is more difficult to recognize the bulb in catagen, because it is somewhere between the anagen and telogen stages and must be tweezed to be observed. What can be observed is that there is a slight reduction in the pigment of the hair, due to a reduction of melanin in the bulb.

Telogen: The Resting Phase

By the time the catagen hair becomes a telogen hair in its resting phase, the follicle is one-third its original anagen size. The base of the hair looks like a club, from whence it gets the name club hair. The bulb is usually white. The now-shrunk dermal papilla is separated from the hair follicle and is attached only by the thin cord of cornified and nucleated epidermal cells. It will be released by the end of the telogen phase, triggering the start of the exogen phase.

club hair
hair that has lost its root structure and that, when shed from the follicle, exhibits a round shape

Exogen: The Shedding Phase

The exogen stage of hair growth has long been recognized in the veterinary world and furrier industry. Any of us with cats and dogs appreciate the aggravation of a shedding pet. There may be minor shedding throughout the year, but as the warmer weather rolls around, the animal's coat seems to shed in handfuls. The shedding process with human hair is more subtle and has therefore been less recognizable as its own phase in the hair growth cycle.

What we once considered a part of the telogen stage, i.e., the hair follicle completely inactive, is only a part of the picture. We also perceived that the hair is simply pushed out by a new anagen hair. New studies now show this not to be the case. The hair sits unattached to the dermal papilla, yet still moored in the follicle by the thin chord of epidermal cells. It has now been determined under microscopic testing and evaluation that during the exogen phase a proteolytic event occurs between the hair and the epidermal cells attaching it to the follicle. The cellular adhesion molecules called desmoglein break down and reduce, thus allowing the hair to shed. This proteolytic action is an event that is its own phase separate from a simple quiescence of the telogen phase. The follicle may sit seemingly and inexplicably empty for a considerable period of time, longer than the typical telogen stage of the hair follicle in that particular area. This may be observed when reshaping eyebrows that had been overwaxed in the center, leaving the area seemingly without active follicles, but when left for some months, follicles begin to produce new hairs. While this shedding phase has not yet been determined or officially labeled a human stage of hair growth, the debate continues.

Hair Growth

Understanding hair growth is still an incomplete science, but there are documented, strong scientific findings that help explain the effects of certain elements on hair growth. Hair grows faster in the summer, for example. Good health improves hair growth. Young people experience more hair growth. In contrast, there is an increase in the number of telogen hairs during illness, after childbirth, and when an individual is experiencing stress. Hair grows at an average of half an inch a month, or approximately half a millimeter per day, again depending on factors of health, age, stress, etc. Table 2–7 gives average measurements of the hair in its various stages in various parts of the body. While not absolutely accurate for any particular individual, this table can help explain what is potentially happening in a hair follicle in a particular part of the body at any given time. Excess androgens may certainly stimulate terminal hair to regrow faster, meaning a shorter telogen phase. Understanding the hair

Table 2–7   Hair Growth Table

Head	% Telogen	% Anagen	% Catagen	% Uncertain	Duration telogen	Duration anagen	No. follicles per sq cm	Hair growth rate	Total no. follicles in area	Depth of terminal anagen
Scalp	13	85	1–2	1–2	3–4 mos	2–6 yrs	350	0.35 mm		3–5 mm
Eyebrows	90	10			3 mos	4–8 wks		0.16 mm		2–2.5 mm
Ear	85	10			3 mos	4–8 wks				
Cheeks	30–50	50–70					880	0.32 mm		2–4 mm
Beard-chin	30	70			10 wks	1 yr	500	0.38 mm		2–4 mm
Moustache Upper lip	35	65			6 wks	16 wks	500			1–2.5 mm
Body										
Axillae	70	30			3 mos	4 mos	65	0.3 mm		3.5–4.5 mm
Trunk	NA	NA					70	0.3 mm	425,000	2–4.5 mm
Pubic area	70	30			3 mos	4 mos	70			3.5–5 mm
Arms	80	20			18 wks	13 wks	80	0.33 mm	220,000	
Legs and thighs	80	20			24 wks	16 wks	60	0.21 mm	370,000	2.5–4
Breasts	70	30					65	0.35 mm		3–4.5 mm

growth patterns greatly aids the electrologist and laser practitioners as they ascertain the early anagen stage of hair growth, which is the preferred stage for successful permanent removal. Understanding these cycles is also helpful to the waxing technician in explaining regrowth to clients.

WHEN HAIR BEGINS TO GROW ON THE BODY

Body hair begins to grow in utero during week 14 of the developing fetus. Coincidently this occurs at the same time reproductive developments take place in the fetus, for example, the development of the prostrate glands in boys and the descending of a girl's ovaries from the abdomen into the pelvis. In women, the link between hair growth and reproduction and reproductive hormones repeat extrauterine during puberty, pregnancy, and menopause. During week 14 of the pregnancy, the lanugo hair forms over the scalp and body, including eyebrows of the fetus, and will continue sprouting until just before the baby is born. The lanugo hair begins to shed soon after birth and is replaced by vellus hair, as well as terminal hair on the scalp. The number of hair follicles that we have as adults were all present at our birth. (See Figure 2–14.)

During puberty the development of the secondary sexual characteristics of hair growth occur, with terminal hair forming around the genitalia and axillae, and in males on the chest and face. This hair growth continues through adulthood with other subtle and not so subtle changes occurring during pregnancy and menopause when women may experience increased facial hair in the same pattern as males during puberty, but may also experience a decrease in body hair in their forties. Men may produce longer coarser hair in their forties onwards, especially as the hair turns grey. Men may also experience hair loss in the form of male pattern baldness.

Hair Density Over the Body

Regardless of gender and ethnicity, we are all born with approximately 50 million hair follicles covering our entire body except the soles of the feet and the palms of the hands. One-fifth of our hair follicles are present on the scalp. It may appear that people from some geographic areas like the Middle East seem to have a greater abundance of hair than people from Eastern Asia, but the reality is that they produce an equal number of follicles. The hair growth appears more abundant in Middle Eastern or Mediterranean individuals as it may be longer, coarser, and more pigmented.

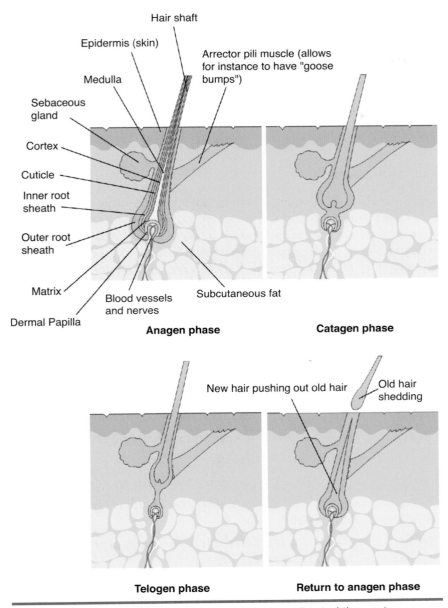

Figure 2–14 The hair growth process is a complicated three step process

The Importance of Hair

Even in utero, the lanugo hair offers protection. Outside the uterus that protective ability is even more important. Hair offers protection from sunlight, trauma, and injury. Hair on the scalp protects the head, eyebrows protect the bony orbital process, and eyelashes protect the eyes. Even nasal hair offers a filter-like protection into the body.

As discussed earlier, the body's thermoregulation is aided by the hair's ability to stand up, causing "goose flesh" and trapping a layer of air on the skin. Hair also offers protection from heat loss. However, we now have the ability to better provide protection with clothing, hats, and sun blocks and can therefore feel free and safe to remove a lot of unwanted body hair.

Conclusion

Understanding the anatomy and physiology of the skin, hair, and hair growth is fundamental for any hair removal specialist, regardless of hair removal method. A good education in the anatomy and physiology of skin and hair is the foundation on which to build all aspects of hair removal training and practice. You should now be able to appreciate the delicate nature of skin and the skin's tremendous capacity to protect itself, heal itself, fight infection, and recover from the many abuses it confronts daily.

TOP 10 TIPS TO TAKE TO THE CLINIC

1. The skin is a dynamic organ that changes daily.
2. Humans shed millions of dead skin flakes every minute.
3. The dermal papilla should not be confused with the papillary dermis.
4. Touch is the first sense to develop.
5. NMF is responsible for the water content in the stratum corneum.
6. GAGs in the papillary dermis are capable of binding up to 1,000 times their weight in water.
7. Hair grows at an average of half an inch a month, or approximately half a millimeter per day.
8. The length of the anagen phase determines the length of the hair.
9. Exogen is the shedding stage of a hair from the follicle.
10. Trimming hair does not have any effect on the root.

CHAPTER QUESTIONS

1. What are the three main layers of the skin?
2. Into which two zones is the epidermis divided?

3. What are the two layers of the epidermis?

4. In which layer are melanocytes found?

5. What are the two layers of the dermis?

6. What is a sudorific gland?

7. What is a Pacinian's corpuscle?

8. Where is the hair matrix?

9. What are three stages of hair growth?

10. Name at least five functions of the skin.

CHAPTER REFERENCES

1. Moore, E. (Ed.) (1999). *Quotation Finder*. Glascow, Scotland: Harper Collins.
2. Gray, J., MD. (1997). *The World of Skin Care*. P & G Skin Care and Research Center. Available at http://www.pg.com
3. American Society of Plastic Surgeons. (2003, December). *2002 Quick Facts On Cosmetic and Reconstructive Surgery Trends*. Available at http://www.plasticsurgery.org
4. Gray, J., MD. (1997). *The World of Skin Care*. P & G Skin Care and Research Center. Available at http://www.pg.com
5. Gray, J., MD. (1997). *The World of Skin Care*. P & G Skin Care and Research Center. Available at http://www.pg.com
6. Spense, A. P. (2004, February 22). *Basic Human Anatomy* (3rd ed.). Available at http://www.sawyerproducts.com
7. Baumann, L., MD. (2002). *Cosmetic Dermatology Practices and Principles*. New York, NY: McGraw-Hill.
8. Baumann, L., MD. (2002). *Cosmetic Dermatology Practices and Principles*. New York, NY: McGraw-Hill.
9. King, D. (2003, November 14). *Introduction to Skin Histology*. Retrieved December 3, 2003, from http://www.Siumed.edu
10. King, D. (2003, November 14). *Introduction to Skin Histology*. Retrieved December 3, 2003, from http://www.Siumed.edu
11. Parsad, D., Sunil, D., & Kanwar, A. J. (2003, October 23). Quality of Life in Patients with Vitiligo. *Journal of Health and Quality of Life Outcomes*, 1(1), 58.
12. King, D. (2003, November 14). *Introduction to Skin Histology*. Retrieved December 3, 2003, from http://www.Siumed.edu
13. King, D. (2003, November 14). *Introduction to Skin Histology*. Retrieved December 3, 2003, from http://www.Siumed.edu
14. King, D. (2003, November 14). *Introduction to Skin Histology*. Retrieved December 3, 2003, from http://www.Siumed.edu

BIBLIOGRAPHY

Bickmore, H. (2003). *Milady's Hair Removal Techniques*. Clifton Park, NY: Milady, an imprint of Thomson Delmar Learning.

Lees, M. (2001). *Skin Care: Beyond the Basics*. Clifton Park, NY: Milady, an imprint of Thomson Delmar Learning.

Milady's Aestheticians Series, Microdermabrasion. (2006). Clifton Park, NY: Milady, an imprint of Thomson Delmar Learning.

Milady's Standard Comprehensive Training for Estheticians. (2003). Clifton Park, NY: Milady, an imprint of Thomson Delmar Learning.

Milady's Standard Cosmetology. (2004). Clifton Park, NY: Milady, an imprint of Thomson Delmar Learning.

Hormones and Hair Growth

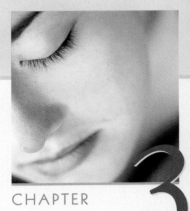

CHAPTER 3

After completing this chapter, you should be able to:

1. Understand the basic functions of the endocrine system, including the endocrine glands and the hormones they stimulate or are stimulated by.
2. Identify the main diseases and disorders caused by any malfunctioning of the endocrine system that relate to the hair removal specialist.
3. Identify the basic causes of hirsutism.
4. Explain the basic causes of hypertrichosis.
5. Differentiate between the two conditions of hypertrichosis.
6. Recognize when a condition may signal the need for further medical evaluation.

INTRODUCTION

endocrine system
network of glands and organs that produce hormones

endocrinologist
one who studies hormones and glands

Hair growth is stimulated by certain glands in the endocrine system, and consequently a thorough understanding of this body system is important for the hair removal specialist. Understanding this body system will help explain the causes of hair growth, the abnormalities of hair growth, and the appropriate times to refer clients to physicians.

This chapter will touch on the highlights of the endocrine system (see Figure 3–1), especially those that pertain to hair growth. Medical diagnosis is outside the scope of the aesthetician's license. Therefore, the information found in the chapter will be directed at the informational needs for the hair removal specialist. It will not discuss in depth the causes, diagnostic processes, and treatments used by physicians. That said, a hair removal specialist may have the need to recommend a specialist or an endocrinologist and, possibly, a reproductive endocrinologist to evaluate a patient. An endocrinologist is a physician who specializes in the treatment of endocrine system disorders.

THE ENDOCRINE SYSTEM

The endocrine system, along with the nervous system, controls and directs the activity of the body's cells. The endocrine system is a network of glands that secrete or excrete chemical substances or messengers, called

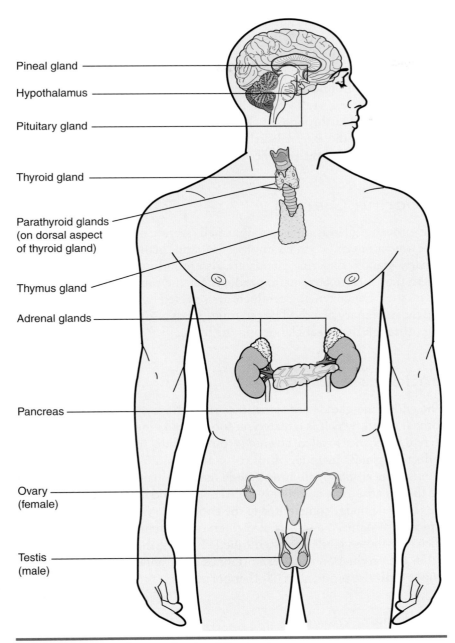

Pineal gland

Hypothalamus

Pituitary gland

Thyroid gland

Parathyroid glands
(on dorsal aspect
of thyroid gland)

Thymus gland

Adrenal glands

Pancreas

Ovary
(female)

Testis
(male)

Figure 3–1 The different glands of the body

hormones, which are released into the blood. These substances regulate growth and development, sexual development, maintaining the body's ability to fight stress, the balance of nutrients, water, and electrolytes, cellular metabolism, and energy. A malfunction in one part of the

hormones
biochemical regulating agents of the body

metabolism
the ongoing conversion of food into energy and the distribution of required biochemicals throughout the body

prostaglandins

substances that resemble hormones

exocrine

secreting externally through a gland

enzymes

proteins that act as biochemical
catalysts

pituitary gland

growth inducing gland found at the
base of the brain; a major endocrine
organ

neurohypophysis

hormone secreting part of the pituitary
gland

adenohypophysis

the anterior part of the pituitary gland

endocrine system often causes another part to malfunction. The endocrine system secretes two types of hormones: amino acid based or steroid.
Prostaglandins are a third category. Prostaglandins are not secreted
from an organ but rather are manufactured from lipids. There are two
types of glands found in the body: endocrine and exocrine. Endocrine
glands are ductless and secrete directly into the blood or lymph. The
cargo is circulated throughout the body. Exocrine glands, on the other
hand, secrete to the external surface: the epithelial. Exocrine glands also
are differentiated by the presence of ducts.

Exocrine Glands

The exocrine glands are generally small, secrete into cavities, and produce mucus or enzymes. Examples of exocrine glands are sweat glands or
salivary glands. Exocrine glands are also found in the digestive system
where they secrete enzymatic products for the purpose of digestion. In
other cases, nonenzymatic products are secreted by the sebaceous glands
and the mammary glands. The exocrine glands also excrete waste material
(e.g., through the sweat glands and the liver).

Endocrine Glands

The endocrine glands are sometimes part of a larger organ such as the
adrenal gland, which is situated on top of the kidney. Endocrine glands
secrete substances called hormones directly into the bloodstream. The
endocrine glands include: pituitary gland, parathyroid glands, adrenal
glands, pineal gland, thymus glands, and the pancreas. Also included
are the gonads, more commonly called ovaries and testes. The hypothalamus is also a major contributor to the endocrine system even though it is
typically recognized as a part of the nervous system. The hormones produced by these glands are often called chemical messengers. They may
aid in the production of other hormones or be antagonistic and work to
stop or slow the production of other hormones.

The Pituitary Gland

The pituitary gland (see Figure 3–2) is found at the base of the brain
and is about the size of a grape. It is divided into two main portions,
the anterior and the posterior pituitary. The anterior is glandular tissue
while the posterior is nervous tissue. The posterior pituitary is also
referred to as the neurohypophysis while the anterior pituitary is called
the adenohypophysis. The pituitary glands produce many of the

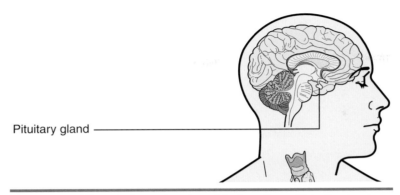

Figure 3–2 The pituitary gland and its location within the body

hormones that we are familiar with, especially several hormones of growth and development.

The Neurohypophysis   The neurohypophysis or posterior pituitary lobe makes two hormones. In the truest sense of the word, however, this lobe does not produce the hormone but simply stores these hormones that are made by hypothalamic neurons. The posterior pituitary is also referred to as the hypothalamus. The hypothalamus is considered to have ultimate control over a major portion of the endocrine system since it stores the hormones produced by the anterior pituitary for liberation into the blood stream.

Those hormones made by the posterior pituitary are oxytocin and antidiuretic hormone. The first hormone is oxytocin, which is released to stimulate the muscles of the uterus to contract during childbirth. It is also actively involved in the process of lactation. The second hormone that the posterior pituitary is involved with is called the antidiuretic hormone (ADH) or vasopressin. Vasopressin causes water to return to the bloodstream; consequently the blood volume becomes greater and the urine becomes more concentrated. ADH also causes the blood pressure to increase by constricting arteries, which is why it is also called vasopressin.

diabetes insipidus
type of diabetes characterized by excessive urine output

hypothalamus
part of the brain responsible for the release of hormones

oxytocin
hormone that stimulates contractions of the womb during childbirth

antidiuretic
affects the volume of urine excreted

vasopressin
hormone that is responsible for blood pressure

The Adenohypophysis   The adenohypophysis or anterior pituitary lobe is also known as the "master gland" of the endocrine system, although this title is somewhat inaccurate as this gland is in turn controlled by the hormones of the hypothalamus. (See Table 3–1.) In fact, although its secretion controls the actions of certain organs, it is in turn affected by the various glands it controls. The adenohypophysis is found in the anterior portion of the pituitary gland and is served by portal veins

Table 3–1   Hormones Produced by the Adenohypophysis

Hormone	Function
Adrenocorticotropic hormone (ACTH)	Controls the adrenal cortex and produces glucocorticoids and sex hormones
Thyrotropic hormone (TSH)	Controls the thyroid gland
Growth hormone (GH)	Affects skeletal development
Melanocyte stimulating hormone (MSH)	Stimulates melanocyte production in the germinating layer of the epidermis Production is inhibited by the hormones of the adrenal cortex
Follicle stimulating hormone (FSH)	Is a gonadotropic hormone that affects the ovarian follicles in women and stimulates seminiferous tissue in men
Luteinizing hormone (LH)	Like FSH (see preceding) is also a gonadotropic hormone that stimulates ovulation and the interstitial tissue in the male testes where testosterone is produced
Lactogenic hormone (LTH)	Stimulates the mammary glands to produce milk; estrogens from the ovaries inhibit LTH production

glucocorticoids
hormones that are involved in metabolism

thyrotropic hormone
hormone that stimulates the thyroid gland

gonadotropic
pertaining to the gonads

luteinizing hormone
hormone that stimulates the corpus luteum

lactogenic hormone
a hormone that induces the secretion of milk; prolactin

pineal gland
secretes melonin

from the hypothalamus. The adenohypophysis produces at least the seven hormones listed in Table 3–1.

The Pineal Gland

The pineal gland (see Figure 3–3) is found in the brain within the third ventricle. The function of this gland is still unknown. The only hormone

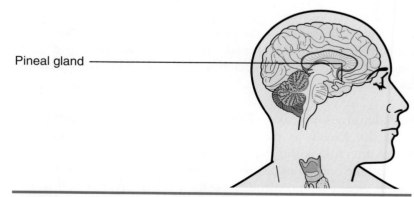

Pineal gland —

Figure 3–3 The pineal gland and its location within the body

that has been found in the pineal is melatonin. This hormone is inhibited by light and is at its maximum blood concentration at night. Melatonin helps to regulate biorhythms. Melatonin is also thought to play a role in the reproduction and maturation of the gonads.

The Thyroid Gland

The thyroid is the most familiar gland in the body. It is found in the neck, on either side of the trachea and larynx. (See Figure 3–4.) It can be felt during a physical examination by a physician. The thyroid gland has two lobes and is responsible for two main hormones: the thyroid hormone or thyroxine and calcitonin or throcalcitonin. Thyroxine is actually two hormones, both with active iodine commonly referred to as T4 and T3. Thyroxine controls many metabolic processes and the basal metabolic rate. Throcalcitonin decreases the blood levels of calcium by sending calcium to the bones.

A deficiency of iodine and an overactivity of the hormone secretions can cause the glands to swell, which causes a condition known as goiter. The underactivity or hypothyroidism of this gland causes a condition called cretinism in children and myxedema in adults, as well as a low BMR and weight gain. Hyperthyroidism produces a condition known as Graves' disease, which causes an increase in the heart and metabolic rates, weight loss, excessive sweating, and the bulging or protruding of the eyeballs from their sockets.

melatonin
hormone responsible for color changes

thyroxine
main thyroid hormone responsible for metabolism and growth

throcalcitonin
thyroid hormone that reduces blood calcium levels, also called calcitonin

goiter
an enlargement of the thyroid gland

hypothyroidism
condition characterized by excessive release of thyroid hormones

cretinism
congenital condition characterized by decreased mental and physical activity caused by reduced thyroid secretions

myxedema
condition characterized by hypofunctioning of the thyroid gland

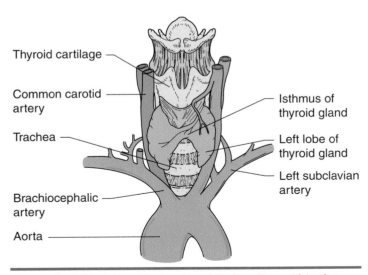

Thyroid cartilage

Common carotid artery

Trachea

Brachiocephalic artery

Aorta

Isthmus of thyroid gland

Left lobe of thyroid gland

Left subclavian artery

Figure 3–4 The thyroid gland and its location within the body

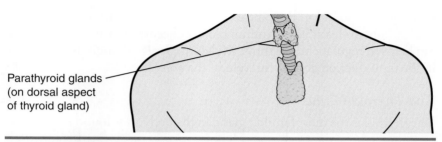

Parathyroid glands
(on dorsal aspect
of thyroid gland)

Figure 3–5 Parathyroid glands and their relationship to the thyroid glands

parathyroid glands
tiny masses of glands found on the
back of the thyroid

parahormone
a chemical substance that has a
stimulating effect, but does not
originate from the endocrine system

thymus
organ responsible for the production of
T cells

thymosin
hormones responsible for the
production of T cells

The Parathyroid Glands   Normally imbedded in the posterior and lateral sides of the thyroid are the parathyroid glands. They are glandular tissue. (See Figure 3–5.) These glands secrete parahormone or PTH. This hormone is important in the regulation of calcium ion, which is intimately involved in homeostasis of the blood. This hormone acts in the opposite direction of calcitonin, which directs calcium *to* the bones. PTH pulls calcium *from* the bones.

The Thymus

The thymus lies behind the sternum. (See Figure 3–6.) It is largest in infancy, growing more slowly than the body and gradually degenerating from puberty onward. It is eventually replaced by adipose tissue. Its importance lies in early development during infancy and youth, when the body grows rapidly and immunity develops. Before birth, the thymus is the major source of lymphocytes, the precursor cells from which the spleen and lymph nodes form. The hormone secreted by the thymus is thymosin, and it affects the growth of lymphoid tissue producing T cells (thymus-dependent cells). The T cells continue to be stimulated by the hormones of the thymus even after they have left it.

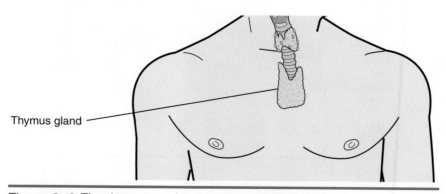

Thymus gland

Figure 3–6 The thymus and its location with in the body

The Adrenal Glands

Adrenal glands sit atop the kidneys like caps, one per kidney. (See Figure 3–7.) The adrenal glands have two sections: the adrenal cortex and the adrenal medulla. The adrenal cortex produces three different types of steroids collectively referred to as corticosteroids: mineralcorticoids, glucocorticoids, and sex steroids. Mineralocorticoids control the mineral and salt content of cellular fluids. Excess mineralocorticoids can lead to the retention of body fluid, called edema. Glucocorticoids affect the metabolism and the amount of blood glucose. They increase in activity in response to stress. They also depress pituitary secretions of ACTH, TSH, and MSH. Sex steroids supplement in weaker degrees the sex hormones secreted by the gonads (i.e., the ovaries and testes). The adrenal medulla not unlike the posterior pituitary develop from nervous tissue. The adrenal medulla secretes two main substances, epinephrine and norepinephrine, together more commonly known as catecholamines or adrenalin. Hypersecretion of corticosteroids results in Cushing's syndrome, often caused by a tumor on the adrenal cortex. Inadequate secretion of glucocorticoids and mineralocorticoids causes Addison's disease.

The Pancreas

The pancreas lies behind the stomach (see Figure 3–8) and contains the islets of Langerhans. The pancreas serves a dual role in the endocrine system since it has both endocrine glands and exocrine glands. The islets of Langerhans are endocrine glands and secrete the hormones insulin and glucagons. The effects of insulin and glucagons on the body are important and too complicated for this text. For our purposes the student should know that together insulin and glucagons help the body to maintain a balanced level of sugar in the blood. A lack of insulin causes diabetes mellitus.

adrenal glands
hormone producing glands situated above each kidney

adrenal cortex
outer portion of the adrenal gland

adrenal medulla
central portion of the adrenal gland

steroids
a group of chemicals that include hormones

corticosteroids
hormonal substances that regulate biochemical reactions to occur at prescribed optimal rates

mineralocorticoids
hormones responsible for fluid balance; steroids that promote the reabsorption of salt and the excretion of potassium in the kidneys

edema
a condition of excessive fluid retention; swelling

epinephrine
hormone that produces the fight or flight response

norepinephrine
important neurotransmitter

Cushing's syndrome
a disease that is caused by a high amount of adrenocortical hormone

Addison's disease
condition in which the adrenal glands fail to produce enough hormones

islets of Langerhans
clusters of cells in the pancreas that are responsible for the production of insulin

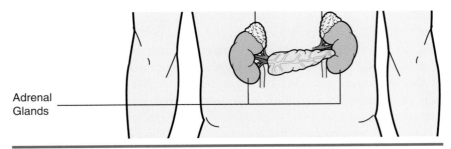

Adrenal
Glands

Figure 3–7 The adrenal glands and their relationship to the kidneys and their location in the body

Diabetes mellitus is a disease that occurs when the islets of Langerhans are not functioning properly. Without insulin, the hormone produced in the islets of Langerhans, the blood sugar would rise to dangerous and most likely fatal levels.

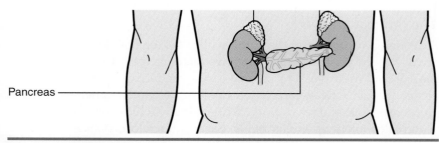

Pancreas

Figure 3–8 The pancreas and its relationship to the rest of the body

glucagons
hormones that have the ability to increase blood glucose levels

diabetes mellitus
type of diabetes characterized by poor production or utilization of insulin

androgens
hormones that promote the production of male characteristics

estrogen
female hormone

progesterone
female sex hormone

corpus luteum
endocrine secreting progesterone

■ THE GONADS

The sex organs located in the groin area are also known as the gonads (testes and ovaries). They secrete the sex steroids that cause secondary sex characteristics in males and females. The sex steroids that are produced in the testes and ovaries are the same sex steroids that are produced in the adrenal cortex. The difference is the source and amounts. In males the sex hormones are known as androgens; in females they are known as estrogen and progesterone. Females also produce androgens in much lesser quantities than males; males likewise produce female hormones in much lesser quantities.

The Female

Female hormones fluctuate in their levels at different stages in the woman's life, such as at the onset of puberty, during the menstrual cycle each month, during pregnancy, and during menopause, when estrogen levels rapidly decline. In the female, hormonal activity is complex and must respond to the possible fertilization, growth, development, and birth of a fetus, followed by lactation to feed and nourish the infant. (See Figure 3–9.) The parts of the female reproductive organs that produce hormones are the ovaries, the sacs, or ovid organs, where the ova or eggs are formed. The ovaries (see Figure 3–10) are found in the pelvic cavity, one on each side. The ovaries do not begin to secrete hormones until puberty. The trigger for the stimulation of estrogen and progesterone is the secretion of the hormones provided by the anterior pituitary. (See Table 3–2.) The hormones estrogen and progesterone produced in the ovaries are responsible for developing the female sexual characteristics. Progesterone creates another structure, the corpus luteum. The corpus luteum is the lining of the empty ovarian follicle. It is an endocrine structure that produces both estrogen and progesterone.

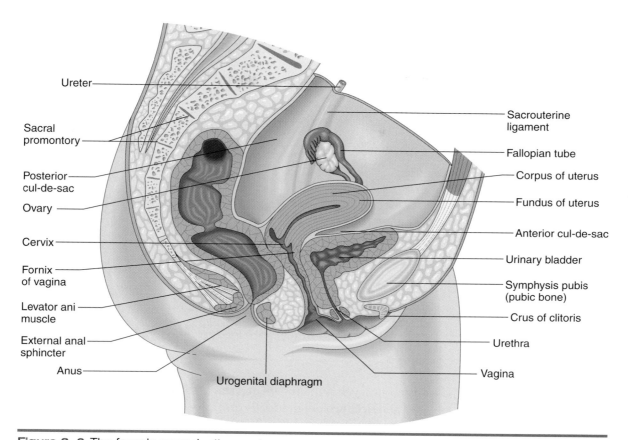

Figure 3–9 The female reproductive system

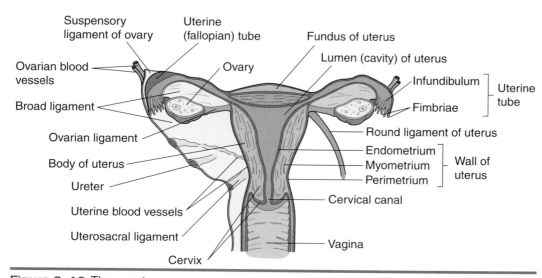

Figure 3–10 The ovaries

Table 3–2   Hormones that Affect Growth and Development

Hormone	Function	Regulated by
Estrogen	Affects the development of the fallopian tubes, ovaries, uterus, and the vagina Produces secondary sex characteristics: • broadened pelvis, making the outlet broad and oval to permit childbirth • the epiphysis (growth plate) becomes bone and growth ceases • softer and smoother skin • pubic and axillary hair • deposits of fat in the breasts and development of the duct system • deposits of fat in the buttocks and thighs • sexual desire Prepares the uterus for the fertilized egg	FSH and LH
Progesterone	Develops excretory portion of the mammary glands Thickens the uterine lining so it can receive the developing embryo egg Decreases uterine contractions during pregnancy	FSH and LH

The Male

Testosterone levels remain high and stable for the most part from puberty onward and decline very gradually and very slightly in men over 50. The male reproductive system (see Figure 3–11) is significantly less complicated with regard to the study of hormones, as the hormones serve to produce the sperm to fertilize an egg. The parts of the adult male reproductive system that produce the male hormones called androgens are the testes (see Figure 3–12) and the interstitial tissue. The testes are paired like the ovaries. They are found in the sac called the scrotum outside the pelvic cavity. Once again, like the ovaries, anterior pituitary produces FSH and LH, which stimulates the testes. There are two compartments of the testes: (1) seminiferous tubules, where sperm forms, stimulated by FSH, and (2) the interstitial fluid, which contains the Leydig cells, which secrete testosterone, the major androgen. The development of the male secondary sexual characteristics is brought about by the stimulation of androgens at puberty.

seminiferous
producing semen

tubules
very small tubes

interstitial fluid
the fluid between cells

Leydig cells
produces testosterone

■ INTRODUCTION TO HIRSUTISM AND HYPERTRICHOSIS

A basic understanding of the endocrine system fosters an understanding and recognition of diseases and disorders that cause excessive and

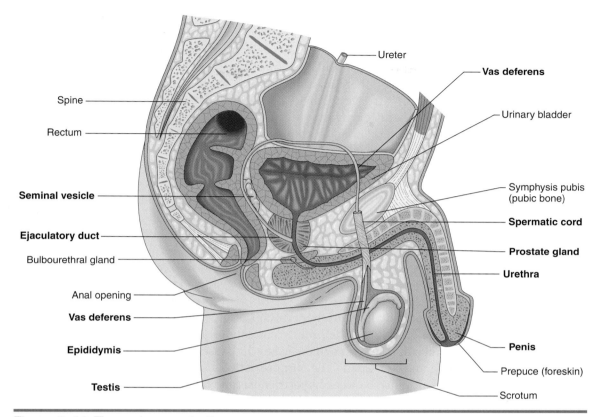

Ureter

Spine

Rectum

Vas deferens

Urinary bladder

Symphysis pubis (pubic bone)

Seminal vesicle

Spermatic cord

Ejaculatory duct

Prostate gland

Bulbourethral gland

Urethra

Anal opening

Vas deferens

Epididymis

Penis

Prepuce (foreskin)

Testis

Scrotum

Figure 3–11 The male reproductive organs

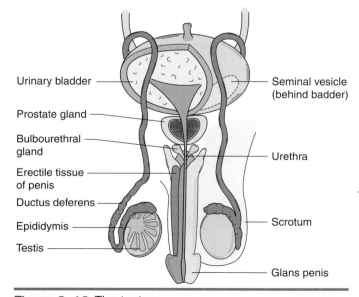

Urinary bladder

Seminal vesicle (behind badder)

Prostate gland

Bulbourethral gland

Urethra

Erectile tissue of penis

Ductus deferens

Epididymis

Scrotum

Testis

Glans penis

Figure 3–12 The testes

unwanted hair. In this section we discuss the concepts of hirsutism and hypertrichosis. Hirsutism is the term for terminal hair growth in women that is caused by excessive male androgens in the blood. Hypertrichosis, on the other hand, is not stimulated by male androgens. It is, however, usually terminal hair but does not grow in the adult-male sexual hair growth patterns as hirsutism. There have been many advances in the field of endocrinology, with many improved and sophisticated readings of hormone levels in the blood, allowing for more accurate diagnosis in diseases that, among other things, cause excessive and unwanted hair growth.

What is considered "excessive" hair growth is subjective. What one person may consider unacceptable another may welcome. For instance, a fair-skinned, blonde woman may consider a few nonpigmented velli along the lip line unacceptable. Another fair-skinned but dark-haired woman might have dark, terminal hair on the upper lip and face in the adult male, sexual-hair-growth pattern and envy the former woman. The former condition may be considered hypertrichosis, the latter, hirsutism.

Hirsutism and hypertrichosis are often grouped, discussed, and treated as the same problem or condition. However, there are some significant differences in regard to the cause of each condition and how each should be treated. The purpose of this discussion is to carefully define and distinguish between hypertrichosis and hirsutism so that the hair removal specialist can understand and recognize the two conditions and the right course of action to treat the offending hair.

■ HIRSUTISM

hirsutism
condition characterized by abnormal hair growth

hypertrichosis
condition characterized by excessive hair

Hirsutism is the definition for terminal hair growth in women that is caused by excessive male androgens. The condition can be caused by the sex hormones secreted in the ovaries or in the adrenal glands, as previously mentioned. The typical areas of excessive growth are the face, chest, buttocks, and groin. (See Figure 3–13.) In the United States hirsutism is found in an estimated 1 in 20 women.[1] Hirsutism is not a disease, but rather a symptom of a disease or problem relating to the overproduction of androgens (see Table 3–3).

■ HYPERTRICHOSIS

The word hypertrichosis stems from the Greek *hyper,* meaning "over," and *trichosis,* meaning "hair"—an overabundance of hair. Hypertrichosis is therefore excess hair growth on any part of the body that is subjectively abnormal for the age, sex, race, and culture of the individual. (See Figure

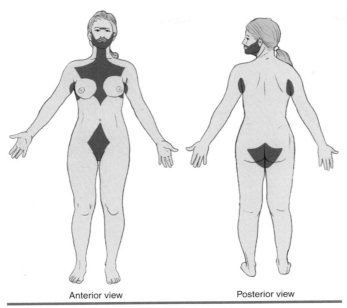

Anterior view   Posterior view

Figure 3–13 Areas of the body that are prone to hirsutism

Table 3–3   Causes of Hirsutism
Stimulation of male androgens at puberty
Drugs affecting endocrine system, increasing the percentage of male androgens
Diseases and disorders of the endocrine system

3–14.) The type of hair in this condition is usually terminal, does not necessarily grow in the adult-male, sexual-hair-growth patterns, and is not stimulated by male androgens. The exact cause of hypertrichosis is unknown, though there are congenital versions of this disease. (See Table 3–4.) Possible causes of the disease might be metabolic changes, drug usage, or anorexia. (See Table 3–5.)

HORMONAL SYNDROMES THAT CONTRIBUTE TO EXCESSIVE HAIR GROWTH

A syndrome is a group of symptoms that, when combined, characterize a disease. Excessive hair growth is no exception. There are several syndromes that have as a symptom excessive hair growth. Included in this list is Cushing's disease, adrenogenital syndrome, Achard-Thiers

adrenogenital syndrome
the stimulation of male characteristics

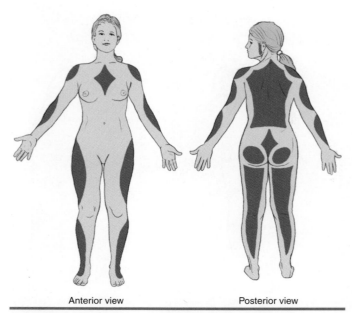

Anterior view   Posterior view

Figure 3–14 Areas of the body that are prone to hypertrichosis

Table 3–4   Causes of Hypertrichosis
Genetically inherited and/or particular to race
Natural life occurrences (e.g., puberty, pregnancy, menopause)
Reaction to certain medical procedures
Result of some cancer treatments
Reaction to certain prescription medications, especially steroids

Stein-Leventhal syndrome
disease characterized by hyperandrogenism and chronic anovulation in women

polycystic ovary syndrome
characterized by high levels of male hormones, lack of menstruation, and cysts on the ovaries

acromegaly
chronic condition affecting middle aged individuals characterized by bone enlargement and thickening of soft tissues

syndrome, and **Stein-Leventhal syndrome**, more commonly known as **polycystic ovary syndrome** (PCOS). Now we know that the sex hormones come from either the gonads (ovaries or testes) or the adrenal glands. Consequently, the origin for these syndromes is usually linked to a problem with one of these glands. Knowing the symptoms of these syndromes will help the hair removal specialist identify potential problems and recommend medical attention. **Acromegaly** is also included in the discussion below as a symptom of this disorder is hirsutism.

Acromegaly

Acromegaly comes from the Greek words "acro" for extremities and "megaly" for great. Acromegaly is caused by the excessive release of

Table 3–5   Common Drugs that Cause Hirsutism and Hypertrichosis

Drug	Hirsutism	Hypertrichosis
Anabolic steroids	XX	
Corticosteroids	XX	
Brevicon	XX	
Ciclosporin (immunosuppressant)		XX
Diazoxide		XX
Dilantin		XX
Loestrin	XX	
Minoxidil		XX
Prednisone	XX	
Premarin	XX	
Provera	XX	
Tagamet	XX	
Tamoxifen	XX	
Thorazine	XX	

growth hormone (GH) by the anterior pituitary gland, usually due to a tumor. In childhood, the excessive release of GH can cause gigantism. Typically, however, the hormonal disorder acromegaly occurs in adulthood, usually middle age. If the body is mature at the onset of the disorder, the result is enlarged hands, feet, and face. Poor vision or blindness may also ensue. Typically the symptoms develop over the course of years and may be difficult to diagnose. Excessive androgen production, associated with this disease can cause hirsutism.

Adrenogenital Syndrome

Adrenogenital syndrome, also called adrenal virilism, results when the adrenal cortex malfunctions and blocks cortisol synthesis and in response causes an overproduction of androgens. The outward symptoms in children are the precocious development of the sex organs, deep voices, and excessive hair growth. In adult women, adrenogenital syndrome causes diminished breast size, an enlarged clitoris, and hirsutism.

Achard-Thiers Syndrome

Achard-Thiers syndrome is a very rare syndrome caused by the combination of Cushing's syndrome and adrenogenital syndrome.

Cushing's Syndrome

Cushing's syndrome develops from chronic excess of cortisol. The normal production of cortisol responds to an exact chain of events, engineered by the body's responses to stress, blood pressure, and cardiovascular functioning, to name a few. It is also involved in the maintenance of blood sugars. The reasons for this overproduction can be complex and beyond the scope of this text. Cushing's syndrome can also be caused by medications such as prednisone or immunosuppression. Finally, it should be mentioned that Cushing's syndrome can be inherited. This is rare and is indicative of a genetic tendency to develop tumors of the endocrine glands.

Outward signs of Cushing's are an enlarged face ("moon face"), neck, and trunk; rounded shoulders; weak abdominals; and hirsutism. The limbs remain unaffected. Women cease to menstruate. Bone and joint pain is not uncommon. The skin is thin and fragile and tends to bruise easily and heal poorly, making it difficult to treat women with this syndrome who have hirsutism. Purple stretch marks may also be present.

Stein-Leventhal Syndrome

Stein-Leventhal syndrome is now more commonly called PCOS. In this syndrome, the polycystic ovary produces excess androgens. The inward signs of this syndrome are irregular or absent menstruation and cystic ovaries. The outward signs of this syndrome are small breasts, sometimes obesity, and, often, hirsutism of the face, neck, chest, and thighs.

Conclusion

What is considered "excessive" hair growth is subjective. What one person may consider unacceptable another may welcome. A female client may present with a condition of considerable hairiness throughout her body but, given the client's race and culture, it may not be considered either a problem or unattractive, and she may be physically very healthy. This is *hypertrichosis*—hairiness that does not follow the adult sexual hair growth pattern. Another female client may present with a beard, and after questioning it is revealed that she has diabetes. Upon thorough examination, an endocrinologist may discover that the client has a rare disorder called Achard-Thiers syndrome. The woman's beard is hirsute and, with medical treatment and hair removal, the condition can be rectified.

The reasons for hairiness and the social response to it are important for the hair removal specialist to understand. Knowledge about the hair growth process, possible diseases associated with hair growth, as well as sensitivity to the potential psychological implications will make the hair removal specialist an expert in this chosen field.

▶▶▶ TOP 10 TIPS TO TAKE TO THE CLINIC

1. Hypertrichosis is hairiness that does not follow the adult sexual hair growth pattern.

2. Hirsutism is terminal hair growth in women that is caused by excessive male androgens.

3. Hirsutism can be caused by several syndromes.

4. The patterns of abnormal hair growth in hirsutism are the face, chest, buttocks, and groin.

5. The patterns of abnormal hair growth in hypertrichosis are the legs, arms, back, and chest.

6. Hirsutism and hypertrichosis should not be grouped, discussed, or treated as the same problem or condition.

7. Understanding the endocrine system gives the clinician insight into potential problems.

8. Certain drugs can cause both hirsutism and hypertrichosis.

9. Medical diagnosis is outside the scope of the clinician. Therefore, clients with potential problems should be referred to the physician before treatment.

10. What is considered "excessive" hair growth is subjective.

CHAPTER QUESTIONS

1. What is the main difference between an exocrine gland and an endocrine gland?

2. Which gland is known as the "master gland"?

3. Hypothyroidism causes what condition in adults?

4. Which two main substances does the adrenal medulla secrete?

5. Does FSH cause the hair follicles to produce terminal hair?

6. List three causes of hypertrichosis.

7. Name the two main causes of hirsutism.

8. Name three common syndromes that cause hirsutism.

9. What is the more common name for Stein-Leventhal syndrome?

10. List the three inward and two outward signs of Stein-Leventhal syndrome.

CHAPTER REFERENCES

1. Goodheart, H. P. (2006, February). *Hirsutism*. Available at http://www.emedicine.com

BIBLIOGRAPHY

Bickmore, H. (2003). *Milady's Hair Removal Techniques*. Clifton Park, NY: Milady, an imprint of Thomson Delmar Learning.

Edsell, L. (1984). *Female Hirsutism, An Enigma*. St. Louis, MO: Pulsar Publishing Co.

Owens, S. (1989). *About That Hair*. Pensacola, FL: Author.

Redmond, G. (1995). *The Good News about Women's Hormones*. New York: Warner Books, Inc.

Senisi Scott, A., & Fong, E. (1998). *Body Structures and Functions*. Clifton Park, NY: Thomson Delmar Learning.

Consultations

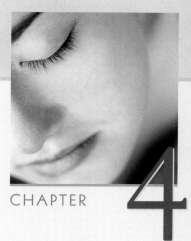

CHAPTER 4

KEY TERMS

body dysmorphic disorder   image business   perception

consultation   impressions   unrealistic expectations

differentiate

LEARNING OBJECTIVES

After completing this chapter, you should be able to:

1. Discuss the consultation process.

2. Create a care plan for the hair removal client.

3. Discuss the components of a consultation that make a relationship successful.

INTRODUCTION

In most businesses, particularly in the medical and luxury spa business, success will be driven by the impressions people have of you and the aesthetic industry. It is an image business. The first impression a new client has of your office and your expertise is based in part on the cleanliness of the office, on the knowledge and friendliness of the staff, and on your appearance. The ability of clients to listen and hear information provided can be affected by how comfortable they feel in the consultation or treatment room. That *comfort zone* includes how medicinal the room appears (which can be intimidating), the seating arrangement, and your professionalism. Professionalism relates to your appearance, knowledge, and ability to communicate. Mastering the skills of friendliness, cleanliness, comfort, professionalism, and communication can all impact the lasting impressions of clients.

Furthermore, the perception clients have of you is one that extends to your physician and his or her partners or the spa director. The impression the client has of you and the facility will determine trust, which is the foundation of any relationship.

The office consultation is the first face-to-face meeting with the client. It is the first and only opportunity to make a positive impression that will cultivate a lasting relationship. Many times, a client's decision to purchase services is made by the time he or she enters the treatment room.

At the consultation appointment, there is a mutual objective between client and technician: improving the client's appearance. The client came to you because he or she has a *need* to look better. You are in your position because through your education and experience you can *fulfill* that need.

Many technicians follow a consultative process modeled from their education or experiences from other jobs. As professionals providing skin consultations, we must differentiate or distinguish ourselves from others in order to be successful.

Differentiation does not mean you should only create comfortable seating areas with televisions, beverages, and snacks. These niceties are really in-house marketing ploys that have little to do with the care delivered to clients. Differentiation means promoting *a change in the process*. A noted difference in care will have an equally notable difference in the client's perception.

So let us turn the consultation process upside down.

▪ THE OFFICE CONSULTATION

On the surface, the objective of the consultation is to determine the client's candidacy for a particular procedure (e.g., laser hair removal). But,

impressions
lasting opinions or judgments of something

image business
type of business in which the way the public views the company is based largely upon how things look, or how they are perceived, more than actual performance

consultation
initial visit with a professional during which the client and the professional both investigate whether a specific treatment or service is warranted or achievable

perception
process by which individuals use their senses to make decisions or gather information

differentiate
to make something stand out or be unique compared to something that would otherwise be similar

we should not, in the process disregard the client's possible concerns or fears. Instead, the focus of the consultation should be to build rapport and begin a relationship. In order for consultation to be mutually successful, the client must be able to communicate his or her fears, concerns, and objectives for the treatment in a safe and trusting environment.

Many individuals are nervous when seeking these services. They have concerns about vanity, costs, and potential problems from unsuccessful treatments. Think of the consultation process as a "scavenger hunt" for information and remember that no scavenger hunt is ever the same. In the same manner, no consultation will ever be the same!

The consultative process introduced in this chapter takes approximately 30 minutes of client time. The consultation includes all necessary and traditional components of a consultation: skin analysis, photographs, and differentiation.

It is important to understand the client's motivation before making substantive recommendations in consultation. To achieve this end, several tactics can be used, including filling out a traditional client information sheet, a skin history sheet, a health history sheet, and the *Help Us to Understand You* sheet. The client should fill out all the documents in the waiting area or at home, if the documents can be mailed in advance, before seeing the technician. Attach the documents to a clipboard in the following order: the client information sheet, the skin history sheet, the health history sheet, and the *Help Us to Understand You* sheet. It is important to ask the client to arrive 15 minutes early so he or she has sufficient time to complete the required paperwork. While it may seem like an inordinate amount of paperwork, the responses to these questions will help guide you through a successful consultation.

The *Client Information Sheet* captures social information, contact information (including e-mail address), and referral sources. The purpose of this form is to learn about the client and how to contact him or her. The form should also capture information about the client's interest in the office, including the procedures about which he or she would like to inquire. Enter this information into the office's computer database so you have access to demographic information on all clients, which will be extraordinarily useful for marketing promotions or direct mail. Because the client information sheet is the source of client referral information, this form is useful when you are thanking or rewarding referral sources and also when you are determining and assessing which form of advertising was the most effective and how best to budget the advertising funds.

The *Skin History Sheet* is a detailed questionnaire about the client's skin. It is important to ask questions in the survey that include past and current skin health. Some of the specific items you will want to know are past and current tanning habits, including history of sunburns (as a child and as an adult), history of skin cancer diagnosis, and locations of skin cancers. Also, ask about moles or lesions that concern the client, including their location. Information regarding past and current acne concerns and use of oral and/or topical acne medications is advisable. It is important to be aware of previous skin treatments, x-ray treatments for acne, PUVA treatments for psoriasis, as well as spa treatments (i.e., facials, body treatments) and problems associated with those treatments. You may want to consider using the Fitzpatrick skin typing to make this information inclusive and complete. Finally, you should inquire about skin condition (oily, dry, normal, sensitive, or combination) and skin type. The skin history sheet will help to understand the client's overall skin health. It will also give a clearer history, not just what the client chooses to tell you verbally.

The skin history sheet can also be used to help describe your clientele. For example, how many of your clients have had a skin cancer? How many of your clients have acne? How many of your clients tan? Keeping a summary of this information will be helpful when creating marketing plans or future promotions.

The *Health History Sheet* asks detailed questions about past and current health status. Included in this document are questions regarding allergies, current and past illnesses, smoking status, pregnancy status, daily medications, and surgical events. The objective of the health history is to obtain a detailed "snap shot" of the client's health in an efficient manner. This form should be set up in a check-box format. While clients may consider some health items to be irrelevant, their responses may help guide care. Therefore, responses to all questions are important. The health history is vital as this is where contraindications may be revealed.

The *Help Us to Understand You* sheet is a communication tool as well as an evaluation tool. The questions on this sheet ask clients to rate their knowledge, communication style, and preferences for skin care. This very important tool will help guide you in providing consultation and instruction sessions in ways in which the client will be more receptive to the information being given. The form distills how the client prefers the material to be presented. It also helps you to understand some of the unspoken concerns the client may have, such as pain, price, and downtime for healing. Once this form is completed, you can begin a meaningful conversation with your client.

Greeting the Client

The paperwork is finished and the client is eager to meet you. (See Figure 4–1.) This is your opportunity to make a positive, lasting impression. Respect for the client should be your first objective. Always take a quick peek in the mirror before you meet someone new to make sure your hair is neat, your face is clean, and your makeup is evenly applied. When you first make contact with the client you should introduce yourself and then

---

The Telephone Interview

The first time you "meet" a client may be on the telephone. Clients often ask questions such as: How many treatments will it take to solve the problem? What products are best for me? Will electrolysis work for me? Obviously, these questions require a face-to-face consultation. Setting an appointment should be the primary objective of the telephone interview.

Help Us to Understand You

Please help us to understand what you would like. The more we know about you, the better we can serve you. We do not want to guess or make assumptions, so please circle the closest number to the statement that matches your feelings or preferences.

I know a great deal about my skin condition	1 2 3 4 5 6	I know very little about my skin condition
I like to be presented with fewer options	1 2 3 4 5 6	I like to be presented with more options
I tend to look at the details	1 2 3 4 5 6	I tend to look at the big picture
I prefer long-lasting solutions that may cost more	1 2 3 4 5 6	I prefer more temporary solutions at a lower cost
I prefer to talk technical terms with my technician	1 2 3 4 5 6	I prefer to talk in nontechnical terms
I like new and modern methods of care	1 2 3 4 5 6	I prefer the tried and true methods of care

Please rate the following from 1 to 6, 1 being the most important and 6 being the least important.

_____ Care in the medical environment

_____ Seeing the same technician at each visit

_____ Being pampered during the procedure

_____ Peace of mind

_____ Rapid improvement

_____ Downtime for healing

Please rate the following from 1 to 6, 1 being the most important and 6 being the least important.

_____ Price

_____ Physical discomfort

_____ Time in the clinic

_____ Personal effort

_____ Fear/anxiety

_____ Other

ask how they prefer to be addressed. The conversation should begin with "Hello, Mrs. Smith. My name is Susan. It is a pleasure to meet you. Do you prefer Mrs. Smith or Lorraine?" Her preference should be documented in the chart. Remember that medical offices can be daunting, even if a client is coming for procedures about which he or she is excited. Take care to explain the physical layout of the facility, location of the restroom, which treatment or consultation room you will be using today, and how to exit the facility. A simple tour usually helps people feel at ease.

Reviewing the Client Information Sheet

The personal information sheet the client fills out is a wealth of important data. It tells where clients reside, where they are employed (if applicable),

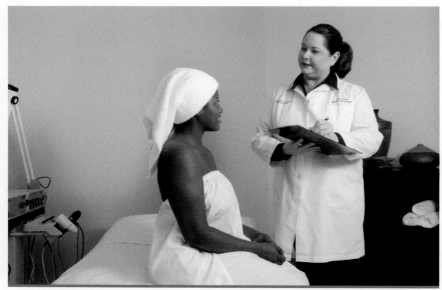

Figure 4–1 Consultation is an important first step in building a long term relationship

what their relationship status is, and what their interests in treatments are. Look carefully at the *Client Information Sheet,* as it will give clues about potential sales and may disclose the primary motivation (e.g., an approaching birthday, a wedding, or being recently divorced or widowed). All of this information is valuable in understanding the client's needs and building rapport with the client.

Reviewing the Health and Skin History Sheets

Make sure the client completely fills out the Health and Skin History sheets. This is a great place to start the conversation. "Mrs. Smith, I am going to take a moment and acquaint myself with your history. Please bear with me a moment while I look through this document." Review the information the client has provided and ask relevant questions to fill in the areas that are incomplete. An incomplete area usually means the answer to the question is "no" but sometimes it could mean the client did not want to give the information or it was unintentionally skipped. Do not leave any blanks. Ask the client to finish completing the document if an area is incomplete. Be sure to review both the Health History and the Skin History sheets. Add anything relevant as you go through documents with the client. Make notes on your consultation sheet, not on the documents that the client filled out. Take this part of the consultation very seriously. This is the time to look for health-related contraindications.

Because people generally like to talk about themselves, reviewing this form is a good place to build rapport with a client. Use this opportunity as an icebreaker to get to know the client. If a client is shy or embarrassed, this technique will help the client become comfortable with you and the informational exchange. If you review this document before seeing the client in the treatment room, you lose this opportunity to build rapport.

Health History Updates

Technicians should inquire regularly about changes in health status and update the clients' medical charts yearly. Relevant changes to health status include: medication changes, new diseases, new illnesses or surgeries, and medical treatments. Updates can be extraordinarily important. Could there be new contraindications? Take the example of a client recently diagnosed with breast cancer or diabetes. Health status changes should cause the technician to adequately reflect about procedures conducted in the spa setting. Does this new information require an updated consultation, evaluation, and examination? The answer should be "yes." Does the new health status demand a reevaluation of the hair removal plan? Health changes do not mean the client must forego her hair removal program; in fact, her treatments may be an important part of her emotional healing as she copes with the disease. But for her safety, the plan needs review.

Evaluating the Client Request

Once you review the *Health History Sheet* and make additions or clarifications, it is time to identify what the client wants to improve and what will be the best approach based on the *Help Us to Understand You* document. This assessment process is accomplished by asking clients what they are concerned about. Although some clients may find the process somewhat intimidating, it is a useful activity if you can encourage them to talk through their concerns and identify perceived problems. This process will give you insight into clients' perceived body image, what is important to them, and what they are willing to do to accomplish the desired result. As you listen to clients talk about their analysis of the problems, try to evaluate if they are being realistic. Watch for signs of body dysmorphic disorder (BDD), which is a pathological preoccupation with an imagined defect of one's body. Technicians should also listen closely to determine if what clients are saying matches their responses on the *Help Us to Understand You* document.

Take notes while clients are speaking to ensure you get all of the information recorded. This will help create useful and complete care plans. Once clients have completed their analyses, technicians should ask

body dysmorphic disorder
psychosocial disease that causes individuals to be inappropriately concerned with their appearance. Those affected with BDD are contraindicated for most aesthetic procedures.

permission to do the same. Asking permission is an important step in building the relationship because it demonstrates trust and respect.

Many times clients do not know what the problem is—they just know they do not like the way they look. It is the job of technicians to identify and elaborate on these issues. Once this process is complete and the client and technician have agreed on the specific areas of concern, it is time to do the formal skin and hair evaluation.

The Skin Analysis—It Is Important for Hair Removal Too

A skin analysis is performed to evaluate the skin condition and determine skin type. This is especially important when considering laser hair removal. Fitzpatrick type will predict the skin's response to treatment, which helps determine what hair removal modality will be best for the client. Technicians should limit skin examinations to the area of hair removal. For example, when giving a bikini wax, technicians should examine only the area that will be waxed.

Before starting the skin examination, have the client change into a wrap or gown. This will allow you a better chance to evaluate the skin without fear of soiling the client's clothing. It is worth noting that hair removal clients are always candidates for skin care. This process allows the opportunity to introduce a skin care program to the client if it has not been discussed previously.

This skin analysis is a standardized process, but for review, we will discuss the steps involved. (See Figure 4–2.)

Cleanse

Once the client has changed and is comfortable on the treatment table, cover the hair with a surgical bonnet or a headband. Using a soft gauze or disposable sponge, gently cleanse the area with a mild cleanser, and pat dry. Be sure to *gently* cleanse the skin. The objective is to take off the makeup, not to stimulate the skin. If the skin is overstimulated, it will be difficult to observe skin irregularities such as telangiectasias. If looking at skin in the groin region or on the legs, be sure to cleanse. You want to remove any body lotions. Furthermore, you want to evaluate whether or not the client is using self tanner prior to evaluating Fitzpatrick skin type.

Analyze and Evaluate

Use a loupe or magnification light to observe the skin. (See Figure 4–3.) You are looking for signs of unwanted hair that has been shaven or waxed

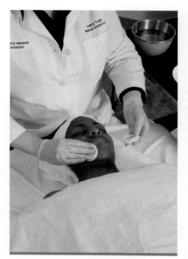

Figure 4–2 A thorough examination of the skin is the first step to understanding skin type and condition

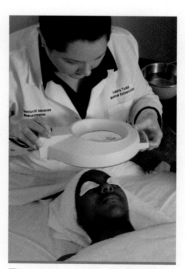

Figure 4–3 Using a loupe allows for a close examination of the skin

and also for visible contraindications. Take note of the skin's sensitivity; for example, did it turn pink during cleansing? Are there areas of hyper- or hypopigmentation? Discuss potential areas of concern that may have been missed in the initial discussion. Hand the client a mirror and point out your concerns. Ask for his or her opinion.

Documentation

After the skin analysis, you should document your findings in the client's clinical chart. For example, if there are scars, document where and how large they are. If the client can elaborate on the history of the scar, document that as well. If there is an area of hyperpigmentation, note its location and color. Make notes about the skin's texture and tone by describing its appearance. Make note of anything that would relate to the outcome of

---

Clinical Care Plan

Patient Name:_____ Phone Number:_____

Clinician Name:_____

Date of Plan:_____

Week Number	Procedure	Clinician	Notes
Visit One			
Visit Two			
Visit Three			
Visit Four			
Visit Five			
Visit Six			
Visit Seven			
Visit Eight			

Long Term Action Plan:
_____
_____
_____
_____
_____
_____

Figure 4–4 Documentation form for hair removal techniques

hair removal. For example, tenderness might make certain treatments more painful than others. Be sure to note the skin type and condition. Any information that you can put on the form will help you over time and at the completion of treatment. Any additional notations made by the technician should be initialized by the client. This affords protection from a client who may later try to claim that a preexisting condition was caused by the technician. The next step is to take photographs.

Taking Photographs

Taking photographs is often overlooked, but is an essential part of client care. Photographs record what the client looked like on the first visit. When dealing with hair removal and hair growth, photographs are very important because it is difficult to recall with accuracy what the client looked like prior to treatment. After two to four treatments technicians and clients often rave about the results, but the photographs tell the real story. Photographs also may protect technicians from potential litigation.

Ideally, technicians should use a digital photography system with computer storage and color printer. If these resources are not available, a sophisticated color Polaroid camera will work. (See Figure 4–5.) To ensure the accuracy and consistency in photography, spas should develop a policy and procedure for technicians to follow. The policy and pro-

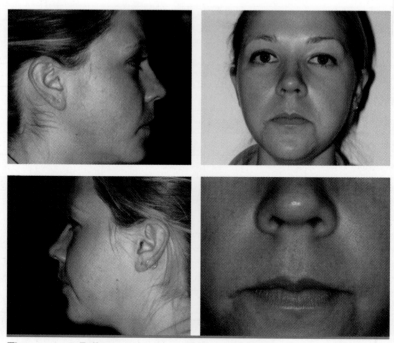

Figure 4–5 Different types and views of photographs

cedure should include topics such as: *Camera Specifics, Care and Maintenance of the Camera, Flash and Lighting Techniques, Focusing and Framing the Shot, Ensuring Accurate Photographs,* and *Troubleshooting the Camera.* For the purposes of this text, we will cover specifically "Ensuring Accurate Photographs" because there are many cameras with variable instructions, and not all specifics can be covered in this text.

It is important to note, however, that some clients may not want to be photographed based on religious grounds, and this must be respected. The hair growth can be documented on paper by counting the hairs in a square centimeter. Others receiving hair removal treatments in private areas may not want photographs taken (e.g., bikini line). It is important to discuss that the main reason for taking photographs is to provide the best possible care. Regardless of the location being treated, photographs are a vital element of treatment, and the client should give signed permission for photographs to be taken.

Standard Policy and Procedure
Company Name
Ensuring Accurate Photographs

Title: Ensuring Accurate Photographs

Policy: All personnel must follow the procedures outlined in this policy.

Purpose: To ensure that photographs are properly focused and framed, providing a documented photographic history.

Scope: All Staff

Procedure:

1. Hold the camera at the approximate distance from the subject for the selected magnification. This can be accomplished by providing a specific mark on the floor for the camera and for the client at premeasured distances.
2. Look through the camera to ensure the client is in the frame and the desired shot is in place.
3. Take the photograph.
4. Review the photograph.
5. Ensure there is a date on the photograph if using the Polaroid camera; if using a digital camera, ensure that an accurate date is being recorded.
6. Take multiple shots of the subject from different angles.
7. Print the photographs that have been taken and make sure client's name appears on each photograph.
8. File the photograph in the chart.

A photo lab with a neutral monochromatic background, appropriate lighting, and distance markers should be in place so that the client is photographed each time with identical variables of light distance and focus.

Policy and Procedures for Accurate Photographs

The necessity for accurate photographs cannot be overemphasized. Having a policy and procedure document that accurately depicts the process is a good start. This process will create consistent qualities in the photographs (e.g., distance, angle of the face, color). When comparing before and after photographs, consistency is critical to detect changes in appearance.

■ CLIENT EXPECTATIONS

Once the documents have been reviewed, missing information has been filled in, and the photographs have been taken, the client may begin treatment. After the technician outlines the plan, minigoals for improvement are established. This plan should be documented in the chart and on a duplicate sheet for the client to take home. It is the technician's job to keep the expectations realistic and to use the care plan as a guide to success. One of the most difficult tasks for technicians is to evaluate and project final results. Even the best technician with years of experience can be surprised by an unexpected result. The best course of action is to "underpromise and overachieve." Technicians should keep in mind that they are not in complete control of situations. However, it is easy for technicians to take too much of the emotional burden of unmet expectations, and they should remember that the client's expectations influence outcomes as well.

Realistic Expectations

I know not all forms of hair removal are permanent. This quote is a sign of a client with realistic expectations and an understanding of the possibilities. Setting and maintaining realistic expectations with your client is an ongoing and fluid process. It is also one of the most difficult tasks for technicians. The best approach is to help clients recognize improvement through three tactics: taking photographs, underpromising, and keeping realistic expectations by not aiming for "perfect" results.

Photographs are the best documentation available to set and sustain expectations. The old saying *a picture is worth a thousand words* is very relevant with these types of treatments. The photographic process should not be disregarded. Be sure to share photographs of progress with clients, which will help them see the changes, allowing for discussion and alterations in treatment modalities.

LASER TREATMENT REPORT

Patient: _____ Date: _____
Clinician: _____

DIAGNOSIS:
Telangiectasia _____ Lentigo _____ Tattoo _____ Capillary Vascular Malformation _____
Excess Hair _____ Treatment Resistant or Complicated Warts _____

INDICATION:
Cosmetic _____ Irritated _____ Causing Functional Disability _____
Other _____

LOCATION:

Forehead	_____	Cheeks R L	_____	Nose	_____	Nostril R L _____
Upper Lip	_____	Peri-Oral	_____	Chin	_____	Neck _____
Ear R L	_____	Scalp	_____	Shoulder R L	_____	Chest _____
Belly	_____	Back	_____	Buttocks R L	_____	Arm R L Up/Lo _____
Hands	_____	Finger(s)	_____	Bikini Line	_____	Thigh(s) R L _____
Calves R L	_____	Feet R L	_____	Underarms	_____	Lower Face _____

Other: _____

SIZE: _____ mm X _____ mm   **NUMBER:**

LASER: Diode _____ Krypton _____ Alexandrite _____

ANESTHESIA: EMLA ___ Lasercaine ___ Ice ___ US Gel ___ Hurricane Spray _____
Other: _____

SETTINGS:
Watts _____ Pulse Duration .2 Interval: .2 _____
Continuous _____ Color: Yellow/Green _____
Total _____

• **DIODE:** PPS _____ Fluence _____ Auto or 30 ms _____

• **ALEXANDRITE:** PPS _____ Joules _____ Total _____

SAFETY: Eye Shields/Goggles: ☐ Patient _____ ☐ Staff
Warnings Signs Posted: ☐
Other _____

COMPLICATIONS: None _____ Yes (explain) _____

POST-PROCEDURE CARE: Verbal/Written Questions Answered _____
Wound Care written information given to patient Yes _____ No _____
Additional treatment or medications: _____

Figure 4–6 Example of a treatment care plan

unrealistic expectations
belief that a certain outcome is
possible, regardless of merit or
circumstance

Unrealistic Expectations

Unrealistic clients are a nightmare for technicians. Those with unrealistic expectations often end up being unhappy and telling friends and family about their unhappiness. To avoid this problem, we should be aware of the common times within the treatment continuum when clients may become unhappy.

First, the consultation process can often reveal if a client has unrealistic expectations. These clients may make statements like, "I want all this hair to go away for good. Will that happen with waxing?" These clients will also argue about potential results. For example, "My friend Sandy had laser hair removal, and she has not had a single hair grow back. I want my face to look like hers." Clients with unrealistic expectations should be educated about the process. If the education does not sink in, then the client should be referred out of the clinic.

Second, once the process has begun, unhappy clients can sometimes become impatient or believe they have not had any results at all. This is where the photographs can be helpful. Use the initial pictures and take pictures on the day of treatment. Show these pictures to the client. Although clients often forget what they looked like before starting treatment, even if it was only a few weeks ago, the "before" pictures can often reveal if there have been any improvements.

Setting Up a Care Plan

The care plan is a road map that helps the technician and the client understand the process to achieve the goal. Clients and technicians alike often forget that the best results for a hair removal program are achieved when the client is conscientious about keeping appointments, as well as about keeping in mind what the pros and cons of each treatment modality are, how the clinical program will progress, and how often treatments will be given, at what intensity, and in coordination with other treatments. These facts and the progression of the process should all be included in the care plan.

Conclusion

First impressions are lasting impressions is a mantra to live by, especially in the spa business. How you behave, how you dress, how you speak to the client, and how well you know hair removal techniques will determine your ultimate success. Clients look to you for your professionalism and knowledge. It is up to you to deliver these qualities. The client has a need, and you have the skills to fill the need. How you impart the information will make the difference as to whether clients hear your advice. The more experienced technicians become at the consultative and communication process, the easier it will become.

Finally, setting the road map of appointments and expectations will help finalize the opportunities for success. Open communication, a quest for knowledge, and the abilities to choose the right programs will set you and your client on the right path.

▶ ▶ ▶ TOP 10 TIPS TO TAKE TO THE CLINIC

1. Be sure to take photographs.
2. Educate your client about the hair removal process.
3. Show the client his or her photographs to demonstrate the long term results.
4. First impressions are lasting impressions.
5. Make sure the treatment room is clean and inviting.
6. Know your subject matter.
7. Be careful to accurately document the health history and contraindications.
8. Use a consultative process.
9. Listen to the client's concerns.

CHAPTER QUESTIONS

1. What makes you different from your competitors?
2. Why is it important to make a care plan?
3. How should a client with unrealistic expectations be handled?
4. What should be done when a client is unhappy?
5. What are the steps of a consultative process?

BIBLIOGRAPHY

Bickmore, H. (2003). *Milady's Hair Removal Techniques*. Clifton Park, NY: Milady, an imprint of Thomson Delmar Learning.

The Tools of the Trade

CHAPTER 5

KEY TERMS

azulene	energy fluence	rheostat
candelilla wax	glycerol ester	rosin
carnauba wax	hard wax	strip method
diathermy	melting points	sugar wax
diopter	muslin strips	thermolysis
eflornithine	Pellon strips	

LEARNING OBJECTIVES

After completing this chapter, you should be able to:

1. Know the factors important for setting up a treatment room.
2. Discuss the pros and cons of hard and soft wax.
3. Explain the devices used for electrolysis.
4. Discuss the different types of lasers.
5. Explain the important safety issues associated with hair removal.

INTRODUCTION

For the technician, having the skill set to perform optimal hair removal procedures involves having a thorough understanding of the procedures, as well as the tools of the trade. For the most part, deciding which tools and devices to use for different procedures will be a matter of preference. However, in order to make an informed decision about the specific tools you will want to use, it is important to know what is available.

Because there are several modalities of performing hair removal, each modality has its own set of devices, tools, and equipment. In this chapter, we will discuss the tools that are used for each modality and identify the pros and cons associated with each. However, the logical place to start the discussion is in the "place" itself, the treatment area. (See Figure 5–1.)

■ THE TREATMENT ROOM

The treatment room is the common denominator for all the treatment modalities. The treatment room should be safe, clean, and aesthetically pleasing. To this effect, it is important to set up the area so that it is safe and comfortable for the client and easy to clean, sanitize, and equip for the technician. A poorly organized and cluttered treatment room may result

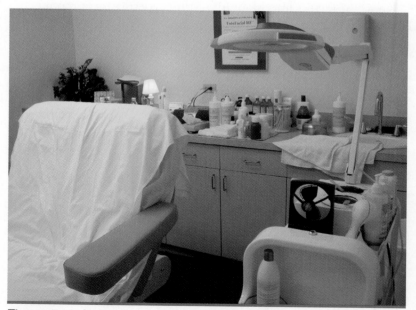

Figure 5–1 A clean and comfortable treatment room will help the client to feel at ease

in a dangerous mishap or poor technique. Electrical cords dangling freely from an epilating unit can be hazardous. Mirrors and other reflective surfaces can be hazardous in a room where laser treatments are performed.

Good lighting is essential in a treatment room. As treatments require privacy, windows are not an option, unless the glass panes are heavily frosted. Fluorescent lights are the closest substitute to natural light and provide the brightest and most economical light. In addition, a movable lamp, loupes, or a magnifying lamp helps light and magnify specific areas to be treated with electrolysis, precision waxing, and tweezing.

The choice of music in a treatment room is important to set a pleasant, relaxing, and professional tone. Music with lyrics should be avoided because lyrics to even the most innocuous songs may upset or offend some clients. For example, a recently divorced client may not want to listen to a love song during an electrolysis session. Selecting music without lyrics gives clients the best environment to relax and minimize discomfort.

The temperature of the room can also affect the clients' comfort during treatments. A client who is chilled and shivering may not want to return; a client who is uncomfortably warm may be agitated and anxious during the treatment. Although it is difficult to please everyone, a thermostat set to a standard 68° to 72°F should be comfortable for most clients. For clients who like to stay warmer, a thermal blanket on the treatment chair or table, or a blanket placed over the client should suffice.

Having a washbasin in the treatment room inspires client confidence, especially when a technician washes his or her hands in the presence of a client. Washing one's hands in front of a client is the foremost way to let the client know that his or her well-being is paramount. (See Figure 5–2.)

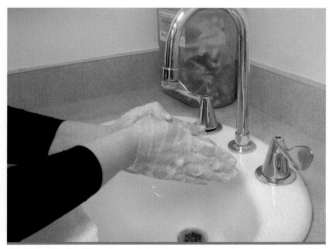

Figure 5–2 Hand washing is an important step prior to treating the client

Basic Equipment for the Treatment Room

Whether providing laser, electrolysis, or waxing service, standard items for a treatment room should consist of the following:

- washbasin for hand washing
- treatment table
- technician stool
- cart
- countertop or cabinet for supplies
- lined trash can
- hooks or hangers for clients' clothes

Other basic items in a treatment room include equipment for laser, electrolysis, or waxing, including necessary attachments. The equipment should be positioned securely on a flat surface and be able to receive good ventilation from all sides. Furthermore, the equipment appendages should be able to move sufficiently without hindrance when performing the service. The equipment should be away from water and free from dangling cords that could cause someone to trip. Equipment should have access to grounded outlets that do not share the same circuitry as other power-drawing appliances.

Hygiene and sanitation supplies include: soap in a pump, paper towels for hand washing, and/or sanitizing gel if there is no hand washing basin in the room. Antiseptic cleaner and towels for wiping counters should be readily available for use between clients. Disposable vinyl gloves should be available for technician and client safety. Washable or disposable paper drapes and disposable panties should be available for client modesty and protection.

Standard items for all hair removal services consist of the following:

- diagrams of skin and hair
- record cards
- release forms
- clipboards
- pens
- handheld mirror
- sanitizing unit filled with disinfectant
- a steel dish and lid for sterilized tools
- eyebrow scissors
- electric buzzer, including extra attachments for sanitation
- tweezers
- sterilized sharp forceps (to remove ingrown hairs)
- ice or cold packs
- Pellon/muslin strips

Consumable supplies that should be available include:

- paper rolls for the treatment table
- hair clips/hair cups/hair bands
- cleansing lotion
- petroleum jelly
- pretreatment lotion/witch hazel
- surgical alcohol
- antiseptic lotion
- tea tree oil (or other preparatory lotion)
- disposable eyebrow brushes
- eyebrow pencils and sharpeners
- tissues
- cotton in a covered receptacle
- soothing lotions and aloe vera gel

Waxing supplies consist of protective collars, multiple size applicators, applicator holder, dusting powder, Pellon strips or muslin strips in at least two sizes (1" x 3" and 9" x 3"), and wax cleaner.

Additional electrolysis supplies include sterilized sharp forceps (for removing hairs treated with electrolysis), an assortment of different sized disposable probes, needle holder caps, and a sharps collection container.

Additional laser hair removal supplies needed are antibacterial wash, aloe, ice packs, disposable razors for shaving (pretreatment), goggles for eye protection, and laser-cooling gel.

Pellon strips
a soft-woven, paper-like strip used for removing wax from the skin

muslin strips
thin, plain-weave cotton cloth strips used for removing wax from the skin

The Patient's Comfort

It is important for clients to feel safe, comfortable, and relaxed during treatments. Privacy is also paramount, especially for clients who must remove clothing; therefore, the treatment room door should have a lock. A lockable treatment room is also important when performing laser hair removal to prevent someone inadvertently walking in during a treatment. A partitioned area for face waxing is acceptable. A step for short clients to get on the treatment table is also helpful.

The Treatment Table

Treatment tables are now available for every budget, from the basic no-frills model for a startup practice on a limited budget (costing several hundred dollars), to a state-of-the-art hydraulic stool or remote-controlled swivel chair for the higher-end budget (costing thousands of dollars). A table is one of four most important purchases for the treatment room. Others include the epilation, laser, or waxing unit, the sterilizing unit, and the magnifying lamp.

When deciding on a treatment table, consider the length of time and frequency that clients will sit or lie on it. (See Figure 5–3.) Can the table facilitate lengthy sessions? Technicians should pay attention to the positioning features of tables and how positions affect the technician's ability to perform treatments efficiently and without straining, leaning awkwardly, or having to keep moving the table and disrupting the service. The table should be at a comfortable height for the technician to work fast and effectively without putting undue stress on the back or posture. Bad posture not only affects the standard of treatment, but can also cause chronic back problems or operator fatigue. The table should have a washable, fitted sheet over it for protection, and a paper liner should always be placed over the sheet for sanitary purposes.

Laser Hair Removal Devices

When purchasing a laser device, there are certain things that must be considered: costs, setup, and maintenance. The costs of the machine will often be a major consideration. If you expect a great deal of volume in

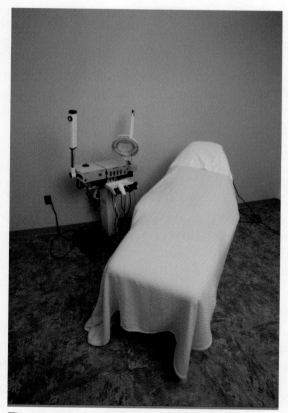

Figure 5–3 A comfortable bed will help the client to relax during the treatment

laser hair removal treatments, it will take less time to recoup your investment. However, the devices themselves are quite expensive. New machines can run anywhere from $75,000 to $150,000. Needless to say, the decision to offer laser treatments should not be made on a whim. Cost comparisons and options ought to be done thoroughly. Remember that costs will include maintenance and repair, so be certain to discuss these considerations with the vendor. We will discuss this topic more in depth later in the text.

Once the decision has been made, and the equipment is purchased, an electrician should check the electrical circuitry. The laser equipment will require an electrical outlet that is grounded and includes proper amperage, power surge protection, and its own circuit breaker. After the setup, the equipment should be serviced and calibrated according to manufacturer guidelines, and preferably maintained by the manufacturer.

The equipment distributor or manufacturer will usually set up the laser equipment. It is a poor idea to buy used laser equipment, unless it comes from a distributor, has been checked and serviced thoroughly, and comes with a use guarantee and a warranty for labor, service, and parts.

There are a number of effective lasers for hair reduction on the market today. The most common of these devices are the neodymium yttrium aluminum garnet, ruby, alexandrite, and diode.

Neodymium Yttrium Aluminum Garnets

Neodymium yttrium aluminum garnets (Nd:YAGs) have a longer pulse, making them more effective for long term and permanent hair removal. The Nd:YAGs use a carbon-based lotion for greater effectiveness. While Nd:YAGs were at one time considered to result in permanent hair removal, published clinical data dispute that claim. Subsequent data collected by operators using this laser with the carbon lotion reported a 27 to 66 percent reduction at 3 months after one treatment. This device, now cleared by the FDA to advertise its ability to produce long term or permanent reduction, is considered by some to be less painful when compared to the alexandrite laser treatment. This is especially true with devices that have cooling ability, and this type of treatment offers fewer side effects than ruby or alexandrite on more pigmented skin.

Ruby

Ruby lasers use shorter wavelength systems. While ruby lasers were cleared by the FDA for hair removal in 1997, clinical research shows that the laser damage does not extend far enough down the hair shafts to result in permanent hair destruction at the dermal papilla. In addition, when used on individuals with dark skin or tans, these lasers sometimes caused hyperpigmentation.

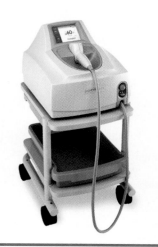

Figure 5–4 A diode laser is commonly used for hair removal

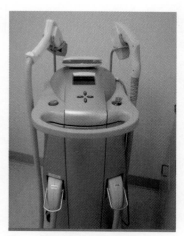

Figure 5–5 An Intense Pulsed Light (IPL) treatment machine

energy fluence
the energy level of a laser; measured in joules

Alexandrite

Alexandrite lasers were cleared by the FDA for hair removal in 1997. Alexandrite lasers are considered by some to be the workhorse of the laser hair removal industry. Yet, some dispute their effectiveness. This is because alexandrite lasers are most effective for treating Fitzpatrick skin types I, II, and III. Hence the effectiveness will depend on the demographic of individual spa/clinic clientele.

Diode

Diode lasers were cleared for hair removal by the FDA in 1997. (See Figure 5–4.) If the diode is high powered, such as the Lumenis 800nm, the results can be significant. The diode laser typically has a cooled tip, which allows for better and safer performance when treating darker skin types than the ruby or alexandrite. The diode laser can provide permanent hair reduction in a significant number of patients with varying skin types. Diode lasers have also been shown to be effective in the treatment of pseudofolliculitis. This treatment is often successful and carries with it a low complication rate.

Intense Pulsed Light

Intense Pulsed Light (IPL) uses full spectrum, noncoherent, and broadband light. (See Figure 5–5.) These lights include blue, yellow, red, and infrared appearing as white light, with low-range infrared-radiation spectrum of approximately 400 to 1200 nm. The operator eliminates and filters out the lower wavelengths to allow a specified range of wavelengths to be used, those that will be most effective in removing hair. IPL is delivered in one to four pulses of 1 to 1200 milliseconds duration, the average being approximately 35 milliseconds and using an energy fluence range of 2 to 7.5 joules/cm^2. During this process, the light is reflected, refracted, scattered, resisted, and absorbable.

This type of treatment was given FDA clearance for hair removal without the designation permanent removal, but allowing the designation of permanent reduction, in 1997. The differences between IPL and laser treatment is that IPL emits every wavelength of light in the visible spectrum, as opposed to lasers that emit only one. The spot handpiece that emits the beam is larger than that of a laser and covers a wide area faster because of its rectangular shape.

It is possible to experience long-lasting and possibly permanent results from this hair removal method. In 2000, the FDA started to allow some manufacturers to make claims of permanent reduction on certain skin types. It is most effective on people with light skin and darker pigmented hairs. It is not suitable as a method on darker skin. Any regrowth often appears as lighter in color and finer in texture.

Epilation Units

Epilation units have evolved significantly since their inception and can be classified in three ways: manual, semimanual, and computerized. (See Figure 5–6.) The units can range from very basic but reliable, doing an adequate job of destroying the dermal papilla with diathermy, to very sophisticated pieces of equipment with many extra features that produce diathermy or galvanic current. Depending upon the features and type of unit, some require substantial training by the distributor. However, once mastered, this type of equipment provides excellent results for clients as demonstrated through records of clients' treatments. Whatever the choice of equipment, the operator must completely understand the equipment, how it works, and all the variables that belong to it so that clients' experience safe and effective hair removal treatment.

diathermy
a treatment accomplished by passing high-frequency electric currents to generate heat; as it pertains to electrolysis, used synonymously with thermolysis

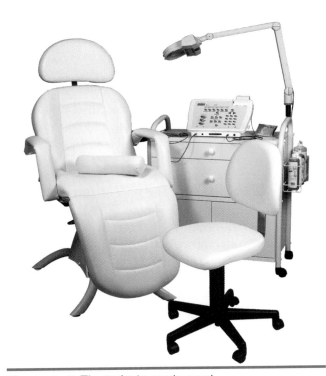

Figure 5–6 Electrolysis equipment

Manual Machines

With the manual thermolysis machine, the intensity of the current is selected and controlled by the operator using a rheostat. The duration of the current is controlled by the foot pedal (or, in some countries like the United Kingdom, a button on the probe holder). The current intensity may be displayed in a sequence of numbers ranging from 0 to 10 or in increments of 10 ranging from 0 to 100. The operator should always refer to the unit's operating manual to accurately interpret the numbering on the dials.

Semimanual Machines

Semimanual thermolysis machines were developed after manual machines, as a result of concerns about the duration of the current. The lengthy and often clumsy use of the foot switch or inaccurate counting with the hand-operated button with manual machines often resulted in the overtreatment of the hair follicle and damage to the skin. To prevent the extended application of current, a dial with an automatic timer was added to semimanual units, allowing the operator to preselect the duration of the current once the foot switch is tapped. The intensity control (rheostat control) is still set on a dial by the operator with semimanual machines.

Computerized Machines

Computerized, or automatic, thermolysis machines can be programmed for galvanic, thermolysis, a blend of galvanic and thermolysis, and pulsing and flash techniques. Computerized units can also be programmed to apply the appropriate amount of current based on the hair type being treated. Some units have additional features, such as features to count treated hairs and features to adjust the flow of current down the needle in the middle of an insertion. Some computerized epilators are also programmed to work in "auto mode," without the use of the foot switch. Another useful feature of computerized machines is their ability to keep clients' files in memory, which enables the operator to continue an effective treatment at the "flick of a switch." A growing number of electrologists claim their clients report feeling less discomfort with programmed treatments and achieve better results than with nonprogrammed treatments. Less discomfort could be due in part to the superflash feature, which is a sequential feature designed with the first "flash" destabilizing and "distracting" the nerve endings that transmit pain, so that when the next actual treatment flash is emitted, it is not felt as intensely.

Considerations for Selecting an Epilator

When selecting an epilation unit for purchase, there are a number of considerations. First, have a clear idea of how to develop the electrolysis business. Is it just going to be small, or will it be a growing entity with five or more full days of treating clients? Will the machine be used by one or multiple operators? Also important are whether or not there are required manufacturing standards for electrolysis machines depending on where the technician lives, and whether or not the equipment meets those standards. The Federal Drug Administration (FDA) regulates electrolysis equipment in the United States.

Second, technicians should consider finances when selecting an epilator unit. What is the cost of the equipment? Is financing offered by the manufacturer or supply company? This may determine whether technicians can purchase the machine that best suits their needs, or whether they have to settle for a less optimal choice.

A third consideration when selecting a unit is the ergonomics of the machine. Is it easy to hold for long periods of time? And in terms of general care several questions are important. Is it clearly labeled and easy to understand? Will it clean easily without wiping crucial numbers and markings off the dials? And finally, what features does it have to make the treatments more effective or comfortable?

Questions should be asked about the manufacturer; for example, does the manufacturer offer additional complementary training with the equipment, ensuring that the operator understands all variables of the equipment and is comfortable with those variables? Another consideration is overall customer service of the company selling the equipment. Does the manufacturer have a toll-free hotline for answering questions and troubleshooting problems? Hotlines help solve problems and avoid having to ship the equipment for repair, which not only saves money but also avoids the loss of time and revenue of not having the machine. In the event of real technical or mechanical problems, it is important to know what the warranty covers, such as parts and labor.

Probes

Probes are tiny hair-like needles, which slide in the hair follicle and emit the treatment energy that destroys the hair follicle. The probes are either reusable or disposable. The primary consideration must always be that the probe is sterile, whether it is a newly opened, disposable sterile probe, or a probe that has gone through complete sterilization. The preferred choice for electrologists and clients today is to use a brand-new, presterilized, prepackaged probe with each client for each visit.

The benefits of electrology:

- Electrolysis is currently the only proven method of permanent hair removal recognized by the FDA.
- Electrolysis can be performed successfully on all types of hair: blonde, dark, gray, straight, curly, vellus, or terminal.
- Electrolysis can be used effectively on all skin types (dry, oily, or mature) and all pigments.
- Electrolysis can be performed on all parts of the face and body, except for the inside of the nose or ear.
- Electrolysis can remove hairs with great precision, one at a time, making it a great choice for shaping eyebrows.

Technicians should open probes in front of clients, to give clients peace of mind and confidence in the professional behavior of technicians. Most clients would willingly pay $1 more per treatment for new, disposable probes. Many packages have visible marks of sterilization and expiration dates. If packaging is damaged in any way, or if the date on the package has expired, discard the probes in the sharps box or by another appropriate method.

Sterilization aside, the probe (of correct diameter size) should be able to enter and slide down the follicle with ease. With all other variables in place, the probe should apply the necessary amount of current to destroy the dermal papilla and/or the sebaceous gland, a process called histolysis.

Many electrologists change probes for fresh ones during extended treatments of 30 to 45 minutes or longer, because the probes bend and weaken with use and tissue debris may adhere to the probe. These issues occur particularly for noninsulated probes if too much treatment energy is used, rendering the probe less effective.

There are only two main types of probes: (1) the one-piece probe, and (2) the two-piece probe (see Figure 5–7). Both types offer variations of length, diameter, tip, and blade.

One-Piece Probes

One-piece probes are fashioned from single, solid pieces of steel. They can have tapers that blend gradually into the blade or tapers that cut more abruptly into the blade. The one-piece probe is generally more rigid and less flexible than the two-piece version, but one-piece probes have enough flexibility to accomplish most electrolysis tasks. The one-piece model bends gently and gradually, and is great for treating coarse hair with deep, straight follicles.

Two-Piece Probes

With the two-piece probe, the blade is attached to the shank by a divot cut most of the way around the shank, called a crimp. This probe is also called a straight or cylindrical probe. The type of probe is generally a little flimsier than the one-piece probe when all other variables, such as length

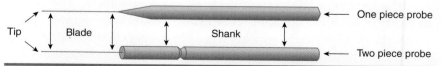

Figure 5–7 (a) Diagram of a one-piece probe. (b) Diagram of a two-piece probe.

and diameter, are equal. Two-piece probes bend and "give" more easily, making it a favorite for experienced electrologists who feel that thinner-diameter probes contour with the follicle as they slide down. Electrologists often claim to "feel" the follicle walls through the probe.

One-piece and two-piece probes alike have several distinct components: (1) The shank, which is the piece inserted into the probe holder. (2) The blade, which is the gold or steel portion inserted into the hair follicle; blades comes in various lengths, diameters, and shapes and are either insulated or noninsulated. (3) The tip, which is the portion in insulated probes where the current is produced in the hair follicle. (4) The taper, which is the graduated link between the shank and the blade; tapers are not present on all probes.

Insulated Probes

Insulated probes are covered two-thirds of the way down with an insulated plastic coating. These types of probes are most effective when using thermolysis modality, because they emit the high frequency current at the tip of the probe. As a result, they produce heat only to the base of the follicle, where heat is most needed to destroy the dermal papilla. According to Dr. James E. Schuster, because the intensity of heat is three to four times greater at the tip of an insulated probe than on a non-insulated probe, the epilator should be adjusted to reduce the treatment energy when using insulated probes.

While there is no electrical reason that insulated probes cannot be used with galvanic current, the lye pattern differs with insulated probes so considerations must be taken into account. Generally insulated probes are not preferred for the galvanic modality or blend method. When using an insulated probe of the same diameter as a noninsulated probe and applying the same milliampere, there will be equal strength but greater density of electrons at the tip of the insulated probe. Furthermore, the energy or heat pattern will be disbursed less densely over the length of noninsulated probes compared to insulated probes. Some also question the durability of the insulation on the probe and whether the lye produced by the galvanic current breaks it down. Consult with the probe manufacturer to determine if the insulation on the probes could withstand the effects of the lye.

Length

When selecting the length of the probe, make sure the probe inserts fully into the follicle so the tip can reach the dermal papilla in its late-anagen stage. Probes are available in lengths that include extra short, short, medium, regular, and long.

Diameter

A general guide is to match the probe thickness to the thickness of the hairs being epilated. Probe sizes come in 0.002, 0.003, 0.004, 0.005, 0.006, and 0.007 (2 to 7 thousandths of an inch).

There are many probes to choose from when selecting the appropriate probe for a task.

For example, if removing vellus with a shallow follicle on the upper lip using thermolysis, a technician would want to use a 0.002 short, insulated probe with reduced-treatment energy, because finer probes generate more heat than thicker probes.

Magnification Tools

Magnification tools include magnifying lamps or optical aids like headband goggles, loupes, or clip-on specs. Most electrologists use circular magnifying lamps with circular fluorescent lightbulbs.

Magnifying lamps have many benefits. As well as the obvious magnification, lamps can provide continuous bright light and serve as an effective shield when working on a client's face. They can be attached to a wall, to an equipment cart, to an aesthetic facial unit, or on a freestanding post for greater mobility. Magnifying lamps that are attached to a wall can be restrictive, often requiring clients to reposition themselves and the technician to move the treatment chair to accommodate the lamp. Sometimes, glare from overhead fluorescent lighting can affect the clear view through the lens. In these cases, the overhead fluorescent light can be switched off using only the magnifying lamp to provide sufficient lighting. Developing eye strain or headaches from magnifying lamps are not likely because the eyes are better able to adapt their degree of focus, which is more difficult when using loupes and other eyewear. Most lamps use 3x, 4x, 5x, or 8x dioptic lenses for magnification (5x being the most common). Some specialized models come with additional lenses for even greater magnification.

Eyewear is a little more complicated and requires a period of adjustment. Technicians claim that, after an initial period of adjustment in which they experienced headaches, they adjusted to the eyewear. Eyewear is available as a loupe that has one lens for each eye and a comfortable headband to keep it securely in place or as a slip-on for regular wear. The technician may flip the lens upward to communicate with the client or to view at distances (e.g., to look at a wall clock or a component on the epilating machine). Also available are binocular loupes that have two lenses for each eye and therefore greater magnification, approximately three times greater at a distance of 14 inches.

Table 5–1	General Magnification Guidelines	
Diopter	**Power**	**Working Distance (in inches)**
2	1 1/2 times	20
3	1 3/4 times	14
4	2 times	10
5	2 1/4 times	8
7	2 3/4 times	6
10	3 1/2 times	4

Table 5–1 illustrates the power that a diopter gives and the working distance in inches that is magnified and in focus. For example, the 2 diopter magnifies to one and a half times better than the natural eye at a distance of 20 inches. If one were trying to use the 2 diopter at more or less than 20 inches, the object would be out of focus.

When removing the eyewear, it is important to focus on something at a distance to exercise the eye muscles that have been focused on a narrow, limited level.

diopter
unit of measurement relating to the power of a lens

Forceps

Forceps come in almost as many shapes and sizes as probes (see Figure 5–8). For technicians, the most important factor when choosing forceps is the ability to withstand frequent sterilization. For this reason, most supply companies offer a wide variety of medically approved steel forceps. The forceps range from 23.4 to 50 centimeters long; most are 41.4 centi-

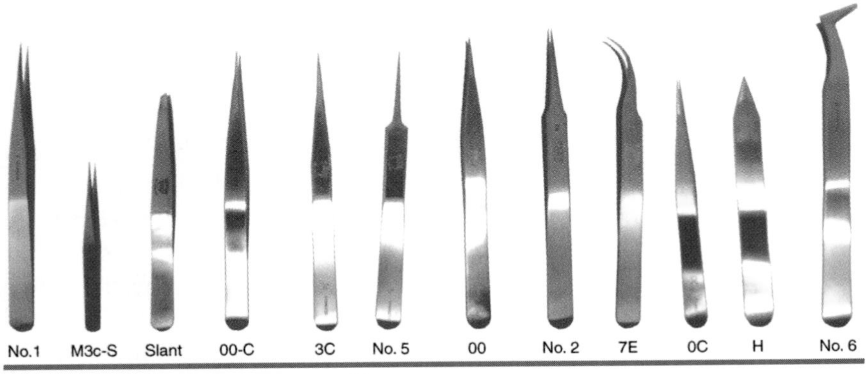

No.1   M3c-S   Slant   00-C   3C   No. 5   00   No. 2   7E   0C   H   No. 6

Figure 5–8 An assortment of forceps

meters long. The 23.4 centimeters forceps fit snugly between the thumb and forefinger of the same hand doing the insertion, and can be moved into place for removing the hair with a quick maneuver or twist of the fingers. The second hand maintains the stretch and offers greater speed and efficiency. Using the forceps in this manner takes practice and experience.

Some forceps are smooth at the tip and shank while others are etched for a better grip. Still others are *electroplated* with minute diamond particles at the tip to ensure better grip of the hair. Most forceps recommended for electrologists have extremely sharp tips to grip the finest hair close to the follicle opening, without snagging or tweezing adjacent hairs. However, some electrologists still prefer the slanted tip, which is suitable in areas where hair growth is not dense.

Some forceps curve or bend at the top, which is an excellent feature for releasing long, embedded, ingrown hairs.

■ WAX

hard wax
depilatory wax used without a strip

strip method
technique of hair removal using a strip over the sugar or wax for removal

sugar wax
a hair-removal product that is made primarily of sugar; technique sensitive

melting points
temperature at which wax begins to liquefy

There are two major methods of waxing for hair removal: hard wax, also known as the nonstrip method, and soft wax or strip method. Soft wax methods include honey-textured waxes and crème waxes. In addition, there are various varieties in between, such as cold wax and sugar wax, and other types with soothing additives. This section covers some of the many types of wax available for hair removal and when each type should be considered.

Wax Types

Pure waxes can be grouped according to the element from which they were derived: animal, mineral, vegetable, or synthetic. (See Table 5–2.) All waxes are insoluble in water and alcohol, and soluble in oils and other organic solvents (such as benzene, carbon tetrachloride, and ether). The nature of these waxes is best defined by referring to their physical properties.

Waxes are usually semicrystalline or amorphous solids that form semiglossy films. Although all waxes are easily molded when in a molten state, waxes vary in consistency from fairly soft and malleable to hard and brittle. The melting points of waxes are generally in the range of 105°F to 212°F (40°C to 100°C). The melting point of depilatory wax must be greater than 98°F (37°C), but less than 165°F (73.9°C). The melting point of wax must be higher than body temperature (98.6°F/38°C), and must be firm enough to grip the hair. A good working temperature for applying hard wax is between 125°F (51.6°C) and 140°F (60°C).

However, it is acceptable to use wax up to 165°F (73.9°C) considering that wax cools at a rate of approximately 7°F (3.9°C) per second.

Because no one wax type meets all criteria, in the cosmetic, aesthetic, and hair removal industries, waxes are often combined with other ingredients to achieve desired properties (e.g., melting point). Honey wax is the most common type, removed with a strip and typically made of beeswax and rosins. Some soft waxes do not actually contain wax, but are made from honey, mixed with glycerol ester of rosin. Other "honey" waxes do not contain honey at all, but are termed this due to their resemblance. To improve the melting point and strength of waxes, gum rosin is often combined with beeswax, candelilla wax, and carnauba wax. However, the rosin causes the wax to adhere to skin, which can cause sensitivity in some clients, particularly to the face and more delicate parts of the body (e.g., bikini area and underarms). Because of adverse reactions to honey wax, especially in clients using alpha hydroxy acids (AHA's) or prescription skin treatments, wax companies now manufacture waxes with azulene, tea tree, and other essential oils to soothe the skin and minimize negative reactions.

Manufacturers have also reintroduced hard, nonstrip depilatory waxes that were popular before honey wax, particularly in Europe. Made mainly from beeswax, hard wax became less popular as honey strip wax proved faster to apply, which allowed salons to book more clients and generate better earnings. Hard wax has made a comeback, however, because it has proven effective on clients who require specialized skin care that would otherwise contraindicate the use of soft wax. The unique properties have also shown hard wax to be preferred for more delicate parts of the body where skin may be thin and fragile, hair coarse (such as the bikini area), or where hair grows in multiple directions in the same area (such as the axillae).

glycerol ester
a refined rosin product that can be mixed with honey to produce a wax-like substance

rosin
a hard, translucent resin derived from the sap, stumps, and other parts of pine trees

candelilla wax
a type of vegetable wax derived from the candelilla plant

carnauba wax
the hardest and most widely used vegetable wax; derived from the leaves of the carnauba palm tree

azulene
an oil that is part of the chamomile essential oil, produced specifically by distillation

Benefits of Nonstrip Hard Wax

Hard wax does not distort the hair follicle because it is removed in the direction of hair growth, rather than against it as with strip wax. As hard wax hardens, it grips the hair tightly, shrinks, and lifts off without adhering to the skin. Thus, nonstrip hard wax causes less irritation than strip wax.

Because of the application of hard wax (applied under and against the growth, following over the top with the growth), the hair is securely gripped from all angles. This method makes it effective in areas where hair grows in multiple directions, and where skin is delicate (such as the axillae and around the labia during a Brazilian bikini wax). As with strip wax, the hair is epilated at the root, which causes the regrowth to be softer and without stubble. Regrowth generally takes 6 to 12 weeks after hard

Table 5-2	Different Types of Wax and the Benefits of Each
Wax Type	**Benefit**
Hard Wax	• Removes hair in the direction of growth and hair growing multidirectionally in the same patch. • Gentle on the skin as it grips hair without adhering to the epidermis, meaning less discomfort for the client and minimal reaction. • Can be used with caution on clients who use AHA products. • Can be used to wax the eyebrows of clients using Retin-A, providing the cream has not been applied to the brow area when done with caution. • Can rewax an area where hair was left behind. • Epilates hair at the root; hair grows back softer.
Soft Wax	• Fast and effective method of waxing, making it most profitable. • Easy to use. • Speed of the application means minimal discomfort to the client. • Warmth of the wax opens pores, which causes hair to slide out easily. • Epilates hair at the root; hair grows back softer.

waxing, depending on the telogen stage of that area. Because hard wax does not adhere to the epidermis, if hair is left behind after removal, it can be waxed a second time, providing there is no visible irritation. Hard wax can also be used with caution on clients who use glycolic acid or other AHA skin care treatments. Eyebrows may be waxed with hard wax if Retin-A or other prescription topical and antiacne medicines like Accutane and Differin are being used, but have not been applied directly to the eye area. Furthermore, using hard wax on clients using these medications should only be done after performing a patch test and after the client is informed of the increased risk of a negative reaction and has signed a release form. Even if clients do not directly apply prescription lotions and creams to the eye area, they can sometimes migrate to the eye area, causing changes in the integrity of that skin. The general rule in the application of hard wax is to first apply it against the direction of growth, coating the underside of the hair, and immediately following over the top in the direction of hair growth; however, one must always check the manufacturer's individual rules for application and removal that can usually be found on the can, package, or accompanying brochure.

Negative Aspects of Nonstrip Hard Wax

The process of waxing with hard wax can be slower and more laborious, taking considerably longer than strip wax (especially for technicians who are new to this process). The amount of time required is greater because the hard wax must cool and set to grip the hair, so it is not preferred for large body areas like the legs and back. The integrity of hard wax is easily altered if left to age in heat and if new wax is not added periodically. Because of inconsistencies in usage by different technicians (e.g., differences in temperature), the wax can become darker or lose its removal properties.

Some consider it more difficult to get good results with hard wax, especially when a female client is menstruating and retaining excessive fluids. This difficulty is thought to be a result of swelling, which tightens the skin and causes the hair to shrink into the skin, making it tough to remove. With hard wax, the hair cannot be "blended" as it can with strip. This may be a good enough reason to use strip wax on areas like the sides of the face or the throat.

Benefits of Soft Wax

There are many benefits to soft wax. It is by far the most popular method of professional hair removal. Soft wax is quick and easy to use, and the technician, with training and practice, can become a "speed waxer," cutting the typical service time in half, which will substantially increase profits. The shorter waxing time means minimal discomfort to the client. Discomfort is also reduced when speed waxing, as the warmth of the wax opens pores and makes the hair slide out easily. Soft wax epilates hair, meaning it removes the hair from below the skin, often at the root, without destroying the root. When the hair grows back, it is often softer. Many clients also experience some reduction in hair growth after multiple wax services.

When the hair is removed at the root or papilla, the new papilla must reestablish itself in the follicle. Not only does this take time, with continual waxing removal it may cause the papilla to weaken and cause extended periods between regrowth, as well as a reduction in hair growth. This is especially apparent with women who have frequently received leg wax treatments, and particularly women who are postmenopausal.

Negative Aspects of Soft Wax

Whereas the negative aspects of hard wax have to do primarily with the speed of the service, the negative aspects of soft wax have to do with the harshness of the rosins on the skin. The rosins can adhere to skin and are therefore the primary cause of irritation. As a result of the way soft wax adheres to the epidermis and lifts a layer of dead skin cells along with the hair, an area cannot be rewaxed immediately. It also means that it is not a

> Blending is a process by which areas with hair and without hair are transitioned by not removing all the hair, eliminating any hard lines.

good choice of wax for people who are receiving glycolic treatments or using alpha hydroxy acids, Retin-A, and other treatments that thin the epidermis. Soft wax is not a preferred method for French or Brazilian bikini waxing for two primary reasons: (1) it can cause injury when used on the delicate skin of the labia, and (2) it is difficult to apply the wax in the hair growth direction and pull away effectively against the growth due to the vaginal opening.

The axilla is another area that does not work well with soft wax treatments due to the multiple hair growth directions in a single patch. Hard wax works better for those areas. The required length of hair is also a negative factor. Hair must be at least 1/4 inch long before waxing. With regular waxing where the pull is *against* the hair growth direction, some distortion of the hair follicles can occur, causing the hair to grow back in an irregular fashion and standing up rather that laying flatter to the skin. Another disadvantage of soft wax applications is that the application process can be messy, leaving thread-like, sticky trails to be cleaned up, which is especially common for novice technicians.

Wax Pots

While hard wax is most commonly melted in wax heating units, new methods of heating and applying soft wax are available that are cleaner and more hygienic.

These systems use disposable applicator heads or rollers that can be sanitized. They also come with prepackaged bottles or tubes of wax.

The disposable applicator used by the professional hygienic disposal system incorporates a backflow valve, which prevents backflow of wax into the tube. Because the wax is heated in prepackaged tubes with the applicator head attached to the tube, technicians can work quickly without having to keep returning to the wax pot. However, these applicators do not work for small areas of the face (e.g., the eyebrows), where the use of a spatula is still the preferred method.

The roller method is portable and convenient because it eliminates the need to keep returning to the wax warming pot. However, the hygienic issues are the same with the roller as with the spatula. The only hygienic difference is if all the wax in a roller bottle is used exclusively for one client. Even when a roller is used, a spatula is still needed for small facial areas.

The self-contained application methods are effective in improving the speed of the service, cutting time, and increasing profits.

Wax should be heated according to manufacturer's specifications, which are usually found on the can of wax or in a brochure accompanying the wax heater. All literature accompanying the equipment should be available for new employees. If possible, use the brand of wax that is recommended for the wax heater. If technicians choose a different brand of wax, then they should use a thermometer to test the wax temperature to make sure it is at the recommended level, and they should make a notation on the warming pot's dial to indicate that appropriate level.

Cleansers, Gauze, Applicators, and Gloves

Applicators can be disposable or nondisposable. Nondisposable spatulas made of teakwood are becoming increasingly popular because they can be used repeatedly. Teakwood spatulas do not hold the heat the way metal spatulas can, which results in less mess and chance for thermal injuries to the client and the technician. The high-gloss finish of nondisposable spatulas prevents the absorption of oils and bacteria. These spatulas can easily be cleaned and sanitized, and are available in an assortment of sizes and shapes.

Disposable wood applicators are available in an assortment of sizes for the various waxing services (see Figure 5–9). Tongue depressors are commonly used, and while they can be cut to different sizes to reduce the number of sticks used, doing so is not recommended because the wood

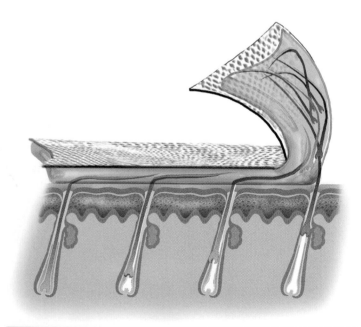

Figure 5–9 A wax applicator

can easily splinter, which may release fine splinters into the wax and risk client injury. The jagged edges of a broken applicator may also scratch the client.

Gloves

As previously discussed, gloves are an important component in technician and client safety, especially when bloodborne pathogens and other bodily fluids are present. Wearing gloves is one of the main universal precautions. (See Figure 5–10.) Available on the market are an assortment of latex and vinyl gloves, with differing attributes. The choice of glove is personal and individual, unless a client has an allergy to latex. During the consultation, question clients about allergies to latex. When clients do have allergies, they are usually aware of it and will mention this when they see the technician donning gloves.

Nonlatex vinyl gloves should be available to wear when working with clients allergic to latex. Some technicians prefer to use nonlatex gloves when performing waxing procedures. Better still, it is worth being or becoming a latex-free practice and avoiding the risks altogether. Another choice with glove selection is to choose gloves that are powder-free, for less irritation, and to avoid airborne allergens from the powder as the gloves are removed. Gloves often run big, so technicians should try one size smaller than their hand size (e.g., those with small hands should try extra small gloves first; for medium hands, try small size; for large hands, try medium, etc.). Gloves should fit snugly to ensure there is sensitivity at the fingertips, which enables the technician to feel any nonpigmented coarse hairs that may not be easily visible. However, the gloves should

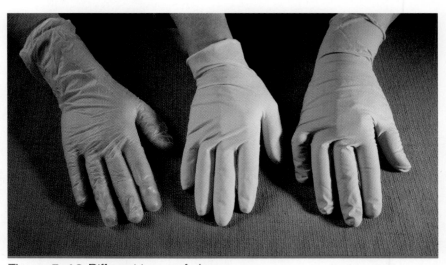

Figure 5–10 Different types of gloves

not be so tight that they restrict circulation. Gloves that are too big buckle and wrinkle and generally afford less sensitivity. Purple gloves are effective at identifying nonpigmented hairs during electrolysis treatments. They make good backdrops for otherwise hard-to-see hairs, as opposed to natural colored gloves, which are too close in color to light-pigmented hair. Gloves should be considered single-use items. A fresh pair should be donned each time the hands have been washed.

■ MEDICATIONS THAT AFFECT HAIR GROWTH

Certain drugs have been known to cause hair growth, usually because they are hyperandrogenaemic, which is defined as causing elevated androgens in the blood. When evaluating clients during consultations, it is important to have any and all medications listed, so it can be determined if the hair removal process will be a lengthy process or straightforward. Some medications may only be temporary, and some hair growth may gradually subside on its own, after the course of medication is complete. Other drugs may be taken long term for chronic conditions, and if a side effect is hair growth due to androgen stimulation, the hair removal process may be considerably longer as hair follicles are constantly being stimulated to produce unwanted hairs. In the case of a lengthier procedure, technicians should advise their clients at the onset to avoid frustration.

Hair Growth Inhibitors

Hair growth inhibitors, sometimes referred to as hair reduction creams, are *not* hair removers. They are designed to extend the time between hair removal treatments, whether via depilatory creams, waxing, or electrolysis. Most effective hair reduction creams are available by prescription and lower dosage products available over the counter. The most common of these is the inhibitor eflornithine found in the popular cream, Vaniqa™. The FDA has approved this product to slow the rate of hair growth by inhibiting the enzyme called ornithine decarboxylase, found in human skin.

eflornithine
chemical substance in the commercial cream Vaniqa™; blocks or inhibits hair growth

Eflornithine blocks metabolic activity in the hair follicle, thereby slowing the hair growth cycle. Prescription strength eflornithine is applied to the area twice a day. This product should be used only on the face and under the jaw because these are areas for which the enzyme was tested and approved. After application, the area should not be washed for at least four hours.

It is worth noting that if a person is receiving electrolysis treatments, his or her goal is most likely permanently eliminating unwanted hair, and using these creams only delays the permanency of electrolysis. However, if the client cannot get in for follow-up treatments on schedule, for example, due to travel or surgery, hair growth inhibitor products are useful. However, creams must be used for 4 to 8 weeks before results are noticeable. Upon terminating use of this product, the hair will return to its previous growth cycle in about 8 weeks. It has not yet been determined if this product is suitable for children or pregnant women.

Pros of Hair Growth Inhibitor Creams

Hair growth inhibitor creams are easy to use and can effectively extend the duration between visits to the hair removal specialist, thereby saving money and time. This is especially true of individuals who want to extend the time between waxing services. However, in the case of electrolysis, where the goal is permanent hair removal, hairs should be treated in their anagen stage and calculated according to the cycle of hair growth for that particular area. Delaying the process therefore does not expedite the desired goal of permanency. If, on the other hand, a client needs to delay electrolysis due to a medical condition, a trip out of town, or financial constraints, then hair inhibitors are useful.

Cons of Hair Growth Inhibitor Creams

With many hair growth inhibitor creams, a prescription is required to obtain these products, which makes it difficult or costly for some to obtain without a prescription plan. Hair growth inhibitors have been known to cause temporary redness, stinging, burning, rash, or folliculitis. Instructions on how to use the product and what adverse reactions to watch for should be given by the medical provider prescribing the product.

Conclusion

A well planned clinic is less likely to be the cause of accidents to clients or technicians, and is easier to maintain and look presentable. The orderliness and cleanliness of the facility will speak to the professionalism and caring of the people who work there. Having the correct tools readily available will ensure that appropriate services can be provided in a timely fashion. Having the correct tools means knowing what services you desire to provide, researching the equipment necessary, and making sure staff technicians are thoroughly qualified and licensed if necessary, in addition to being well trained on that particular model of equipment. Following those guidelines will ensure a safe and profitable business.

▶ ❯ ❯ TOP 10 TIPS TO TAKE TO THE CLINIC

1. Music should be soft, relaxing, and without lyrics.
2. A comfortable treatment table equals more comfortable services.
3. A treatment table at the correct height will allow technicians to provide fast efficient services with minimum discomfort.
4. If possible, avoid latex gloves.
5. Clients should sign a release prior to every waxing service.
6. Disposable single-use probes are the standard for electrolysis.
7. Hard wax is preferred for multidirectional hair in one area.
8. Careful documentation of client medications is very important prior to any hair removal treatment.
9. Anyone doing or receiving laser treatments should always wear ANSI-approved protective eyewear, and proper signage should be posted to indicate that a laser is in use.
10. Laser and electrolysis equipment should have grounded outlets and their own circuit breakers.

CHAPTER QUESTIONS

1. List two benefits of hard wax.
2. List two benefits of soft wax.
3. What are the four main types of laser?
4. List three important safety considerations for the treatment room.
5. List three important safety considerations for the laser equipment.
6. List three important laser safety considerations for the operator.
7. List three important laser safety considerations for the client.
8. List three benefits of electrolysis.
9. What is the main active ingredient in hair reduction creams?

BIBLIOGRAPHY

Bickmore, H. (2003). *Milady's Hair Removal Techniques*. Clifton Park, NY: Milady, an imprint of Thomson Delmar Learning.

Milady's Standard Comprehensive Training for Estheticians. (2003). Clifton Park, NY: Milady, an imprint of Thomson Delmar Learning.

Milady's Standard Cosmetology. (2004). Clifton Park, NY: Milady, an imprint of Thomson Delmar Learning.

Skin Typing and Hair Removal

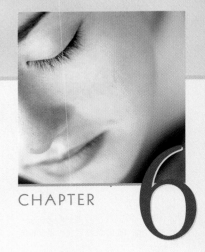

CHAPTER 6

KEY TERMS

Fitzpatrick Skin Typing

melanocytes

postinflammatory
hyperpigmentation

skin condition

skin typing

LEARNING OBJECTIVES

After completing this chapter, you should be able to:

1. Discuss Fitzpatrick Skin Typing.
2. Know how different skin types will respond to treatments, especially laser hair removal.
3. Be able to use a Fitzpatrick Skin Typing scale.

INTRODUCTION

The response to skin therapies is different from patient to patient because of biological variables. For example, when we speak of recommended drug doses, we calculate the dose based on the individual's weight. To determine the "who, when, how, and why" of the skin, we also need to have criteria to help predict suitability and effectiveness of a specific procedure. A variety of classification methods have been developed to assist us, the simplest of which is the classification of skin condition (normal, oily, dry, sensitive, or combination). While important, classifying skin condition is not vital in the assessment for laser hair removal or other hair removal therapies and consequently will not be discussed in this text. A different type of skin classification that we will discuss, however, is skin typing.

■ FITZPATRICK SKIN TYPING

It goes without saying that one person will not respond to a treatment exactly the same as the next person. Therefore, technicians need to understand how individual skin types respond to different treatments, specifically laser hair removal. Analysis of skin type allows technicians to understand which clients can receive aggressive treatments and which require greater caution

Many years of clinical research have shown that several factors regularly and consistently affect the skin's response to injury. These factors include: genetics, eye color, hair color, ethnic background, and natural skin color. In 1975, Dr. Thomas Fitzpatrick created a classification system, which became known as Fitzpatrick Skin Typing. (See Tables 6–1 through 6–6.) This method of analysis is perhaps the most widely used skin typing classification applied today to predict response to a variety of therapies. The method also assists technicians in determining which clients have a greater risk of complications such as scarring and pigmentary problems from various treatments. The specifics of the classification and the means to determine a client's type are discussed at length below.

The Fitzpatrick Skin Typing scale is presented in its simplest form in Table 6–1.

To derive these classifications, technicians must ask clients a number of questions in combination with the examination. Tables 6–2, 6–3, and 6–4 list some important questions.

Add up the total scores for each of the three sections for the Skin Type score, as shown in Table 6–5. This will give you a better evaluation of the client's skin type.

---

skin condition
fundamental skin classification in which an individual's skin is grouped according to the degree of moisture retention and/or its reaction to products or environment

skin typing
a more detailed skin classification that gives indications as to how a certain skin type will react to various treatment conditions

Fitzpatrick Skin Typing
method of skin typing that considers skin's complexion, hair color, eye color, ethnicity, and the individual's reaction to unprotected sun exposure

---

Several factors regularly and consistently impact the skin's response to injury: genetics, eye color, hair color, ethnic background, and natural skin color. The skin's responses to these factors define the Fitzpatrick Skin Typing System.

Table 6–1   Fitzpatrick Skin Typing Scale

Skin Type	Skin Color	Hair & Eye Color	Reaction to Sun	Common Ethnic Considerations
Type I	White	Blond hair & green eyes	Always burns, freckles	English, Scottish
Type II	White	Blond hair & green/blue eyes	Always burns, freckles, difficult to tan	Northern European
Type III	White	Blond/brown hair & blue/brown eyes	Tans after several burns, may freckle	German
Type IV	Brown	Brown hair & brown eyes	Tans more than average, rarely burns, rarely freckles	Mediterranean, Southern European, Hispanic
Type V	Dark Brown	Brown/black hair & brown eyes	Tans with ease, rarely burns, no freckles	Asian & Indian, some African
Type VI	Black	Black hair & brown/black eyes	Tans, never burns, deeply pigmented, never freckles	African

Table 6–2   Genetic Disposition[1]

	0	1	2	3	4	Score
What color are your eyes?	Light blue, gray, green	Blue, gray, or green	Blue	Dark brown	Brownish black	
What is the natural color of your hair?	Sandy red	Blond	Chestnut/ dark blond	Dark brown	Black	
What color is your skin (nonexposed areas)?	Reddish	Very pale	Pale with beige tint	Light brown	Dark brown	
Do you have freckles on unexposed areas?	Many	Several	Few	Incidental	None	
					Genetic disposition total	

Once the results have been calculated, a further analysis can be made into the categories within the typing matrix. (See Table 6–6.)

Skin Color

Skin color is essentially an inherited racial and ethnic characteristic. But even within the same race and ethnicity, there is variability. (See Figure 6–1.)

Table 6–3   Reaction to Sun Exposure[2]

	0	1	2	3	4	Score
What happens when you stay too long in the sun?	Painful redness, blistering, peeling	Blistering followed by peeling	Burns sometimes followed by peeling	Rare burns	Never had burns	
To what degree do you turn brown?	Hardly or not at all	Light color tan	Reasonable tan	Tan very easily	Turn dark brown quickly	
Do you turn brown with several hours of sun exposure?	Never	Seldom	Sometimes	Often	Always	
How does your face react to the sun?	Very sensitive	Sensitive	Normal	Very resistant	Never had a problem	
					Reaction to sun exposure total	

Table 6–4   Tanning Habits[3]

	1	2	3	4	5	Score
When did you last expose your body to sun (or artificial sunlamp/tanning cream)?	More than 3 months ago	2–3 months ago	1–2 months ago	Less than a month ago	Less than 2 weeks ago	
Did you expose the area to be treated to the sun?	Never	Hardly ever	Sometimes	Often	Always	
					Tanning habits total	

Table 6–5   Scores[4]

Summary	
Total for genetic disposition	
Total for reaction to sun exposure	
Total for tanning habits	
Skin Type score	

Table 6–6   Fitzpatrick Skin Type[5]

Skin Type Score	Fitzpatrick Skin Type
0–7	I
8–16	II
17–25	III
25–30	IV
Over 30	V–VI

Caucasian

Within the Caucasian classification group, it is important to remember that *white* can come in a variety of shades, and this will impact whether the client is a Fitzpatrick I or II or even III. In the Fitzpatrick I category, the ethnic considerations are English, Scottish, Irish, Norwegian, Swedish, and Icelandic. Individuals will present with very fair skin, freckling, green or light blue eyes, and light hair colors. If their hair is dark, they are

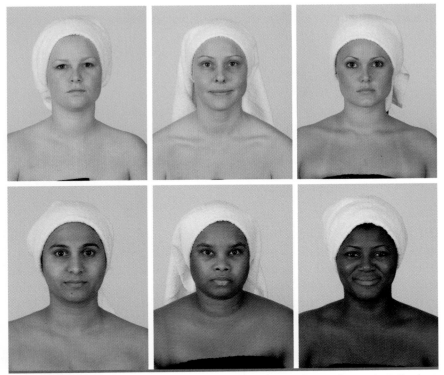

Figure 6–1 Skin color is an inherited racial and ethnic characteristic, but even within the same race and ethnicity, there is variability

great candidates for laser hair removal, with potentially few complications. An example would be the dark hair in the armpit.

Non-Hispanic Caucasian

The non-Hispanic Caucasian category of skin type has darker hair, mainly dark blond and brown. This category can also present several variations on the shades of darker whites and brown skin. These individuals will probably fall into the Fitzpatrick III and IV categories. Eye color is blue, dark blue, and brown, and the ethnic background is usually Mediterranean and Southern European, which would include Greeks, Middle Easterners, and Italians. These individuals are also good candidates for laser hair removal with few complications. While the skin is darker, so is the hair. The possibilities for machine settings should be considered.

Hispanic

The Hispanic skin category has darker skin, darker hair, and darker eyes. (See Figure 6–2.) Hair is dark brown or black, and eyes are brown. These individuals will generally fall into the Fitzpatrick IV and, perhaps, V categories. Their ethnic background is Spain, Mexico, South America, and Cuba. These individuals have darker skin and dark hair. They may sometimes be a challenge for laser treatment since they have the potential for postinflammatory hyperpigmentation.

African American

The skin types of Africans or African Americans are darker. (See Figure 6–3.) However, skin will vary from light brown, like Hispanics, to very dark to a blue black color. Their hair is always naturally black, but eyes can be brown to black. In the darkest color, this skin type is the Fitzpatrick VI, but these individuals also can be Fitzpatrick V as well. Their ethnic background is African.

Asian/Pacific Islander

These skin types are light brown to brown in color; often the hair can be light brown or sometimes a dark red to dark brown. (See Figure 6–4.) Eyes are brown and sometimes dark brown. These skin types have an ethnic background of Japan, China, and the islands of the South Pacific to mention a few. Typically these skin types will be types IV and V.

American Indian or Alaskan Native

Skin types are light brown to brown, and hair color is brown to black. (See Figure 6–5.) These people are found in differing parts of the United States. Typically these individuals will be types IV and, possibly, V.

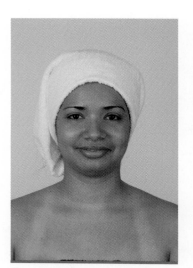

Figure 6–2 Hispanic skin generally has darker qualities with darker hair and darker eyes

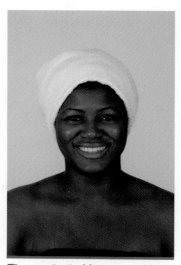

Figure 6–3 African or African Americans are darker, but the skin will range from light brown to very dark, almost a blue black color

Choosing Skin Color

So let us learn to choose skin color at a glance. In the clinic, as you begin the analysis of the skin, use these three easy steps. First, choose three areas of the body to evaluate. Begin with the face, under the breast or abdomen, and with the forearm. The face needs to be void of makeup. Next, look for freckles, telangiectasia, and skin tone. Finally, decide on a skin color based on what you see.

Eye Color

Eye color is determined genetically, just like the skin. (See Figure 6–6.) Eye color seemingly is straightforward, but there are some considerations. There are three basic eye colors: blue, brown, and green. These colors are further expanded into light blue, blue, blue-green, hazel, light brown, brown, dark brown, or black. Obviously, the degree of color is determined genetically but also relates to the skin tone. If you are struggling to assess the correct Fitzpatrick Skin Type, look at the eye color because it will help you to make the decision. Usually the eye color is the most helpful in analyzing Fitzpatrick I and Fitzpatrick II. These two skin types have varying colors of blue and green eyes, which can be confusing even to experienced technicians. If clients wear colored contact lenses, they should be asked to bring their lens case to the consultation, so the contacts can be removed for further evaluation.

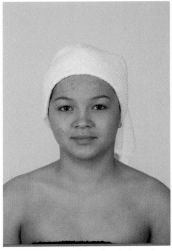

Figure 6–4 Pacific Islander or Asian skin is light brown to brown. The hair can be light brown or sometimes a dark red to dark brown.

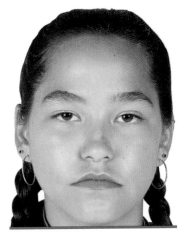

Figure 6–5 American Indian skin types are light brown to brown, and hair color is brown to black

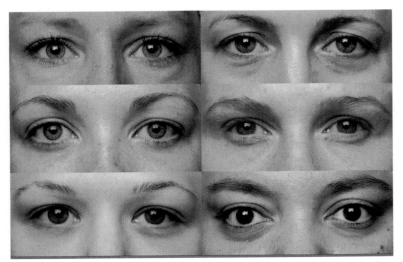

Figure 6–6 There are three basic eye colors: blue, brown, and green. These colors are further expanded into light blue, blue, blue-green, hazel, light brown, brown, dark brown, or black.

Hair Color

Hair color is probably the most difficult to appraise. (See Figure 6–7.) Most women color their hair to some degree, whether it is highlights, full color, or a combination of both. Hair color can be determined at the roots, but what if the client just had her hair colored? Also, the comparison of the colored hair against the natural hair can be deceiving. Maybe the eyebrows are worth looking at, but these can also be colored, bleached, or otherwise altered. If your client's hair color is altered, have her/him try to describe her/his natural color. Hair color is an indicator that you may or may not factor in, depending on the potential for error.

Response to UV Light with SPF Protection

Aside from identifying the skin type based on your skin analysis, the color of the eyes, and the color of the hair, evaluating the skin's response to UV light is *the* most important indicator of skin type. How you ask about the client's response to UV light is critical to the accuracy of the answer. This question requires clients to be entirely honest, which is sometimes evaded. You want to know how the skin responds to the sun *without* sun-

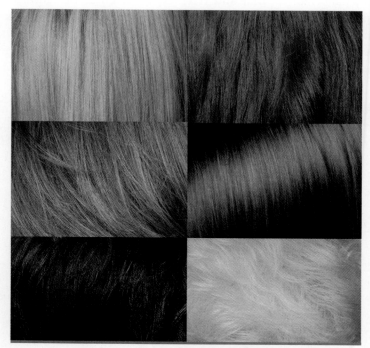

Figure 6–7 Hair color is probably the most difficult to appraise, since men and women color their hair

screen. The problem is that no one wants to admit he/she goes out in the sun without sunscreen. Usually the client will respond, "I never go into the sun," or "I never go in the sun without sunscreen." The best question to ask is "did you have a sunburn as a child?" If the answer is yes, get the details. For example, you want to know if the sunburn produced blisters and, if so, where on the body. If it did not produce blisters, can the client remember how long it was sore or red? If she cannot remember, probe a little bit further. "As a child did you vacation at the beach? How did your skin respond at the beach? As a child did you swim during the summer? How did your skin respond at the swimming pool? Did you sunbathe in college? Did you use baby oil to sunbathe? What happened to your skin?" The next question to ask is whether or not she has had a glycolic or tri-chloroacetic acid (TCA) peel. If the answer is yes, ask for details. What strength was used, how long was the peel left on, and what were the results of the peel? Were there any complications from the peel? Remember, Fitzpatrick analysis tells us how the skin responds to advanced skin care products and treatments.

Using the System

Now that you have collected all of the information, you make an analysis of Fitzpatrick Skin Type selection by using the following specific definitions. Your determination is based on what you see: the ethnic heritage (geographic origin of forbearers), eye color, and response to UV light. You should also factor in hair color if it is the natural color. There is a natural tendency to primarily evaluate skin color when we are typing the skin. Teach yourself to look at all of the characteristics associated with the Fitzpatrick Typing chart. The more difficult skins to type will be differentiated by the details of eye color and the skin's response to sun (especially as a child).

1. *Fitzpatrick I* is the *very fair* skinned individual. This person usually has very blond or red hair, light blue or green eyes, and burns within 10 to 15 minutes of being in the sun when exposed without sunscreen. This person tans by freckling. Good examples of Fitzpatrick Skin Type I are the Irish, English, or Scottish.
2. *Fitzpatrick II* is the *fair* skinned individual. This individual has blond hair, sometimes "dishwater blond," with blue or green eyes. He or she may tolerate a slightly longer period of time in the sun before burning, perhaps 30 to 40 minutes. This individual still freckles a lot and has difficulty tanning. Good examples of Fitzpatrick Skin Type II are Northern Europeans: Swedish, Finnish, or Norwegian.
3. *Fitzpatrick III* is still *white* but tans more easily than Fitzpatrick I and Fitzpatrick II. This person will have fewer freckles than the

The Fitzpatrick Skin Typing System has six categories. Your determination is based on what you see and the questions you ask.

Fitzpatrick I and II. His/her hair can be blond, but is more likely to be a light brown to moderate brown color. The eye color is usually dark blue to brown. This individual can be in the sun 60 to 70 minutes without sunscreen before beginning to burn. Examples of Fitzpatrick Skin Type III are German, Northern Italian, and French.

4. **Fitzpatrick IV** is *brown* and tans easily, usually without freckling. This individual can be in the sun without sunscreen and will rarely burn. The hair color is usually brown to dark brown, and the eyes are brown. Examples of Fitzpatrick Skin Type IV are Greeks, Southern Italians, some Asians, and some Hispanics.

5. **Fitzpatrick V** is *dark brown*, tans easily, and generally does not have freckles. This person can be in the sun without sunscreen and will not burn. The hair is usually brown or black with brown eyes. Examples of Fitzpatrick Skin Type V include some Asians, some Hispanics, some Africans, and Middle Eastern Indians.

6. **Fitzpatrick VI** is *black*, tans with ease, does not freckle, and is deeply pigmented. The hair is black, and the eyes are brown or even black. Examples of Fitzpatrick Skin Type VI are Africans.

Identifying skin types is as much a science as an art. Usually one component of the skin's characteristic will be more dominant than others, which will be a determining factor in the skin type. Many times clients simply will not fit into one category; they seem to have attributes of several categories, making them a Fitzpatrick I+ or a Fitzpatrick III–, for example. How do we make the decision of where they fit?

Mixed Skin Colors

As people have become more mobile, the world has become a smaller place and skin colors have become mixed. Mixed skin color is an important factor as technicians evaluate for skin typing (see Figure 6–8) and also makes the task more challenging. Therefore, it is incumbent on the technician to ask questions about the ethnic and racial heritage of clients. Most clients are proud of their heritage and understand that genetics impact their appearance. But, before you begin asking clients questions about their ethnic makeup, explain why you need to know. Begin by explaining that genetics impact their skin color, and ask about their heritage. Even though they may look like one parent more than the other, it is helpful to know the heritage of both parents if possible.

What if your client is adopted? Unless they happen to know the heritage of their birth parents, this piece of information is lost. In this case, it will be really important to ask enough questions about the previous sun exposure to give you an understanding of the skin type. What if they

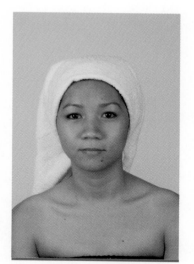

Figure 6–8 An example of mixed skin colors

know only one parent? Ask extensively about the known parent, which will help evaluate if the patient resembles this parent. Then, as with adopted clients, you will need to use your clinical skills to come to an accurate conclusion. What you observe and your analysis of what you see will guide you in these situations.

Pigment Changes

Pigment changes are changes related to skin damage, sun exposure, and aging. When skin is exposed to the sun, pigment changes are likely. The pigmentation will present as tan and freckles, as well as subsequent damage causing lentigines, telangiectasia, and premature aging. Some pigment changes, however, are secondarily related to the sun and primarily related to medication or pregnancy. (See Figure 6–9.) The origin of the pigment change is not specifically noted in the classification. If you are using this classification, you will want to note the origin of the dyschromia. Dyschromia is an irregularity in color, hyperpigmentation or hypopigmentation, that occurs on the skin. In a more subtle way, pigment also refers to the dull, sallow appearance of the skin that is created over time.

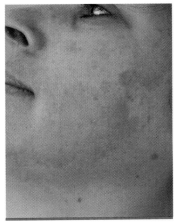

Figure 6–9 Melasma is a condition that occurs with pregnancy or birth control pills

■ HYPOPIGMENTATION

Melanocytes reside between the epidermis and the dermis. They secrete pigment known as melanin, which gives skin, hair, and eyes their color. The relative number of melanocytes is the same for men and women and for all races. The major contribution to the depth of skin color is melanocyte *activity* rather than quantity. Hypopigmentation occurs when melanocytes no longer produce melanin, which leaves areas of the skin without pigment. This condition can occur from disease processes such as vitiligo or from injury such as those associated with phenol peeling or CO_2 laser treatment. (See Figure 6–10.) Unfortunately, this phenomenon also occurs when a laser hair removal treatment is mishandled. When hypopigmentation occurs, the maltreatment injures the melanocyte, which causes a malfunction or lack of function prohibiting the melanocyte from performing properly. While hypopigmentation is an uncommon injury, it can occur with all types of skin treatments including peels, ablative and nonablative laser, light treatments, as well as laser hair removal.

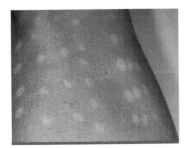

Figure 6–10 Hypopigmentation as a result of hair removal treatments

melanocytes
melanin-forming cells

■ HYPERPIGMENTATION

Hyperpigmentation results from the increased deposition of melanin that causes the skin to be darker in patches. Hyperpigmentation is especially common in darker skin types, typically Fitzpatrick IV, V, and VI. The irregular patchy pigmentation has origins in solar exposure, pregnancy, medications, birth control, and dermatological skin diseases. But just like hypopigmentation, hyperpigmentation can also occur when skin has been damaged through aggressive treatment.

The treatment for hyperpigmentation varies depending on the probable cause. In general, a bleaching cream of prescription strength such as hydroquinone 4%+ is necessary, often physician recommended with the use of tretinoin, and, of course, the use of sunscreen is recommended. Some patients will be under the misguided assumption that using the bleaching cream will be enough to solve the problem. Technicians need to help patients understand the importance of sunscreen, because without it, the area of pigmentation that the hydroquinone is supposed to target is vulnerable to further UV damage, rendering the bleaching process pointless.

Postinflammatory Hyperpigmentation

postinflammatory hyperpigmentation
dyschromia associated with injury to the skin

Both injury and inflammation can cause increases in melanin production. Such injury is known as postinflammatory hyperpigmentation and is a recognized complication of microdermabrasion, peeling, IPL treatments, and laser hair removal. (See Figure 6–11.)

Once the skin has been typed, it is important to ascertain whether the client has had a history of postinflammatory hyperpigmentation. Asking the client about previous injuries and how the healing process progressed is important. Those with postinflammatory hyperpigmentation will report a period of time with dark sustained pigment after the wound closed. It may have taken months for the pigment to fade. In fact, in some cases, the pigment remains darkened indefinitely if left untreated.

In cases of laser hair removal, treatment of postinflammatory hyperpigmentation should begin prior to clinical treatment. Most physicians recommend the use of hydroquinone twice a day to the area. After the client has received the laser treatment, a combination of hydroquinone and prescription strength topical cortisone is recommended. This application should be applied on the treated area twice a day and should continue for one week.

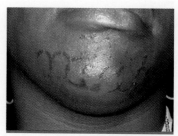

Figure 6–11 Hyperpigmentation as a result of laser hair removal

■ SKIN TYPE AND ELECTROLYSIS

Skin type, whether it is dry or oily, hydrated or dehydrated, ethnic or nonethnic, can have an effect on the electrolysis treatment and results of that treatment.

Dry skin is not the same as dehydrated skin. A dry skin lacks the production of sebum that an oily skin has an abundance of. A dehydrated skin lacks the moisture in the form of water that a well hydrated skin has. Understanding these differences enables the electrologist to appropriately adjust treatment energy levels. Sebum acts as an insulator and therefore warrants a slight increase in treatment energy, whereas water, or in this instance hydration, is a conductor of current, and therefore a well hydrated skin would warrant a reduction in the treatment energy. These factors are not just specific to certain individuals for skin type, but are also specific to body areas. An individual with a combination skin may have hydrated but non-oily skin on the cheeks and sides of the face requiring a lower treatment energy than the oilier area on the chin. A forearm or lower leg that is constantly exposed to extremities may be dehydrated, whereas the axilla or groin area may be well hydrated, all requiring adjustments in the treatment energy.

Ethnicity plays a role in skin type for the person considering electrolysis, but it is not as important as it is with laser hair removal regarding skin pigmentation and the need for evaluation according to the Fitzpatrick typing. As long as the guidelines for dry versus oily and hydrated versus dehydrated are followed, electrolysis can be performed on all ethnic skin types. There is a lower level of risk for scarring on a Caucasian than an individual of African descent, but *when correctly applied,* electrolysis is not dependent on or restricted by pigmentation issues the way laser hair removal is. However, ethnicity affects the type of hair growth. People of African descent present with tight curly hair that descends down into a curved follicle. This impacts the electrologists' choice of modality, whether it be thermolysis, galvanic, or a blend of the two. This is discussed in more depth in the chapter on electrolysis, but, in general, straight hair follicles are quickly and effectively treated with thermolysis as the probe can slide down to the hair bulb and target it directly with the high frequency current. As a straight probe cannot turn a corner, curved and distorted follicles benefit from being treated with the galvanic current or a blend of the two, creating sodium hydroxide that bleeds down to the hair bulb for effective destruction, regardless of whether the probe tip can reach the hair bulb or not.

SKIN TYPE AND WAXING

The condition of the skin is especially important for an effective waxing service. This is particularly true of soft wax, which adheres to the surface of the skin, and less so for hard wax, which does not. Skin that is dry may present with scaly patches of dead skin cells that may benefit from the exfoliating properties of soft waxing, but the dry skin may also trap multiple hairs that should be released with exfoliation prior to the service. Very moist or hydrated skin can also be problematic as the moisture inhibits the wax from adhering to the skin and from being left behind during the removal process. Continuous dusting with powder during the service helps alleviate the problem.

Where skin typing can have a more far reaching effect is ethnicity and the skin's response to injury from a poorly administered waxing service. Caucasian skin that has been injured resulting in scabbing can hypopigment, and skin that has been exposed to UV light while still in a state of erythema from waxing can become hyperpigmented. With people of African descent, the hypopigmentation can be even more dramatic and problematic. This can be especially true with overly aggressive facial waxing of coarse curly hairs with curved follicles that are difficult to epilate with waxing. Hair follicles may produce ingrown hairs and become infected, a condition known as pseudofolliculitis barbae. The result of this inflammatory condition is both hyperpigmentation and hypopigmentation.

SKIN TYPE AND LASER HAIR REMOVAL

The key to successful laser hair removal is to accurately assess and type the skin and hair according to the Fitzpatrick Skin Typing, and by following the treatment parameters suggested for that type by the manufacturer of the equipment used. Failure to follow those guidelines and parameters can mean at best an ineffective treatment with a poor end result and a dissatisfied customer, and at worst a serious and disfiguring injury possibly followed by a malpractice lawsuit.

Conclusion

Now we understand the method by which all professionals collect information about hair and skin color, skin type, and aging. Thorough analysis will help technicians choose the appropriate treatment method for their clients. The skin color analysis reveals not only who will tolerate moderate treatments and who will tolerate aggressive treatments, but also how to protect the patient against postinflammatory hyperpigmentation.

Skin typing is an important element in the overall success of hair removal treatments. While mastering the Fitzpatrick Skin Typing System can initially be challenging, it is worth the effort. Whether the treatment is laser hair removal, electrolysis, or waxing, skin typing will play a role in the overall success of the treatment, of the appearance of the skin, and ultimately in the client satisfaction with treatment outcomes.

▶▶▶ TOP 10 TIPS TO TAKE TO THE CLINIC

1. The Fitzpatrick Skin Typing process is a commonly accepted method of measuring the skin's response to UV light.

2. The Fitzpatrick Skin Typing process can help predict the skin's response to chemical peeling, laser hair removal treatments, and microdermabrasion.

3. The Fitzpatrick Skin Typing method should be used on every patient seen to ensure the proper treatment plan has been selected.

4. Technicians must inquire about ethnic history and sun exposure history to find the right Fitzpatrick assignment.

5. Eye color and natural hair color are indicators for Fitzpatrick assignment.

6. Generally most skin types are "mixed" and require study to ascertain the correct typing.

7. Asking questions about the skin's response to the sun as a child will help determine the accurate skin type.

8. Knowing the Fitzpatrick Skin Type will help determine which skin types need to be pretreated for postinflammatory hyperpigmentation.

9. Skin typing will exclude certain clients from laser hair removal treatments.

10. Skin typing will assist technicians in predicting potential problems, regardless of the hair removal process.

CHAPTER QUESTIONS

1. What is Fitzpatrick Skin Typing?
2. Why do we skin type before treating a client for any type of hair removal process?
3. How do you identify the skin type of someone who is tanned?
4. How do you identify the skin type of someone with colored hair?

CHAPTER REFERENCES

1. Fitzpatrick Skin Typing Chart (Part 1—Genetic Disposition). Used with Permission of the Medical Procedure Center, P.C., and adapted from multiple sources.
2. Fitzpatrick Skin Typing Chart (Part 2—Reaction to Sun Exposure). Used with Permission of the Medical Procedure Center, P.C., and adapted from multiple sources.
3. Fitzpatrick Skin Typing Chart (Part 3—Tanning Habits). Used with Permission of the Medical Procedure Center, P.C., and adapted from multiple sources.
4. Fitzpatrick Skin Typing Chart (Part 4—Scoring). Used with Permission of the Medical Procedure Center, P.C., and adapted from multiple sources.
5. Fitzpatrick Skin Typing Chart (Part 5—Your Fitzpatrick Skin Type). Used with Permission of the Medical Procedure Center, P.C., and adapted from multiple sources.

BIBLIOGRAPHY

APA Optics, Inc. (2004, March 18). *Personal UV Monitor*. Available at http://www.apaoptics.com

Bickmore, H. (2003). *Milady's Hair Removal Techniques*. Clifton Park, NY: Milady, an imprint of Thomson Delmar Learning.

D'Angelo, J., Dean, P., Dietz, S., Hinds, C., Lees, M., Miller, E., & Zani, A. (2003). *Milady's Standard: Comprehensive Training for Estheticians*. Clifton Park, NY: Thomson Delmar Learning.

Deitz, S. (2004). *Milady's The Clinical Esthetician*. Clifton Park, NY: Thomson Delmar Learning.

Genetree. (2004, February 28). *Genetree Eye Color Inheritance Chart*. Available at http://www.genetree.com

Institute for Medicine, Physics, and Biophysics. (2004, February 27). *Definitions* (Working Group UVR).

Parks, J., MD, & Pierce, P. A. M. (2002, May). *Effectively Treating Ethnic Skin*. Available at http://www.skinandaging.com

Science Education Partnership. (2004, February 28). *The Genetics of Human Eye Color*. Available at http://www.seps.org

Thomas, C. L., MD, MPH (Ed.). (1997). *Taber's Cyclopedic Medical Dictionary* (Vol. 18). Philadelphia, PA: F. A. Davis Company.

Lasers and Hair Removal

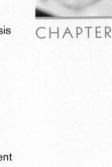

CHAPTER 7

LEARNING OBJECTIVES

After completing this chapter, you should be able to:

1. Explain how lasers work.
2. Describe the effects of laser light on human tissue.
3. List the treatment parameters of laser hair removal.
4. List all the important safety issues.

143

INTRODUCTION

Nobel-prize-winning physicists Albert Einstein and Max Planck first defined the theory of "stimulated emission" in the 1920s. Since then lasers have been known throughout the world. Lasers are now seen in everyday life, such as in CD players, grocery store scanners, and surgical tools to name a few. (See Figure 7–1.) Lasers have the strength to pierce nature's hardest substance, the diamond, to perform orthodontic procedures on the gums, or to conduct delicate procedures on the eyes. The clinical use of lasers began in the early 1960s. In 1965, Dr. Leon Goldman began work with lasers in earnest, removing tattoos and superficial vascular lesions.[1] In 1980 the laser was first introduced as a method of hair removal. This actually happened quite by chance and was noted during the treatment of birthmarks. When certain types of lasers were used, the hair that was present ceased to regrow. In 1996, the first laser devices to be used for hair removal were cleared by the FDA. Initially CO_2 and argon lasers were used for hair removal. Over time newer technology was introduced. Today several lasers and lights are used for hair removal. The hair removal lasers include ruby, alexandrite, diode, and neodymium yttrium aluminum garnet (Nd:YAG).

Regardless of the technology used (see Table 7–1), the degree of hair follicle destruction is not complete. Typically, though, some follicles have an irreversible destruction. Histological examinations, performed after laser treatment, have shown damaged follicles dispersed among intact follicles randomly, questioning the exact mechanisms of hair destruction by

argon

a chemical element in the form of an inert gas used in the creation of early lasers

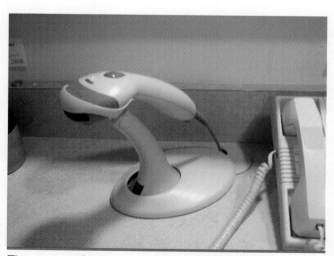

Figure 7–1 Store scanning devices are lasers

Table 7–1   Lasers and Their Uses

Type of Laser	Applied Use
Alexandrite	Hair removal (veins)
CO2	Ablative skin resurfacing
Continuous dye laser	Photodynamic therapy
Copper bromide	Dermal rejuvenation, telangiectasia, rosacea, pigmentation
Diode	Hair removal, vein therapy, & dermal rejuvenation
Erbium:YAG	Ablative skin resurfacing
Krypton	Pigmentation spots
Nd:YAG	Hair removal, vein therapy, & dermal rejuvenation
Potassium titanyl phosphate (KTP)	Telangiectasia, pigmentation spots
Intense Pulsed Light (IPL)	Hair removal, dermal rejuvenation, telangiectasia, rosacea, pigment irregularities
Ruby	Hair removal

laser. Nevertheless, improvement cannot be denied, and with the billions of dollars invested in the laser industry for hair removal it is a technology that will be around for a long time to come.

But before we delve into hair removal and the specific applications of technologies that are used, it is important to review the concepts of light and laser light. An understanding of traditional light and the difference between coherent, monochromatic, and intense light is valuable for the laser technician.

■ LASERS AND LIGHT SOURCES

Let us begin with a discussion of the different characteristics of light. (See Figure 7–2.) Natural light is polychromatic; that is, it contains all colors and wavelengths of the visible light spectrum, including ultraviolet and infrared. Laser light, on the other hand, has two differences: (1) it has low divergence (spreading), and (2) it is monochromatic (single wavelength and single color). Light with these two characteristics is known as coherent light. Coherent light itself is not laser light, rather a laser is amplified coherent light.

Natural light waves go in all directions, lighting the surrounding area according to strength. Light from most sources diverges rapidly. The

photodynamic therapy
a chemical reaction activated by light; this reaction selectively destroys tissue

polychromatic
consisting of light of multiple wavelengths, appearing as different colors

monochromatic
light of one wavelength, which therefore appears as one color

The term *laser* is an acronym for light amplification by stimulated emission of radiation.

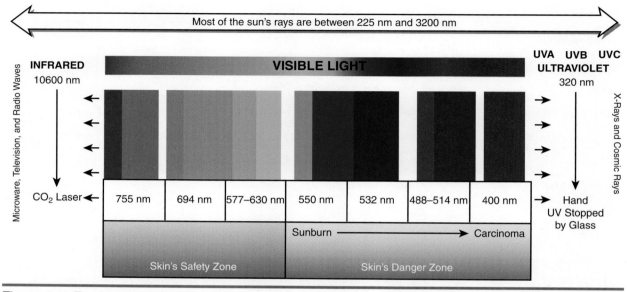

Figure 7–2 Traditional light waves go in all directions, lighting the surrounding area according to strength

farther natural light moves away, the dimmer it gets; the closer it gets, the brighter it gets. Light from a flashlight, for example, fans out quickly and fades after a short distance. Examples of natural light are the sun (our strongest natural light source), a light bulb, or a candle.

For a device to "lase," it must produce light waves that have characteristics that are monochromatic, coherent, and intense. Lasers are also differentiated by the delivery system and the characteristics of the beam. Delivery systems speak to the handpiece, which is sometimes articulated, or the fiber optics. Examples of beam characteristics are Q switch, pulsed, or continuous.

Coherent Light

Coherent light waves travel in perfect unison. They are parallel and in the same direction, which is called "in phase" or "in step." These beams of light are like people marching together in line and in the same direction, as opposed to crowds bustling randomly on a busy street. Because coherent light travels in straight lines, it does not appear to dim as it moves away. Holograms are recorded with coherent light.

Monochromatic Light

Monochromatic literally means a single color. In this case, it is used to describe the type of laser light. Laser light has its own color, which determines its single wavelength. During hair removal, the color of the laser

---

fiber optics
a delivery system for lasers; the light runs through small glass cables inside a handpiece

coherent light
light waves that travel in parallel and in the same direction

There are four main kinds of lasers, which are defined according to the active medium:
1. solid-state
2. semiconductor
3. gas
4. dye

Table 7–2   Lasers and the Efficacy on Hair Removal, Adapted from *Lasers and Lights*, Volume 2[2]

Laser or Light	Skin Type	Hair Color	Type of Hair
Pulsed Diode	I–IV	Black to light brown	Prefers coarse
Ruby	I–III	Black to light brown	Fine and coarse
Normal mode Nd:YAG	I–VI	Dark	Prefers coarse
Q switch Nd:YAG	I–VI (temporary removal only)	Black to light brown	Fine and coarse
Alexandrite	I–IV	Black to light brown	Fine and coarse
Intense Pulsed Light	I–VI	Black to light brown	Prefers coarse

light determines how the laser will react with the pigment in the hair and skin. All lasers react to different chromophores depending on the wavelength. This is why there are so many different lasers, each with a different purpose. (See Table 7–2.)

Collimated Light

Collimated light refers to a very thin beam of laser light, in which all rays run parallel. Collimated light is often formed between two mirrors as is the case with lasers. Collimated light is said to be focused in infinity. Examples of collimated light are the stars.

Intense Pulsed Light

Intense pulsed light is polychromatic and broadband. The clinical use of polychromatic light is achieved through filters that affect the wavelength. Typically, the wavelength is between 400 and 1,000 nm. The filters that are used create wavelengths that selectively target different skin structures: hair, pigment, or vessels. Intense pulsed light, while not specifically a laser, does behave like a laser from the perspective of photothermolysis. Lasers treat one chromophore with one monochromatic light while intense pulsed light can target multiple chromophores.

   IPL has recently enjoyed popularity in the treatment of facial lines and wrinkles. The mechanism of this treatment is thought to be a thermal denaturation of dermal collagen, which leads to collagen synthesis.[3]

Effects of Laser Light Absorption

As the light hits the skin, it is managed in one of four different ways: reflection, absorption, scattering, or transmission. Reflection is simply the bouncing of light off the skin. Absorption of light into the skin

chromophores
the elements that laser light is attracted to; blood, hair color

collimated light
refers to a very thin beam of laser light, in which all rays run parallel

Stimulated emission of radiation or laser light is made possible when electrons of high energy atoms absorb energy, forcing them to move away from the nucleus. As the electrons begin to move back toward the nucleus, a photon of light is emitted. Simply put, high energy atoms are stimulated to release light. When billions and billions of atoms do this at once, they produce a beam of laser light.

All types of lasers share four main components:

1. Active medium: a solid, gas, liquid, or semiconductor that contains an atom that can be excited by an external energy source
2. Means of excitation: the energy source that excites the active medium
3. High reflectance mirror: a highly reflective surface that reflects 100% of all light
4. Partial reflectance mirror: a mirror that reflects less than 100% of all light

depends on several factors, among them intensity, penetration, and length. Scattering occurs because the collagen in the dermis is similar in size to the molecule of visible light, and there is forward scattering and backscattering. Transmission is the residual light that is transmitted through the skin to the subcutaneous tissue. The effects of laser light absorption are directly related to the wavelength of the light, the energy, and the chromophores. Those who work with hair removal lasers should be aware of these laser light absorption processes and how the skin will be impacted.

Reflection

It is said that up to 6 percent of the light applied to the skin via a laser or light device is reflected off of the stratum corneum.

Absorption

Without absorption of light into the tissues, there cannot be effective treatment. As such, the calculated and organized specifics of light intensity, penetration, and length are the variables that produce a result.

Scattering

Scattering of light is due to the size of collagen molecules in the dermis and the wavelength of light. There are two types of scattering: forward scattering (toward the epidermis) and backscattering to the deep dermis. This concept is important because if too much scattering occurs there will not be enough energy fluence to impact the target, in this case the hair follicle.

Transmission

Transmission speaks to the light destination. Depending on the amount of scattering and wavelength, the light will transmit to the target. Residual light (light that is not scattered) will find its way to the subcutaneous tissue.

Chromophore

Atoms and molecules of various substances selectively absorb photons of light from specific laser devices. That substance is a chromophore. Because different lasers operate at different wavelengths, the substances (e.g., hair or skin) will be chromophores attracted to one wavelength but not to another. Chromophores allow for selective targeting. (See Figure 7–3.) For example, the Nd:YAG is one of several lasers that target melanin in hair (the chromophore), which absorbs the photons of light, converting them to thermal energy or heat that destroys the hair. This is why

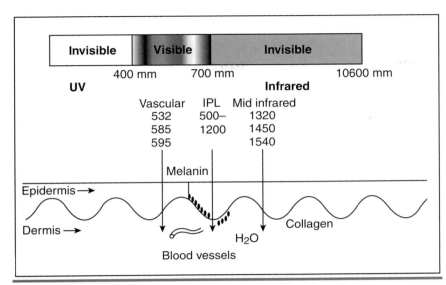

Figure 7–3 Light and the chromophores that they target

very blond hair or gray hair does not respond well to laser hair removal. Other laser wavelengths are attracted to the chromophore in blood, making them a treatment mechanism for birthmarks or spider veins.

Physics of Laser Hair Removal

The most common process of laser hair removal is based on the principle of selective photothermolysis. In this case the damage is achieved by selectively targeting an area using a specific wavelength to absorb light hair sufficient to cause damage while allowing the surrounding area to remain relatively untouched. When the focus is on hair with natural dark pigment and, in particular, the dark pigment of the matrix close to the dermal papilla, the light is absorbed by the pigment. It heats the pigment and vaporizes the dermal papilla. The result is hopefully a severely damaged if not destroyed dermal papilla. Other less common methods of laser hair removal include mechanical and photochemical injury to the hair follicle.

A typical laser has three main parts. They are the energy source, the active medium, and the optical cavity, also called a resonator. To understand how laser light is produced, consider a laser hair removal device using a ruby rod for the active medium, making it a ruby laser. The energy source is a device that supplies energy to the active medium in a process called pumping. Lasers, particularly for hair removal, use electricity as the energy source. Electricity, as the energy source, pumps and excites the atoms of a substance that normally exist in a state of lowest

selective photothermolysis
the selective targeting of an area using a specific wavelength to absorb light into that target area sufficient to damage the tissue of the target while allowing the surrounding area to remain relatively untouched

wavelength
the distance between two consecutive peaks or troughs in a wave

energy source
the device in a laser that supplies energy to the active medium

active medium
the part of a laser that absorbs and stores energy

optical cavity
the part of the laser that contains the active medium

resonator
another term for "optical cavity"

pumping
the process whereby the energy source supplies energy to the active medium

ground state
the condition of a physical system in which the energy is at its lowest possible level

excited states
the conditions of a physical system in which the energy level is higher than the lowest possible level

singlet state
a state of higher energy of atoms arrived at upon excitation

metastable
in an apparent state of equilibrium, but likely to change to a more truly stable state if conditions change

photons
miniscule units of electromagnetic radiation or light

spontaneous emission
the process whereby an excited atom, after holding extra energy for a fraction of a second, releases its energy as another photon, then falls back to its grounded state

amplification
the creation of a new photon of light, resulting from a chain reaction involving the collision of other photons

stimulated emission
the process whereby a newly created photon of light (generated through amplification) acquires energy equal to the photons that created it and travels in the same direction

in phase
a property of light characterized by waves traveling in parallel and in the same direction

energy, called ground state (atoms can also exist in higher energy states called excited states). Atoms in ground state considerably outnumber those in excited states. When atoms in ground state are "excited," they arrive at a higher-energy state, called a singlet state. After the singlet state has been reached, some of the atoms immediately begin to drop back to an intermediate level, called the metastable state. Some, not all, of the atoms arrive at the metastable state. The atoms that can sustain the metastable state are capable of lasing. As the atoms in the metastable state return to their ground state, they emit energy in the form of photons of light, which are minute units of electromagnetic radiation. The photons of light are reflected, absorbed, transmitted, and scattered. Excited atoms can hold extra energy for only a fraction of a second before releasing their energy as other photons and falling back to ground state. This process is called spontaneous emission. Some atoms store energy for relatively long times in excited states, up to 2 seconds, which is much longer than most excited states, which are 1/1,000 of a second. As long as the energy source is applied, a continuous chain reaction occurs. The photons of light strike other atoms in the metastable state. This collision causes the atoms to return to the ground state and, in so doing, creates another photon of light in a process called amplification. This second photon has an equal amount of energy and moves in the same direction as the original photon. This process is called stimulated emission. All the activity produces photons of light colliding with each other that are of the same energy levels, parallel, of the same wavelength in the visible color spectrum, and in phase. The result is a photon cascade. The optical cavity contains the active medium, in this case the ruby rod. At either end of the ruby rod are mirrors: one that is fully reflective on one side and another two-way, partially reflective on the other (like the one-way mirrors used in police interview rooms) that reflects the light back into the active medium. The photon cascade crashes back and forth in the ruby rod, reflecting off the mirrors and becoming stronger until enough energy is produced to cause the photon cascade to blast through the two-way mirror (called an output coupler) in the form of a narrow beam of laser light.

■ SAFETY IN THE LASER TREATMENT ROOM

Even though it may be used for other treatments as well, the room used for laser treatments or IPL treatments should be set up following the strictest guidelines associated with laser equipment. Specific to laser hair removal, the room should have no windows or should have windows blacked out with protective coverings. In addition, no large mirrors or

Benefits of Laser Hair Removal vs Other Treatment Modalities

- Offers a fast, long-lasting hair removal
- May produce some permanent or complete results
- Can treat large body areas with greater speed by treating multiple hairs at once, unlike the hair-by-hair method of electrolysis
- No risk of disease transmission via blood
- Not considered as uncomfortable as electrolysis, though subjective
- Regrowth can be finer and lighter

Downsides of Laser Hair Removal vs Other Treatment Modalities

- Costly, requiring an average of three to six or more treatments
- Safety and effectiveness concerns over the long term
- Ineffective on light and nonpigmented hair, like blonde, red, or gray/white
- Generally ineffective on dark or tanned skin
- Safety concerns for the eyes and need for protective eyewear
- Mild discomfort
- No guarantee of satisfaction
- Inadequate and inconsistent state regulatory controls and guidelines

artwork housed in glass should be hung on the walls. This will minimize the risk of unwanted reflective damage. The laser treatment room should have a door that can be locked during the treatment and/or a warning light or sign (see Figure 7–4) outside indicating treatment is in progress to prevent or warn others from entering. Protective eyewear should be available for individuals to put on before entering a treatment room.

The equipment distributor or manufacturer will usually set up the laser equipment. In preparation for the arrival of laser equipment, an electrician should check the electrical circuitry. The laser equipment will require an electrical outlet that is grounded and includes proper amperage, voltage, a surge protector, and its own circuit breaker. After the setup, the equipment should be serviced and calibrated according to manufacturer guidelines. It is a poor idea to buy used laser equipment, unless it comes from a distributor, has been checked and serviced thoroughly, and comes with a use guarantee and a warranty for labor, service, and parts.

photon cascade
excited, parallel photons of light of the same energy, wavelength, and in phase

Lasers used in hair removal target the melanin. This is why it is easier to treat dark haired fairer skinned individuals.

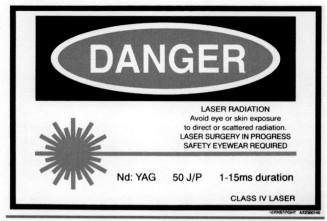

Figure 7–4 A sign should be on the outside of the door indicating treatment is in progress to prevent or warn others from entering the room

Safety Issues for Technicians

The technician should be well trained and qualified in the use of a laser hair removal device. Technicians should also be protected by insurance in case of accident and malpractice claims. Prior to conducting a hair removal treatment, the technician should remove all reflective clothing and jewelry, and should be dressed sensibly and professionally with a lab coat and comfortable shoes (preferably with closed toes). The technician and other individuals in the room must wear ANSI-approved protective eyewear to prevent risk of laser blindness. At the conclusion of the treatment, the technician should make sure the key is removed from the laser equipment. The key should *never* be in the equipment when not in use. The technician should also make sure the laser tip is regularly cleaned to prevent carbon buildup and contamination.

The treatment room itself ought to be well ventilated. The vaporized hair shafts smell of sulfur. In large quantities, the smell can be irritating to the respiratory tract. Having proper ventilation will be beneficial to both the client and the technician.

▪ PATIENT SELECTION

There are four main categories that excess hair growth will fall into: hypertrichosis, hirsutism, hair bearing flaps, and, finally, cosmetic concerns. Hypertrichosis, as we know, is increased hair growth that is not

Prior to the laser hair removal treatment, the client should have received:

- a detailed and thorough consultation and patch test
- precare and postcare instructions
- pertinent information to be able to make an informed choice regarding laser hair removal
- information that adequately describes the benefits and risks of treatment
- instructions to remove all reflective clothing and jewelry
- a pair of ANSI-approved protective eyeglasses and instructions to keep the eyewear on throughout the entire treatment

androgen dependent. Typically, it is a result of medications or disease processes. Hirsutism is androgen dependent and can be accompanied by other diseases. (See Figure 7–5.) Hair bearing flaps are the result of surgeries where skin flaps have been used in the reconstructive process. While surgeons always try to be careful about turning flaps with unwanted hair, this can still happen. In this case a patient may seek hair removal laser to remedy this situation. A cosmetic concern is by far the most common reason for seeking hair removal. Primarily this is an issue of unwanted hair in areas such as the legs, bikini line, face, and back.

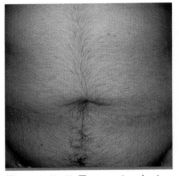

Figure 7–5 Excessive hair growth on a female client

An important consideration in patient selection will involve patient expectation. Managing a patient's expectations ensures an optimal outcome for both the technician and the client. The first and most important conversation should be about the topic of permanency. Clients that seek laser hair removal should know the difference between temporary hair removal, permanent hair reduction, and complete hair removal. Temporary hair removal is a short term (up to 3 months) reduction in hair. Permanent hair reduction is longer termed, but the probability of the hair follicle to recover is great. Complete hair removal involves the complete obliteration of the hair follicle beyond recovery. While it is a possibility that some candidates will experience complete hair loss, most will experience only permanent hair reduction. Once a client has been educated about the topic of permanency, the subject candidacy can be evaluated. A client is the best candidate if the skin is light and the hair is dark, the skin is not tanned, the endocrine status is normal, and waxing or plucking is not being done on the area. Furthermore, a potential client should understand and be able to accept the possible risks and complications that can occur with laser hair removal treatments.

As a client is evaluated for laser hair removal, the clinician should remember that there are several conditions that would be considered contraindications. These conditions include open wounds in the area to be

Table 7-3	Partial List of Contraindications for Laser Hair Removal
Pregnancy
Epilepsy
Tanned or sunburned skin (or any previous thermal injury resulting in hypopigmentation or hyperpigmentation)
Open wounds
Birthmarks, moles, or beauty spots on the area to be treated, unless treatment is approved by a physician
History of keloid scarring
Certain oral and topical medications known to cause photosensitivity or photoallergic reactions (especially oral antibiotics used to treat acne—i.e., doxycycline or minocycline)

treated, pregnancy (see Table 7–3), epilepsy, and the use of photosensitizing medications. Consideration should also be given to those who develop cold sores if the treatment is taking place on the face. In this case the client should be pretreated with an antiviral for protection from a herpes simplex I breakout.

EFFECTS OF LASER ON SKIN TYPE

While all skin types have a great deal in common, such as the number of hair follicles (whether or not they actively produce terminal hair), thickness of the epidermis and dermis, and components found in layers, they have other characteristics that set them apart. As previously discussed, skin color is important in the candidacy of a potential client. There are many different skin types as defined by the Fitzpatrick scale (see Table 7–4), but let us look at the skin types in relationship to laser hair removal.

Caucasian European

Caucasian Europeans have the most varied skin type and hair and eye color variations, as determined by heredity. In most cases this ethnic group has lighter skin, but the hair can range from very light (Norwegians) to darker (Germans). Typically, this is a good ethnic group for laser hair removal.

Table 7-4   Skin Type and Laser Hair Removal

Fitzpatrick Skin Type	Description	Laser Hair Removal Considerations
Type I	Very fair skin accompanied by blond or light-red hair and blue or green eyes. Never tans, always burns.	May not be good candidates because of lack of contrast between hair and skin color.
Type II	Fair skin accompanied by light-brown or red hair and green or brown eyes. Occasionally tans, always burns.	Good candidates for laser hair removal.
Type III	Medium skin accompanied by brown hair and brown eyes. Often tans, sometimes burns.	Good candidates for laser hair removal.
Type IV	Olive skin, accompanied by brown or black hair and dark-brown or black eyes. Always tans, rarely burns.	Good candidates for laser hair removal. Best done by experienced practitioners.
Type V	Dark-brown skin accompanied by black hair and black eyes. Rarely burns	May not be good candidates because of lack of contrast between hair and skin color. If performed, use only YAG lasers. Best done by experienced practitioners.
Type VI	Black skin accompanied by black hair and black eyes. Rarely burns.	May not be good candidates because of lack of contrast between hair and skin color. If performed, use only YAG lasers. Best done by experienced practitioners.

Eastern Asian and Pacific Islander

Eastern Asians include the Chinese, Japanese, and Koreans. This group of people generally has the least amount of facial and body hair. In terms of laser hair removal, they are good candidates due to their dark hair. But their skin can be dark, so care must be taken when treating these individuals to avoid skin injury.

Middle Eastern and Mediterranean

Middle Eastern and Mediterranean people tend to have the darkest and coarsest hair on face and body.

Skin color varies from dark white to medium brown. Individuals with lighter skin as always are the best candidates for laser hair removal. There is an increased risk of causing hyperpigmentation on the skin of this ethnic group.

Treating Ethnic Skin

With dark brown skin, African, African American, African European, and African Caribbean people are typically poor candidates for laser hair removal. This is because the laser light absorbs into the skin pigment before it reaches the hair follicle. Unfortunately, this can cause burns and scars, including keloids if the client is predisposed to this problem. However, newer hair removal lasers used on the proper settings can safely treat these clients with only minimal risk. When treating a patient of this ethnic background, it is important to proceed slowly.

The Consultation

The primary objectives of the consultation are education and the determination of candidacy. After it is determined that the client is a good candidate for laser hair removal, give the client a brief and basic overview of laser hair removal, including the variables affecting treatment. It is important that the client understand the three stages of hair growth. Because the hair grows at different times and in different follicles in the same area, this impacts the number of treatments. Generally, 3 to 6 treatments are needed for optimal, long-lasting reduction. The client should be aware of the time commitment and the financial commitment before entering into a treatment relationship. Clients may have questions about information that they have researched on the World Wide Web or read about in magazines. It is the role of the clinician to debunk the inaccurate information for the client. Because there is so much information floating around about hair removal, it is not uncommon for some of it to be inaccurate or misleading.

The client should also be educated about the acceptable methods of hair removal while undergoing laser hair removal. This should be discussed at length to ensure client cooperation. Cease all methods of hair removal other than shaving or depilatory creams at least 4 to 6 weeks before treatment. Removing the hair from the follicle by tweezing, waxing, or electrolysis throws the hair follicle into a resting stage, delaying the effectiveness of the laser hair removal. Shaving or clipping may be done up to two days before treatment. By shaving two days before the treatment, the technician can ascertain the percentage of growing hairs as they will grow up from the skin leaving the dormant hairs flush with the skin and will then shave the area before the treatment. This is a point of education that should not be missed.

Finally, it should be acknowledged that while laser hair removal is not as costly as it once was, it is still expensive and for some a stretch for their budget. The clinic's financial requirements should be discussed during the consultation to avoid any misunderstandings or embarrassing situations at the first treatment.

Laser hair removal, because it is considered cosmetic, is not covered by insurance. Each laser treatment is separate and usually incurs a separate charge unless a specific treatment package is arranged.

If possible, the consent should be signed at the consultation if the client makes the commitment to move forward with treatments. And if the laser is available at the time of the consultation, a patch test should be done. In this way, when the client arrives for the first treatment, an analysis of the patch test can be made and the treatment can proceed without delay. (See Figures 7–6 and 7–7.)

Patch Testing

A patch test is important for two reasons (see Figure 7–8). First, it gives the technician an opportunity to gauge clients' tolerances to the treatment and to select the appropriate fluence levels. Second, it gives clients an opportunity to experience the laser and to perhaps relieve some of the anxiety that might be associated with the treatment. An initial, single pulse should be performed at a test site near the treatment area and observed for damage to the epidermis in the form of blistering or an epidermal separation caused by lateral pressure on the skin, called the Nikolski sign. If such a reaction occurs, lower the fluence by 5 to 10 J/cm^2. Record the test results on the record form.

Nikolski sign
a condition on the skin characterized by blistering or epidermal separation, caused by lateral pressure on the skin

■ THE LASER HAIR REMOVAL TREATMENT

Take photos of the area to be treated. These photos are visual evidence of treatment progress. Prior to treatment, a consent form must be signed. This informs the client of the treatment process, the possible risks and complications, and the anticipated outcome. The consent also protects the clinician and the facility by ensuring that the client has been properly informed of all of the issues surrounding the treatment that has been elected. As previously noted, the hair color, hair coarseness, skin color, and any health issues should be discussed and documented. The client should have been informed at the time of the consultation to avoid plucking and waxing. (See Table 7–5.) Hopefully, the client has complied and the area to be treated has only been shaved. Assuming this, the next step is skin cleansing, preparation, and numbing if required. The client's skin

Laser Hair-Removal Consultation/Record Form

Name _____ Date ___/___/___

Address _____

Telephone Home (___) _____ Work (___) _____ DOB ___/___/___

Attending physician _____

Medical History: Allergies _____ Keloid scars _____

Infectious diseases _____ Cancer/melanoma _____

H/L blood pressure _____ Heart disease/pacemaker _____

Hormone therapy _____ Thyroid condition _____

Herpes _____ Nervous disorders _____

Epilepsy _____ Laser resurfacing _____

Diabetes _____ Pregnant _____

Lupus _____ Vitiligo _____

Scleroderma _____ Other _____

OB/GYN History _____

Medications and herbal supplements currently and recently taken _____

_____

Area(s) to be treated _____

Natural color of hair: ☐ brown ☐ blonde ☐ red ☐ gray/white   Hair pelosity: ☐ coarse ☐ medium ☐ fine

Skin tone

☐ Very fair: Always burn, never tan, blue eyes   ☐ Fair: Mainly burn, sometimes tan

☐ Medium/olive: Mainly tan, rarely burn   ☐ Dark: Never burn, dark hair, dark eyes

☐ Tattoos or permanent makeup   ☐ Gold and salt injections

Previous Hair Removal

Temporary means of hair removal _____ Frequency _____

Permanent means of hair removal _____

Date began _____ Last treatment _____ Approximate number of treatments _____

I, the undersigned, do hereby certify that the answers to the above questions are correct to the best of my knowledge.

Signature _____ **Date** _____

Signature of parent/guardian if under 18 years of age _____

Figure 7–6 Laser Hair Removal Consultation/Record Form (front)

should be clean and free from dirt, perspiration, deodorants, perfumes, and cosmetics that could impede the laser or aggravate the skin posttreatment. The cleanser should be mild and gentle and have the capacity to rinse clean away, leaving the skin dry, nonirritated, and unstimulated. For larger body areas, the client can shower before the appointment with a simple antibacterial soap.

Date	Laser Device	Area(s) Treated	Fluence	Pulse Width	Spot Size	Additional Comments

Figure 7–7 Laser Hair Removal Consultation/Record Form (back)

Skin Preparation

The client's skin should be close shaven; however, if the client has opted to use a topical anesthetic, then shaving ought to be done a day or two prior to treatment to allow any superficial scrapes or irritations to resolve themselves. This can be done prior to the appointment, particularly for

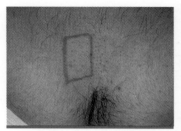

Figure 7–8 A patch test enables the technician to gauge a client's tolerance and gives the client an opportunity to experience the laser and relieve any anxiety associated with the treatment

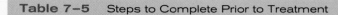

Table 7–5 Steps to Complete Prior to Treatment
Instruct the client to remove all necessary clothing, and provide a gown and drapes. Leave the room, and knock before reentering.
Take photos if none were taken during the consultation.
Cleanse and free the area of lotions, deodorants, perfumes, and cosmetics.
Shave the target area.
Cool the skin before treatment to help reduce side effects.
Give the client the safety goggles to wear.

the first treatment. However, with subsequent visits, the practitioner may choose to assess the hair growth pattern and have the client come to the office unshaven.

Topical Anesthesia

With continually improving laser devices, cooling heads, and gels, anesthesia of any kind is often unwarranted and unnecessary for most clients for most treatment areas, but there are exceptions. For those individuals who have difficulty with the pain of laser hair removal, there are choices of anesthesia. However, complete pain blockage is not appropriate, because feedback from the client will help determine if the treatment power is too high. Typically, clients can purchase a numbing cream from the clinic or be supplied with a prescription from the physician. (See Figure 7–9.) The client should be instructed on the use of the numbing cream and should follow the instructions carefully. This is a powerful medicine and can have harmful adverse side effects. In the United States, the most popular prescription-required topical anesthetic used by clients today is a mixture of local anesthetics. It is important to note that topical anesthetics cause vasoconstriction in the area where it is applied, making the area look blanched. This can cause the clinician to misinterpret the status of the skin if the blanching was not noted in advance.

Many topical anesthetics are now available without prescription. Over-the-counter products from the local drugstore in the first-aid section usually contain 2 percent lidocaine and come in a cream, spray, or gel. The practitioner can now provide an assortment of numbing products in the form of creams, liquids, gels, and sprays and provide retail products like LMX™, Topicaine™, or Laracaine™, to name a few. They usually contain 4 percent lidocaine or 20 percent benzocaine as the active ingredient. Do not use these products around the eyes. Liquids and sprays

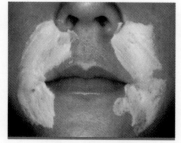

Figure 7–9 Using a numbing cream will help the client to be more comfortable during the treatment

should not be used around the ears. It is also not recommended to use spray anesthetic on the face unless the eyes are well protected. Instead, spray cotton until it is well saturated with the numbing solution and apply it to the area. When using a numbing cream purchased from the

Performing Laser Hair Removal Treatments

Follow all treatment steps in their entirety for a safe, effective, and comfortable treatment.

Communicate with the client throughout the treatment to monitor her/his level of comfort.

1. Unlock the laser device.
2. Don safety goggles.
3. Set the treatment parameters according to manufacturer's guidelines or charted settings from previous treatment for the area, hair, and skin and according to the response at the test site.
4. Perform the treatment at the highest fluence the skin can tolerate and in accordance with the manufacturer's recommendations for the most effective hair reduction. The time needed to cover the area depends on the spot size of the beam and the scanning pattern of the handpiece.
5. Compress the skin firmly with the handpiece to disperse the oxyhemoglobin (a chromophore that competes with melanin) away from the treatment area. Doing so, which allows for greater absorption of the laser light, reduces the risk of epidermal damage as well as maneuvers the dermal papilla closer to the surface, which makes for a more effective treatment.
6. During the treatment, between some of the pulses, clean the handpiece with a mild cleaning solution to free it of the carbonized hair that collects on the window. The buildup makes the window feel hot and impedes the flow of the laser beam.
7. Client comfort level is affected by the treatment fluence and treatment time.
8. Adjust either according to the client's tolerance if other attempts, like topical anesthesia and cooling remedies, have not reduced the discomfort.
9. At the end of the treatment, turn off the laser device and remove the key.
10. Because the handpiece contacts the skin, wipe it clean with a disinfectant between treatments or soak distance gauge in bleach water overnight.

> It is important to note that extreme caution must be used with topical anesthetics. Make sure that the client is made aware of the importance of following directional use as prescribed by a physician.

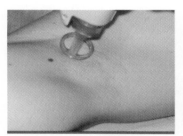

Figure 7–10 A laser hair removal treatment in progress

thermal storage coefficient
the measure of heat stored in a chromophore

cryogen
a substance used to produce extremely low temperatures

practitioner, the client must be cautioned to follow the manufacturer's directions and understand the warnings.

It should be noted that topical anesthetics can be dangerous and can cause death and injury. These medications should not be handled frivolously. Large areas should be numbed in sections and never occluded. If for some reason the skin blisters and is open or potentially open, the clinician should *never* reapply numbing cream to the area. The medications can be absorbed systemically causing severe problems. In short, be careful with numbing cream.

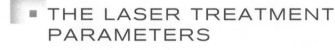

THE LASER TREATMENT PARAMETERS

Once the area is shaved and numbed, it is time to begin the treatment. (See Figure 7–10.) Some clinicians use a treatment grid to ensure that they have covered the treatment area evenly with the laser. If a grid is not used, it is important to use a specific pattern to avoid missing spots or, worse yet, double treating spots in the area. Refer to the patch test before starting the treatment. Examine the area and discuss it with the client to get any relevant feedback. Remember, each machine will have varying wavelengths, pulse durations, fluence, and other considerations that will affect the outcome of the treatment. Several technical issues will have an affect on the overall result of the hair removal process. Among these issues are spot size, energy fluence, cooling the skin, pulse duration, thermal storage coefficient, and thermal relaxation time. While many lasers today are so computerized that the need for this information is almost unnecessary, it behooves the clinician to have an understanding of the theories and processes used to achieve hair removal. As such, the following sections provide a brief description of each.

Cooling the Skin

Cooling the skin allows for a higher and more effective fluence. There are different means of cooling the skin during treatment. Among the different types of cooling include cryogen *spray,* which is used before and after each laser pulse; a *gel* that is chilled and applied to the skin; *contact cooling,* where cold water circulates through a window on the laser head, cooling the skin on contact; and a *chilled tip,* which is one such device, like the diode laser, and uses a cold sapphire window on the handpiece to cool the epidermis before, during, and after each laser pulse. The cooling not only helps prevent epidermal tissue damage, it reduces the discomfort of the treatment. Cooling the skin is widely accepted and recommended when doing hair removal laser.

Spot Size

The spot size, measured in millimeters, is the size or width of the beam effecting treatment.

The larger the laser beam's spot size, the less fluence. A spot size of 12 to 18 mm is considered acceptable for laser hair removal. Spot sizes smaller than 12 mm lose depth of penetration, causing less controlled damage to the hair follicle and yielding a poorer result. The spot size can be affected by dermal scattering, which affects the relationship of the spot size deeper in the tissue due to its size on the skin's surface (i.e., the spot size is smaller deeper in the tissue and gradually becomes larger on the surface). The spot size also affects penetration depth.

Wavelength

Described in nanometers (nm), the wavelength of a laser is on a spectrum, ranging from 400 to 1,200 nm. The greater the wavelength, the deeper it will penetrate. The wavelength is specific to the type of light source used. For example, a diode laser has a wavelength of 800 nm, whereas an Nd:YAG laser has a wavelength of 1,064.

Energy Fluence

Choosing the highest tolerable fluence will ensure that the best results are achieved. Used in pulsed lasers, energy fluence is measured in joules per square centimeter (J/cm^2). (See Figure 7–11.) The larger the laser beam's spot size, the more fluence that is necessary to produce the same effect. Lower fluences have been observed to cause higher rates of double hairs in regrowth. Fair skin types I to III traditionally can take a fluence level of 25 to 40 J/cm^2. As noted above, by cooling the epidermis a higher fluence is possible, and consequently achieves a better result.

Thermal Storage Coefficient

The *thermal storage coefficient* (Tr2) is the storage of heat in a chromophore. When a chromophore is heated beyond its Tr2, the heat spills over and is diffused into the surrounding tissue. Hair has a higher Tr2 than the epidermis. Coarse hair has a higher Tr2 than finer hair. To minimize damage to surrounding tissue by not exceeding the Tr2 of the

spot size
the width of a laser beam

dermal scattering
the change that occurs between the laser's spot size at the surface of the skin and the spot size deeper in the tissue

nanometers
each is one billionth of a meter

joules
units of energy or work

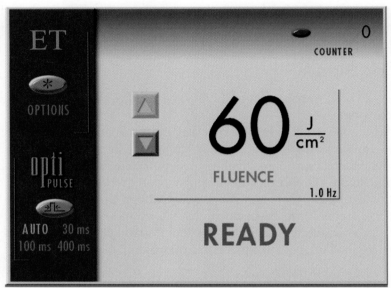

Figure 7–11 The laser machine will show a readout of the J/cm²

chromophore, the laser technician should understand this principle and follow the recommended guidelines of pulse duration and energy fluence.

Pulse Duration

Pulse duration (or **pulse width**), which is measured in milliseconds (ms), is the timing of light energy, or how long the laser is actually on the skin. The pulse duration should match the fluence needed to damage the target hair follicle. A longer pulse duration is generally required for melanin in the hair than for fragile capillaries in the epidermis. Typically coarser hair will require a longer pulse duration. Longer pulse widths are considered more effective with fewer side effects because they allow for more skin types to tolerate higher fluences. This should be particularly true of dark skin. The pulse should also be longer than the thermal relaxation time of the epidermal tissue but shorter than the thermal relaxation time of the hair follicle, keeping the heat in the hair follicle. This is aided by the use of cooling agents or mechanisms applied to the epidermal tissue.

Thermal Relaxation Time

Thermal relaxation time (TRT) is the time it takes for 50 percent of heat energy to be dissipated from the target tissue. It can be registered in

pulse duration
the duration of an individual pulse of laser light; usually measured in milliseconds; also see "pulse width"

pulse width
see "pulse duration"

thermal relaxation time
the amount of time it takes a substance (e.g., dermal tissue), after heating, to return to its normal temperature

milliseconds. For skin it is between 600 and 800 milliseconds. Because the TRT of the hair follicle depends on the follicle's diameter, the laser source must have a range of pulse widths capable of damaging different size follicles. Knowing the TRT and making the necessary adjustments in the treatment of different size follicles in different areas minimizes collateral thermal damage to the dermal tissue, or skin tissue not at the surface of the skin.

HAIR GROWTH FOLLOWING LASER TREATMENT

As we know, hair follicles have four stages of growth. The hair vulnerable to the laser is in the early anagen phase of growth. Because of this, multiple treatments are necessary to catch and injure the follicles in the early anagen stage of growth. Any subsequent hair growth in the laser treated area is the result of newly active follicles coming into the anagen stage. The number of needed treatments depends on the pattern of hair growth, hormonal influences, and plucking or waxing done before the laser treatment. If hormonal imbalances or medications are influencing hair growth, maintenance will be necessary to treat new hairs as they appear. Laser can only remove hair that is present and growing in the follicle, not hair that will develop. As previously stated, this is information that the client should be made aware of and that the clinician should clearly communicate to the client.

Spacing the Return Visit

The spacing for a return visit is dependent on the clients' previous methods of hair removal. If the area has been previously waxed, forcing the telogen stage, the practitioner can anticipate when the new anagen hairs will come through based on the telogen stage of the hair follicles in that area, and schedule the follow-up session accordingly. The key is to treat a high percentage of terminal hair in the anagen (preferably early anagen) stage. Typically the client is asked to return every 3 to 4 weeks.

When to Stop Treating

A few clients have little or no success with laser treatments. These clients are called nonresponders, and there is no way to predict which patients will be nonresponders. Even with all optimal conditions, such as hair in the anagen phase and melanin in the hair shaft, laser is still unpredictable.

Posttreatment in the Clinic

Posttreatment procedures will help minimize client discomfort and prevent adverse posttreatment reactions. A client should never leave the facility without appropriate aftercare.

1. Use ice in a vinyl surgical glove for aftercare. Use cold packs, aloe vera, or any other cooling preparation to ease temporary, mild burning.
2. Apply a total sunscreen (SPF 30 or greater) if the area will be exposed to ultraviolet light.
3. Apply makeup as long as the skin is not broken. Makeup also serves as additional sunscreen. Use new, uncontaminated makeup product, and apply it with a clean sponge.
4. Advise the client to return within 4 to 12 weeks, depending on the telogen stage of hair growth for that area of the face or body. Ensure that any hair follicles that were in the resting stage during the initial treatment are in a growing stage at the time of follow-up.

At Home Care

Encouraging the client to follow the recommended home-care guidelines will promote faster healing and prevent adverse reactions like hyperpigmentation and hypopigmentation.

Make sure that the client fully understands her/his responsibility in following the guidelines.

1. Recommend quick, warm showers. If areas other than the facial area are treated, advise no hot baths for 24–48 hours.
2. Place additional clean, cold packs on the treatment area. Bags of frozen peas, as long as they are protected with a clean cloth work well.
3. Apply a soothing, healing ointment like Aquaphor™. Keep the area lubricated to prevent tissue crusting or scabbing.
4. In the event of blistering, apply a topical antibiotic cream or ointment and cover with a nonadhering dressing. Have the client notify the technician and/or physician overseeing the laser treatment.
5. Advise clients to avoid the sun for 1–2 weeks following Nd:YAG treatments and 4–6 weeks following alexandrite or diode treatments to avoid hyperpigmentation. Also advise them to avoid tanning if they are planning to have follow-up treatments.
6. Apply a sunscreen of at least SPF 30 to any area that could be exposed to ultraviolet light as long as there is an erythema. If further treatment is needed, have the client commit to staying out of the sun. Sun exposure creates certain minor complications, which should be discussed fully with the client.
7. Apply makeup and lotions the next day or when signs of irritation or erythema have subsided and if the skin is not broken. Use uncontaminated makeup, and apply it with clean fingers or a new, clean sponge.
8. Instruct the client to contact the facility and the technician or physician if there are any concerns or questions.
9. For areas prone to friction, like the abdominal area or inner thigh area, advise the client to avoid tight clothing in those areas to prevent infection and irritation.

If after several treatments the client is not responding, the treatments should be discontinued. That said, it may be that the hair is returning but at a slower rate.

Treatment Consequences

Treatment consequences are a predictable outcome of the procedure that occurs in a reasonable percentage of people having the procedure. An example might be a patient has a light peel and superficial "rug burns" result. In the case of laser hair removal treatment, consequences might include swelling and redness, perifollicular edema. Clients should expect to see tiny black spots in the follicles over a few days. These "singed" hairs, called splattering, will gradually and naturally expel from the skin and can be wiped away. (See Table 7–6.)

▪ SIDE EFFECTS

Side effects are "….an action or effect of a drug or treatment other than that desired, such as nausea or vomiting."[4]

In the case of laser hair removal care, an example might be crusting, temporary redness (lasting longer than 2 hours), or skin discoloration (hyperpigmentation). Hyperpigmentation may be treated with 4 percent hydroquinone, which is skin bleaching cream. (See Figures 7–12 and 7–13.) Clients must strictly adhere to follow-up instructions to provide comfort and protection and to minimize these potential problems. (See Table 7–7.)

Complications

Complications are untoward events that occur following a normally applied procedure. For example, a patient has a peel and a scar results.

splattering
the appearance of tiny black spots, which are singed hairs, in hair follicles; caused by laser treatments

hydroquinone
a white, crystalline compound used in skin bleaching

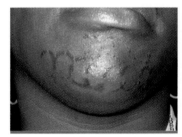
Figure 7–12 Hyperpigmentation after laser hair removal

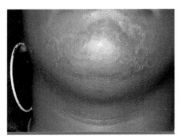
Figure 7–13 The same hyperpigmentation after a period of fading

Table 7–6   Treatment Consequences of Laser Hair Removal
Erythema and edema, most of which subsides within 20 minutes to a few hours
Longer wavelengths produce tiny bumps resembling "goose bumps" also known as perifollicular edema and additional edema, which should appear in a matter of hours
Singed hair called splattering

Table 7–7	Side Effects of Laser Hair Removal
Herpes simplex	
Bacterial infection (very low risk)	
Crusting	
Extended redness	
Hyperpigmentation	

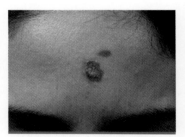

Figure 7–14 Blistering after a laser hair treatment

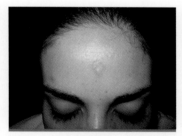

Figure 7–15 The blister after it has healed

In the case of laser hair removal a complication is defined as epidermal separation or blistering. (See Figures 7–14 and 7–15.) Other complications include hypopigmentation, scarring, intense itching, and hives. Also, it has been noted that respiratory irritation can occur if the plume of smoke secondary to the hair is significant. Failure to recognize and respond to a negative or adverse reaction is negligent and could result in serious repercussions, including a possible malpractice lawsuit. In the event of an adverse reaction, the treatment should end immediately, and appropriate medical intervention should be initiated by a qualified medical professional. (See Table 7–8.)

▪ STATE LICENSURE

There exists a great deal of variation between states with regards to licensure requirements. Some states require only cosmetology certification for authority to operate a laser device for hair removal, whereas some states require that only a physician may operate a laser device. Still, most states allow aestheticians to operate laser devices for hair removal. It is important that you consult your state's regulating agency to find out the specific requirements for laser device operation. The rules and regulations for licensure not only vary, but they are also subject to frequent revision;

Table 7–8	Complications of Laser Hair Removal
Blistering	
Hypopigmentation	
Scarring	
Intense pruritus and urticaria	
Respiratory irritation due to inhalation of *plume*	

therefore, staying abreast of legislative amendments affecting your practice, within your state, will help you stay within the boundaries of the law.

Conclusion

According to the American Society of Plastic Surgeons, laser hair removal is among the top five nonsurgical procedures performed each year. In fact, there are more laser hair removal procedures done each year than Restylane treatments. The removal of unwanted hair can make a huge difference in the self-esteem as well as the appearance of an individual. The positive results of laser hair removal cannot be denied, and with more understanding of hair biology the results just keep getting better.

▶ ⟩ ⟩ TOP 10 TIPS TO TAKE TO THE CLINIC

1. Know the phases of hair growth.
2. Know the rules of laser safety: no mirrors or windows, lock the door, and wear the proper goggles.
3. Short lived erythema is a treatment consequence of laser hair removal.
4. Laser light is attracted to the color of the hair to destroy the follicle.
5. There are different kinds of laser and not all work for laser hair removal.
6. There are four reasons someone might seek laser hair removal.
7. Patient selection and education is important to the long-term success of the hair removal process.
8. Patients should never be tanned when hair removal laser is performed.
9. Patients who are pregnant or have epilepsy are not candidates for laser hair removal.
10. Cooling the skin allows for a higher fluence and as such a potentially improved result.

CHAPTER QUESTIONS

1. For what does the acronym "laser" stand?
2. What are the four main types of laser?
3. What are the three main components of a laser?
4. What is the scientific term for the substance that acts as a target to the laser light absorbing it?

5. List three important safety considerations for the treatment room.

6. List three important safety considerations for the laser equipment.

7. What are the three steps of pretreatment?

8. What are the three components of treatment?

9. What are four steps of postcare?

CHAPTER REFERENCES

1. Barlow, R. J., & Hruza, G. J. (2005). Lasers and Lights Tissue Interactions. In D. J. Goldberg (Ed.), *Lights and Lasers* (Vol. 1). Philadelphia, PA: Elsevier Saunders.
2. Dierickx, C. C., & Grossman, M. C. (2005). Laser Hair Removal. In D. J. Goldberg (Ed.), *Lights and Lasers* (Vol. 2). Philadelphia, PA: Elsevier Saunders.
3. Marmur, E. S., & Goldberg, D. J. (2005). Nonablative Skin Resurfacing. In D. J. Goldberg (Ed.), *Lights and Lasers* (Vol. 2, pp. 29–41). Philadelphia, PA: Elsevier Saunders.
4. Thomas, C. L., MD, MPH (Ed.). (1997). *Taber's Cyclopedic Medical Dictionary* (Vol. 18). Philadelphia, PA: F. A. Davis Company.

BIBLIOGRAPHY

Milady's Standard Comprehensive Training for Estheticians. (2003). Clifton Park, NY: Milady, an imprint of Thomson Delmar Learning.

Milady's Standard Cosmetology. (2004). Clifton Park, NY: Milady, an imprint of Thomson Delmar Learning.

Bickmore, H. (2003). *Milady's Hair Removal Techniques.* Clifton Park, NY: Milady, an imprint of Thomson Delmar Learning.

Barlow, R. J., & Hruza, G. J. (2005). Lasers and Lights Tissue Interactions. In D. J. Goldberg (Ed.), *Lights and Lasers* (Vol. 1). Philadelphia, PA: Elsevier Saunders.

Thomas, C. L., MD, MPH (Ed.). (1997). *Taber's Cyclopedic Medical Dictionary* (Vol. 18). Philadelphia, PA: F. A. Davis Company.

Dierickx, C. C., & Grossman, M. C. (2005). Laser Hair Removal. In D. J. Goldberg (Ed.), *Lights and Lasers* (Vol. 2). Philadelphia, PA: Elsevier Saunders.

Waxing Basics

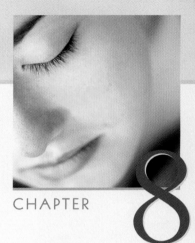

CHAPTER 8

LEARNING OBJECTIVES

After completing this chapter, you should be able to:

1. Understand the differences between hard and soft waxes.

2. List the benefits and downsides of hard depilatory wax.

3. List the indications and contraindications of hard wax.

4. List the benefits and downsides of soft wax.

5. List the indications and contraindications of soft wax.

6. Understand when to best utilize either wax for any given area or situation.

171

INTRODUCTION

Different waxes have different properties that, as a result, require different guidelines for their usage. Understanding the different waxes that are available, and the benefits and downsides to each, as well as how to use them is important in providing the most suitable and effective waxing service for the client.

For the purpose of hair removal there are two main types of wax, hard wax, also known as the nonstrip method, and soft wax, also known as the hot wax or strip method. As more sophisticated skin care treatments have been made available to clients over the years, and as clients have expressed dissatisfaction with unsightly redness following treatment, there has been a bigger demand to improve the wax by making it less irritating. (See Figure 8–1.)

To this effect, soft waxes have become more varied to meet these ever-changing needs and demands of the clients. The variations include the honey-textured waxes that are effective for speed waxing and larger body areas and crème waxes or waxes with soothing additives like tea tree oil for the face. In addition to hard and soft waxes, there are various varieties in between, such as cold wax and sugar wax, and many with soothing additives. Home waxing kits are also gaining popularity. In this chapter, we will introduce the types of wax available for hair removal in a professional environment and also indicate when one type of wax should be considered over another.

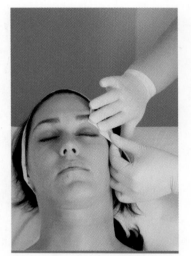

Figure 8–1 A client being waxed

Why Wax When We Have Laser

There are four main reasons that one would select waxing over laser: The first reason is the skin color and hair color combination as indicated by the Fitzpatrick skin typing scale, which is discussed in more depth in Chapter 5. The ethnicity indicates that either the skin is too dark or the hair is too light or both. If there is not sufficient pigment in the hair, the laser light will not heat up the hair shaft down to the dermal papilla, and the treatment will be ineffective. (See Table 8–1.) In this case alternative methods of hair removal should be recommended, including waxing as a possible alternative. Another reason for selecting waxing over laser hair removal is when there is an established contraindication to laser hair removal, for example, lupus. Laser may simply be cost prohibitive for the client. If economics is the reason, waxing, while not offering permanent reduction, is an affordable alternative. Last, a deep-seated fear of laser technology may prevent the client from moving ahead with this method of hair removal. The client may benefit from having laser tech-

Table 8–1 The Benefits of Waxing over Laser

Unsuitable skin/hair color combination as indicated by the Lancer Ethnicity Scale
Contraindications to laser hair removal
Economics; laser may be cost prohibitive
Fear of laser technology

nology and how it is applied to hair removal explained in easy to understand terms, and perhaps, if the client is amenable, a patch test can be offered to demonstrate. At the end of a consultation when all questions have been answered, if the client still has a fear of laser hair removal, waxing, although temporary, offers a solution that will satisfy the client for at least a number of weeks at a time.

■ HARD WAX

Hard wax was the original depilatory wax that vanished into relative obscurity when the quick and efficient soft wax came to the forefront in salons. Because time is of the essence to the technician, soft wax with the strip is more practical for large body areas, but in recent years hard wax has reemerged, making a strong comeback. This comeback has been due in part to the advances in skin care. There has never been a time of more concern to the waxing practitioner than now as clients seek advanced antiaging and antiacne skin care treatments from aestheticians, dermatologists, and plastic surgeons. Even home skin care regimens that also have the ability to effect more dramatic changes in the skin are causing concern for those who provide facial waxing. With the increase in use of retinoids and AHA's came an increase in incidents of skin lifting during an eyebrow, lip, or other facial waxing service. It became apparent that the hard wax of decades past caused less injury to clients receiving specialized skin treatments, as it does not adhere to the skin. This section focuses on the use of hard wax in hair removal, including the benefits and downsides of using hard wax; the areas where hard wax is most effective and the preferred method of hair removal; and the times when hard wax use is contraindicated.

Until the 1980s, skin care consisted of three basic steps, cleanse, tone, and moisturize, with the occasional addition of a mask. Ultraviolet lamps were used to treat acne. With the growing popularity and use of many antiacne and antiaging facial treatments, such as glycolic peels and microdermabrasion and products like Retin-A® and alpha hydroxy acids,

Retin-A®
A topical medication originally used to treat acne; now also used to treat lines, wrinkles, and discolorations of the skin

comes the increased risk of problems for clients with regard to face waxing. Strip wax came onto the market before AHA's, Retin-A®, microdermabrasion, and other products and treatments now commonly used for antiaging. Now depilatory hard wax is making a strong comeback for use on delicate and fragile skin due to these problems and to hard wax's ability to lift up and off the skin as it hardens, leaving the skin intact while still gripping the hair.

This is a time for technicians to be more vigilant than ever when waxing a client's face. However, where strip waxing would ordinarily be contraindicated, there are now gentle but effective hard waxes available for use on delicate skin. The next few pages discusses the correct method of applying hard wax to the various parts of the face and body, as well as tips for a successful service and ways to troubleshoot some of the most common mistakes.

Hard Wax Basics

As previously discussed, hard wax should be soft in the pot and easily spreadable on the skin, but should not burn the skin. Once on the skin it should quickly solidify but without becoming brittle. In order for all this to take place, the melting point of a depilatory wax must be greater than 98°F/37°C but less than 165°F/73.9°C. Because the body temperature is around 98.6°F/38°C, if the melting point were lower, the wax would not solidify. In addition, the wax must be sufficiently firm to grip the hair. Therefore the temperature for hard wax should be between 125°F/51.6°C and 160°F/71.1°C. Wax cools rapidly, at approximately 7°F/3.9°C per second, so one will need to work quickly to achieve maximum efficacy from the wax. As no one wax meets these criteria, depilatory waxes are often combined with *beeswax, candelilla wax,* and *carnauba wax,* to modify their melting points and increase strength (see Figure 8–2).

Strip wax is much hotter and has more of a liquid consistency on application. As it is applied to the skin, it more readily runs to the base of the hair shaft. Because the application temperature of hard wax is somewhat lower and therefore thicker, when it is applied to the area, it sets faster. Applying most hard waxes initially in the opposite direction of hair growth gives the wax the chance to get to the base of the hair first while the wax is still warm. The wax then starts to shrink as it cools and sets. Gliding the wax back over the top of the hair, like frosting a cake, allows for thorough coverage of the hair shaft, which means a good, tight grip to even the coarsest hairs. Although the wax is usually removed against the hair growth, hard wax can also be removed in the direction of hair growth, especially when it is used on vellus hair, without distorting the hair follicles.

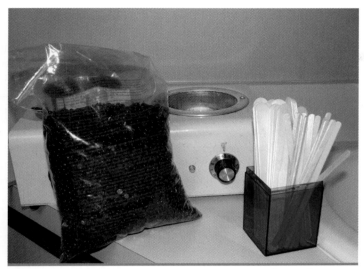

Figure 8–2 Hard waxing requires a variety of supplies

Benefits of Hard Wax

The benefits of hard wax are predominately due to its unique properties and qualities for providing a relatively gentle and safe method of hair removal. Hard wax does not contain resins and does not adhere to the skin, but lifts up off the skin as it cools and sets, so while loose dead skin cells may be exfoliated during the wax service, live skin cells are left in place and intact, causing less irritation than strip wax. Not only does hard wax cause less irritation and erythema it also does not distort the hair follicle, because it can be removed in the direction of hair growth, not against it, like soft wax. This means that with continued waxing with hard wax, the hairs will not change their angle of growth, grow deeper into the dermis, or grow straight up out of the skin in an unruly and obvious fashion.

Hard wax is especially effective in areas in which the hair grows in multiple directions in the same patch, like the axilla. This is because of the ability of hard wax to grip each individual hair tightly the entire length of the shaft that protrudes from the skin, which means that regardless of the direction of the pull, the removal should be effective. The gripping ability of the hard wax and lack of adhesion to the skin make this the most effective wax for using around the labia during the Brazilian bikini wax, where the hair is coarse and grows in multiple directions, and the skin is delicate. If hair is left behind after removal, it can be waxed a second time with the hard wax, providing there is no visible irritation. As mentioned previously, because hard wax does not adhere to the skin it can be used with caution on clients who use glycolic acid or other AHA skin care treatments. Eyebrows may also be waxed with hard wax if Retin-A® or other prescription topical and antiacne medicines like Accutane® and Differin® are being used but have not been applied directly to the eye area. This is possible only if a patch test has been performed, if the client has signed a release, and if the client is aware of the increased risk of a negative reaction. Prescription lotions and creams still migrate somewhat to the eye, causing changes in the integrity of the skin in that area.

The final benefits are shared with strip wax, that regrowth with hard wax is softer and lacks stubble. Also, as the hair follicle is forced into the telogen stage, the regrowth generally takes 6 to 12 weeks after hard waxing.

Downsides to Hard Wax

Perhaps the biggest downside to the use of hard wax is the process itself. Waxing with hard wax is slow and laborious, especially for the novice technician, and takes considerably longer than soft wax, so it is not the preferred method for large body areas like the legs and back. Hard wax is also not as stable as soft wax. If hard wax is left to age in heat and new wax is not added periodically, the old wax may become brittle and lose its removal properties. The wax may also become visibly darker.

Many believe that hard wax is more difficult to get good results with when a client is menstruating and retains excessive fluids. This is thought to be because the swelling tightens the skin, which in turn causes the hair to shrink into the skin, making it tough to remove.

With hard wax, the hair cannot be "blended" in the way it can with wax already on a strip that snags a portion of longer hairs while leaving behind shorter hairs. This may be a significant enough reason to use the strip wax on areas like the sides of the face or the throat.

Indications for Hard Wax

Hard wax is an excellent choice for facial waxing, especially if the client has used Retin-A®, Accutane®, or AHA's, which would prohibit the use of hot wax, although caution should still be exercised, the client informed of the possible adverse reactions, and a release signed. It is also the preferred wax for areas where the hair grows in more than one direction in the same patch, for example, the axilla and bikini areas, especially for French and Brazilian style bikini waxing. If a client wants her forearms waxed for the first time for a special occasion and it is something she does not want done on a regular basis, hard wax is an excellent choice and worth taking the additional time to do. This is because the hair can be removed in the direction of growth and the regrowth is less likely to be wispy, growing straight up rather than lying flat and closer to the skin.

Contraindications for Hard Wax

Generally, the *extensive* use of Retin-A® and other prescription topical antiacne medicines like Accutane® and Differin® or glycolic acid or other strong exfoliating treatments contraindicate facial waxing due to the risk of extreme irritation and the lifting of skin; *however,* if none of these products have been directly applied to the eyebrow area or upper lip, it is possible to successfully wax those areas with hard wax. Any inflamed or irritated skin should not be waxed. Moles, skin tags, and warts should not be waxed; nor should scar tissue, including keloids. Skin disorders (for example, eczema, seborrhea, and psoriasis) should not be waxed when the skin is broken, but waxing with hard wax over the areas of flakiness will exfoliate some of the dead skin cells, leaving living cells intact. Circulatory disorders that cause easy bruising (for example, phlebitis and thrombosis) contraindicate hard wax as does epilepsy, if the medication causes easy bruising. Varicose veins should be avoided during the waxing service, although surrounding areas may be waxed. Depending on degree of severity and the degree of healing, diabetes contraindicates hard wax. Fractures and sprains should not be waxed until completely healed. Hemophiliacs should not be waxed as the risk of bleeding, even minor, is still there and can be serious. Clients with an active outbreak of herpes or herpes simplex areas (cold sores) (see Figure 8–3) should not be waxed until the virus has become dormant. The client can take a prophylactic medication prior to the waxing appointment. Lack of skin sensation always contraindicates waxing services in the area of numbness. Pregnant women should avoid lying on their backs for more than 20 minutes, so any service of that time or longer should wait until after the baby is delivered.

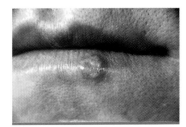

Figure 8–3 Cold sores are a contraindication to waxing until the cold sore is healed

The medications that contraindicate waxing are discussed above in more detail but include tetracycline, Coumadin®, warfarin, Retin-A®, Differin®, and Accutane®.

Techniques for Hard Waxing

When first learning to wax with hard wax, it is much easier to start with small sections, even on large body areas. The sections or strips of wax should be applied no more than 2 inches wide by 4 inches long. With experience and competency, the technician can gradually increase the length of the area to 12 inches for large body areas. A strip should not extend beyond 12 inches long, and the width should remain at 2 inches. The application should always be about 1/8 inch thick on the face to

1/4 inch thick on larger body areas, or between three to five coatings of wax. The strip of wax should have a clean, even edge all the way around for a clean removal and be somewhat thicker at the edge, where it will be lifted during removal. Failure to have a clean edge means that little pieces of wax will be left behind, and their removal can annoy the client. Wax will appear shiny and wet and will feel sticky when first applied. When the shine diminishes and the wax looks opaque and maintains a fingerprint, it is ready to lift off. Allowing wax to set for too long causes the wax to become brittle. Such wax breaks and becomes difficult to remove, and it also breaks the hair.

Hard wax should not be overheated. Instead, keep it on a thermostatically controlled timer. It should also not be heated continually for 24 hours. Overheating the pot causes the wax to lose its epilation properties. The wax hardens and becomes brittle too quickly.

SOFT WAX

Soft wax, using a strip for removal, is currently the most popular method of hair removal and has been since its inception in the 1970s. However, as mentioned previously, with the ever-evolving skin care treatments, products, and regimens, it has posed a problem, particularly with regards to facial waxing. Therefore, it is important to know when soft wax is the preferred choice of hair removal and when it may not be the most suitable method.

Soft Wax Basics

This kind of wax, which has a liquid-honey consistency, is so popular because it is a much faster method of waxing than the hard wax and is more effective in the hair it removes, clearing virtually every hair of the appropriate length in its path. When used correctly, soft wax causes limited discomfort.

Larger body areas, such as the legs and back, benefit from being waxed with this choice of wax because of the speed and effectiveness. Manufacturers are now recognizing the concerns of skin sensitivity, particularly on the face, but also on other body areas, due to the more sophisticated treatments and products, particularly for antiaging and antiacne, and as a result are producing many other types of soft wax for the more sensitive skin and for skin that sports the stubbly coarse hair that still requires the soft wax strip method. These new waxes have a more opaque, creamier texture and can achieve a thin, liquid consistency at a lower temperature. They may also contain azulene, chamomile, or tea tree oil for their soothing and calming properties. (See Figure 8–4.)

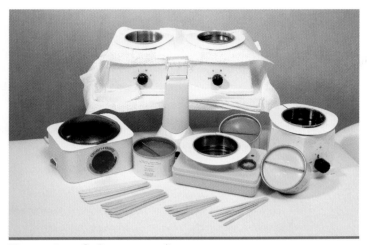

Figure 8–4 Soft wax supplies

Benefits of Soft Wax

The biggest benefit to soft wax is that it is quick and easy to use, which helps make soft waxing a good profit maker with a relatively low cost out- lay. The profit margin is increased when the technicians are proficient in speed waxing. Performing faster services allows more clients to be treated. A shorter waxing time also means minimal discomfort to the client so he or she will be more inclined to return. Client comfort is also aided by the temperature of the wax. With this higher temperature wax, the warmth of the wax opens the pores, allowing the hair to slide out more easily. As with hard wax, the soft wax epilates hair, meaning it removes it from the der- mal papilla, causing it to take longer to grow back because the papilla must regenerate and reestablish a new hair in the follicle. When it does so, it feels softer as it is new fine tipped hair rather than coarse or blunt razor trimmed hair. Many clients claim to experience some reduction in hair growth after multiple wax services. This is especially apparent in the hair growth on frequently waxed women's legs as those women reach menopause.

Downsides to Soft Wax

The most obvious downside to soft waxing is the degree of irritation that is often caused. This is because the rosins in soft wax can adhere to the skin, causing epidermal tissue to be removed during the removal process. Because of the epidermal tissue that is lifted on removal, the area cannot be rewaxed immediately. Hair must also be 1/4 inch long before rewaxing for effective hair removal. (See Table 8–2.)

Table 8–2   Contraindications to Soft Wax

Do not wax inflamed or irritated skin.

Do not use soft wax on clients who are receiving laser resurfacing treatments, glycolic treatments, microdermabrasion treatments, or other peels that are strong exfoliators or that thin out the epidermal tissue.

Do not use soft wax on clients who use products or prescriptions that contain Retin-A® or topical antiacne medicines such as Accutane® and Differin®.

Do not wax clients with circulatory disorders that cause easy bruising (e.g., phlebitis and thrombosis).

Do not wax clients receiving chemotherapy and radiation for cancer treatment as these may cause increased sensitivity. Wait until six weeks after the last cancer treatment.

Do not wax clients with epilepsy, unless the physician approves and the medication does not cause easy bruising.

Do not wax clients with diabetes without physician approval for the degree of healing, and never wax the lower extremities.

Do not wax areas of fractures and sprains until completely healed.

Do not wax hemophiliacs.

Do not wax individuals with active herpes and herpes simplex (cold sore). They should be instructed to take appropriate prophylactic medication before waxing appointments.

Do not wax clients with a lack of skin sensation.

Do not wax moles, skin tags, and warts.

Do not wax pregnant women in the last six weeks of pregnancy if the areas needing to be waxed take more than 20 minutes of the pregnant client lying flat on her back. In these cases waxing should wait until after the birth of the baby.

Do not wax over scar tissue, including keloids.

Do not wax over sunburned areas; wait until completely healed.

Do not wax over skin disorders (e.g., eczema, seborrhea, and psoriasis) or where the skin is broken.

Do not wax over varicose veins, although surrounding areas may be waxed.

Do not wax clients who routinely take medications including tetracycline, now found in birth control pills, because it can cause an adverse reaction with soft wax; blood thinners like Coumadin® and warfarin; and drugs that treat epilepsy, because they cause easy bruising.

Strip wax is not the best choice to use on areas with multiple hair growth directions in the same path as the application rule is to always apply with the growth and remove against the growth. Any deviation from the rules of application will not ensure a clean removal of hair. Hairs going in different directions within a patch often snap and appear a day or two after the service, to the dismay of the unsatisfied client. Soft wax is not the best choice of wax when doing a Brazilian bikini wax because it is impossible to apply the wax in the hair growth direction and pull away effectively against the growth due to the vaginal opening. Hard wax is the preferred method in this area. Regrowth after strip waxing is often irregular. Where the hair, albeit unsightly, once lay uniformly in a certain direction and close to the skin, after removal with the strip it tends to grow back irregularly, standing more upright, in the way it would if one had goose bumps. This is because the hair is removed against its natural growth direction and the follicles that grew at a 20-degree angle become distorted by the pull and start to grow at a deeper angle. When vellus facial hair is removed in this manner, those distorted follicles receive a richer blood supply with an increased percentage of androgens, from deeper in the dermis, and as a result produce hair that is coarser and pigmented. Facial hair is easily stimulated as the area is a secondary sexual characteristic and therefore is targeted by the chemical messengers of androgens in the blood. Removing the hair against the growth also increases the risk of ingrown hairs, another downside to waxing in general and especially with the soft wax. Until a technician is skilled with the use of soft wax, it can be messy, leaving thread-like, sticky trails to be cleaned up.

Indications for Soft Wax

Soft wax is the best choice of wax for large body areas, such as the back and legs, especially when large patches of hair are found growing in the same direction. The skilled waxing technician can develop speed waxing skills and remove hair from larger body areas quickly, reducing the length of the service and minimizing the discomfort.

▪ TECHNIQUES FOR SOFT WAXING

The wax should be heated according to the manufacturer's specifications, which are usually found on the can of wax or in a brochure accompanying the wax heater. All literature accompanying the equipment should be kept and made available for new employees. If possible, use the brand of wax that is recommended for the wax heater. If the technician chooses to try a different brand of wax, then a thermometer should be used to test the temperature of the wax and make sure that the wax is heated to the recommended level. A notation should be made on the pot's dial indicating that level.

Soft wax should be thin enough to run off the spatula easily; its edge should glide along the client's skin, leaving a thin film on the skin.

Even though the wax heater may be thermostatically controlled, it is wise to always test the wax first, on the inside of the lower arm where the skin is more sensitive and where there is no hair. If the wax is the correct consistency and a comfortable temperature, it is safe to use. If the wax is too cool and thick, it will not glide easily onto the skin, and it may bruise and possibly lift the skin. It will also be tougher to remove.

The Do's and Don'ts

Do's
- Know your state's regulations for waxing, and follow them.
- Always wash hands before and after touching a client.
- Wear gloves for wax services.
- Use a full pot for large surface areas so that a larger surface area of spatula is covered when dipped into the wax.
- Use the edge of the spatula.
- Hold the skin taut when applying the wax.
- Always hold the skin taut at the free edge end of the strip before pulling.
- To ease the client's discomfort, have the client take a deep breath while rubbing over the strip and blow out during the pull.
- Always apply pressure quickly after each pull—gentle pressure for the face and firm pressure for the torso and limbs.
- Tell the client not to use makeup or perfume, to avoid exercise immediately after, and to avoid tanning and hot tubs for at least 24 hours after the service or until any signs of trauma and irritation have been completely eliminated.

Don'ts
- Do not apply wax to an area that is longer than is going to be immediately removed.
- Do not apply wax to an area that has just been waxed.
- Do not overlap with hot wax.
- Do not wax the areola of the breast.
- Do not wax inside the ear or nose.

Do's of the Soft Wax Method

Before waxing a client, one of the most important "do's" is to always question the client about any changes in skin care since the consultation or previous wax service. Also, have the client sign a release. Another important "do" is to wash hands before and after touching a client. This prevents cross contamination and the spread of germs and viruses. Wear gloves for the service to prevent coming into contact with even trace amounts of blood. Make sure a full pot of wax is available for large surface areas so that a larger surface area of the spatula is covered when dipped into the wax. Always test the temperature of the wax on the inside of the arm to prevent burning the client. When applying the wax, it is important to use the edge of the spatula so that the wax gradually slides off the spatula onto the skin. Soft wax is always applied in the direction of hair growth and removed against the direction of hair growth. It is always important to hold the skin taut at the bottom edge of the strip before pulling and to keep the skin taut during the pull. This allows for a swift clean pull. The tension on the skin will also prevent bruising. If the skin is not held taut enough, the pull will be slow and sluggish, causing the skin to drag with the pull, producing bruises to the skin as well as considerable discomfort to the client. To ease the client's discomfort, have the client take a deep breath while rubbing over the strip and blow out during the pull as if blowing out a group of candles. Another way to minimize discomfort is to always apply firm pressure on the waxed area immediately after each pull on any body area, and apply gentle pressure in the form of a tap for the face. Doing this will stop the lingering sensation of pain. At the end of the service another important "do" is to give the client home care instructions, including reminders not to use makeup or perfume, as these will irritate the skin, to avoid tanning, as the client will be more likely to burn, and to also avoid hot tubs for at least 24 hours after the service or until any signs of trauma and irritation have been completely eliminated. Last, it is important for the technician to be familiar with the state's regulations for waxing and to follow those regulations.

Double Dipping

Double dipping is the process of repeatedly using the same applicator on a client, returning it to the pot after each application. The Centers for Disease Control (CDC) does not view double dipping as a health threat. However, it is important for the clinician to realize that the possibilities exist for bacterial cross contamination. If even one client is harmed by double dipping, it is one too many. Technicians should take it upon themselves to create a safe environment for their clients, and this includes the avoidance of double dipping. Many state regulatory boards prohibit double dipping, and consequently technicians are required to follow those regulations.

Don'ts of Soft Wax

Unless one is a speed waxer, discussed below, do not apply wax to a larger area than is going to be immediately removed. If the wax gets too cool, it makes the removal of the hair more difficult as the pores close. The hair is also more likely to break, and there is also an increased risk of the skin lifting off. One should also not apply the wax to an area *longer* than will be removed by the strip, as the excess wax will gather and hang from the end of the strip, creating a sticky mess. To prevent injury, do not apply wax to an area that has just been waxed, and also do not overlap with soft wax. Finally, do not wax inside the ear or nose or on the areola of the nipple, although it is acceptable to wax the hairs that grow around the outside of the areola. (See Table 8–3.)

◾ SPEED WAXING

Speed waxing is a technique in which soft wax is applied to an entire area and removed rapidly with the same strip or a small number of strips. Developing a good speed waxing technique is financially more profitable, as treatment times are shortened and the technician is able to book more clients. (See Figure 8–5.) It is also beneficial for the client to receive the service in a more timely manner and with a shorter period of discomfort, which can result in a greater inclination to rebook. To be an effective speed waxer, the technician must be well organized and have the service protocols thoroughly worked out and understood. Placement of the treatment table and easy access to the wax is also important. Drips and spills must be avoided, as the time it takes to clean up the threads and drips of wax is time that could be spent working on clients. To be an effective speed waxer, one must clearly know the start point and follow the same rehearsed routine for each body part with each client. Thinking about where to go next is time lost. The same is true not only with the wax application but also with the application of precare and aftercare products.

The fronts of both legs can be misted at once top to bottom followed by a quick wipe down with a paper towel in each hand. Dusting powder can be sprinkled quickly and rubbed in, again with both hands in unison. These are the kinds of protocols that save considerable time. When misting the fronts of the clients' legs, they can even be asked to raise their legs

Table 8-3   Waxing Problems and the Potential Causes

Hard Wax

Problem	Cause
Hard wax breaks occurred during removal process.	1. Wax was too old or was not "refreshed" with new wax. 2. Wax may have been overheated or kept hot for 24 hours or more. 3. Wax may have been allowed to get too cold during application. 4. Wax may have been applied too thinly.
Too many bits of wax were left on the skin after removal.	Wax was not applied with clean even borders.
Client experienced small pustules a few days after a lip wax.	Area was not sufficiently cleansed of makeup and dirt. Aftercare lotion massaged in transported microorganisms into the vulnerable follicle or client failed to observe home care instructions properly.

Soft Wax

Problem	Cause
Skin lifted off during eyebrow or lip wax.	1. Client used a skin altering product like Retin-A®. 2. A poor waxing technique was used—the strip was pulled up too high during removal, rather than parallel to the skin, and the skin was not held taut.
Wax stayed on the skin and did not come off with the strip.	1. Client's skin may have been damp. 2. Client's skin may have been dry. 3. Client's skin may have been too cold. 4. Client's skin was not held taut. 5. Wax strip was not rubbed properly by the technician.
Bruising occurred in the bikini area.	1. Wax was applied over the femoral ridge, and not up to it, crossing two plains. 2. Skin was not held taut.
Too much hair was removed from the eyebrow.	1. Too much wax was applied, which "bled" into the brow line when the strip was rubbed. 2. Hairs growing downwards at the point of arch may have accidentally got caught in the wax and removed. 3. A strip with wax already on it may have been reused.

one at a time so the backs can be misted and prepped at the same times the fronts are, instead of repeating the step when they turn over. When speed waxing the legs, the wax can be applied completely up one side of the front of the leg, knee to ankle, and removed quickly the entire length

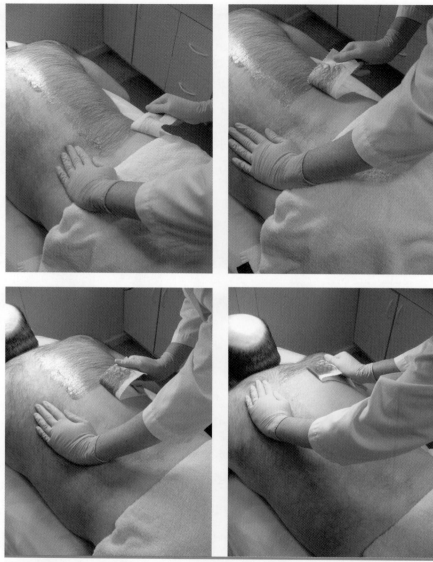

Figure 8–5 Speed waxing can increase the aesthetician's revenue and is more efficient for the client

> Speed waxing is a technique in which soft wax is applied to an entire area and removed rapidly with the same strip or a small number of strips.

with the strip. Only one or two firm rubs with the strip is necessary. More rubbing than that is also a waste of "valuable" time.

Blood Spots

Blood spots may appear postwaxing and are to be expected. This is due to the fact that a rich, healthy blood supply was feeding the hair at the root.

Because the hair was removed at the dermal papilla, the blood that was feeding the dermal papilla now gathers in the follicle until it realizes that there is no longer a hair there to "feed," at which time it reabsorbs back into the dermis. Blood spots, therefore, are always *good* signs. Certain areas are more likely to produce visible blood spots, like the axilla, bikini area, and back. As these areas are obvious, technicians routinely wear gloves. However, with any waxing service where even the slightest pink bumps are apparent, there could well be blood-borne pathogens present, so it is important to always wear gloves, particularly if the technician's skin is not intact. Even a hangnail is considered nonintact skin.

Ingrown Hairs

One of the side effects to soft waxing is an increase in ingrown hairs. This occurs mostly in the bikini area; however, many people are prone to ingrown hair regardless of their method of hair removal.

There are many good products available for the technician to recommend and sell to clients as well as use during the service to help keep ingrown hairs to a minimum. These products usually contain a high percentage of AHA or salicylic acid. Many ingrown hairs can also be removed manually. It can be a long and tedious process for the technician to remove a lot of ingrown hairs, so the client can be asked to release *but not remove* as many hairs as possible at least four days before the waxing service. The hairs should be released as close to the follicle opening as possible by sterile needle-pointed tweezers and should not be tweezed away but left sticking out of the opening, allowing time for the follicle to heal and normalize around the hair. If the skin is broken and the hair is completely removed, the opening will scab over, a new anagen hair may become trapped under the scab, and it will become ingrown, perpetuating the problem.

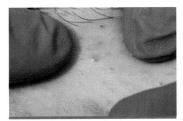

Figure 8–6 Sample black-head type of ingrown hair

If the ingrown hair looks like a blackhead (this is particularly apparent in the bikini area), then it usually has a follicle opening and can be extracted gently and fairly easily before the service by the client. If the technician is going to remove the ingrown hair(s), gloves should be worn and the prewaxed area wiped with an antiseptic first. The "blackhead" should then be gently squeezed using the *sides* of both forefinger nails, *not* the nail tips, until the hair extracts (see Figures 8–6 and 8–7). Once the hair is extracted, it can be wiped away. Because the skin was not broken, the follicle opening was not compromised and does not need time to heal and normalize.

For embedded hair that is visible under the skin as a thin line, the technician can release the hair after the waxing service by again wearing gloves, wiping the area with alcohol, and using sterile sharp-pointed

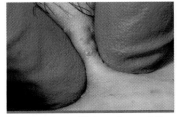

Figure 8–7 Extraction of the blackhead type of ingrown hair

tweezers. A magnifying lamp can make this procedure much easier. The tweezers should be sharp enough to break the skin as minimally as possible. The hair is released by sliding the tweezers' point underneath it as close to where the follicle should be as possible. The client should be instructed to leave the hair protruding for as long as possible up to four days, allowing the follicle to heal and normalize around it, for the reasons mentioned above. The hair may then be tweezed away days later, when it is healed. Needle-pointed tweezers or lancets used to break the skin are critical items and must be sterilized and treated as surgical instruments.

REGROWTH AND RETURN VISITS

It is important to let the client know what to expect in the way of hair regrowth and when to expect it. This will prevent the first time client from being disgruntled if expectations were not met. Many first time clients leave the salon or clinic after a waxing procedure believing that the waxed area will remain completely hair free for a full six weeks. Although waxed hairs usually take from six weeks to three months to reappear after waxing, depending on the area, it is important to tell clients what to expect with regrowth and when to expect it. Explain to the client that a percentage of hairs that were at a different stage of hair growth and not present for the waxing procedure may start to appear a few days or weeks after the procedure and that it is not due to any shortcoming of the waxing service. These hairs were new growing (anagen) hairs lying just below the skin at the time of waxing.

As soon as the hair is removed, the hair follicle goes into its resting phase. Therefore, it is wise to ask the first time clients to come back after a few days to a week to remove new hairs that have recently grown out to remove as many hairs as close to the same cycle as possible.

This will also be true of clients who book their waxing services monthly. Hairs that were waxed away two treatments prior will appear soon after a waxing service. By clarifying this ahead of time with clients, clients will not view this as an excuse for a bad waxing service. Many clients have a hard time keeping a six-week or two-month calendar and like to book their waxing services monthly. Therefore, they should be prepared to experience regrowth from previous services. For clients who are prepared to wait six weeks to two months between services, it is beneficial to return a week after their first waxing services to wax away new, visible, anagen hairs. This may force more hair follicles into the same telogen stage as the hairs waxed in the previous week, enabling the client to experience a greater percentage of hair-free areas over longer periods of time.

Conclusion

As skin care has advanced, so must we change how we perform our waxing services now, especially for face waxing. If a client is not a suitable candidate for a waxing service, it should not be performed. If there is another viable option available, the technician should advise the client of the option or options. As manufacturers continue to try to create waxes that are gentler to use on more delicate areas, technicians should in turn be aware of the waxes and associated products, and how and when to effectively use them. This will ensure that the technicians can offer the best possible waxing service to their clients. With the improved waxes, when protocol and procedures are followed, negative incidences and reactions are considerably reduced, and the waxing services will be successful and satisfying.

With continued practice and mastery in the use of strip wax, the technician can become a speed waxer, someone who offers a great temporary hair removal service in a short time and with little discomfort to the client. Speed waxers quickly earn the loyalty and continued patronage of clients who appreciate skill and speed. Their business will grow in leaps and bounds through referrals and positive word of mouth.

▶ ＞ ＞ TOP 10 TIPS TO TAKE TO THE CLINIC

1. Hard wax is generally applied initially against the direction of hair growth, then immediately in the direction of growth.
2. Soft wax is applied with the growth and removed against the growth.
3. The safest and most suitable wax for a French or Brazilian bikini wax is hard wax.
4. The temperature of the wax should be tested on the technician's wrist.
5. Blood spots indicate that the hair was *epilated.*
6. Regrowth takes 6 to 12 weeks depending on the telogen stage of the hair follicle.
7. Embedded hairs should be released by the client four days prior to the service or by the technician after the service.
8. Technicians should wash hands before and after each client.
9. Gloves should be worn for waxing services.
10. Contraindications must be learned, understood, and observed.

BIBLIOGRAPHY

Milady's Standard Comprehensive Training for Estheticians. (2003). Clifton
   Park, NY: Milady, an imprint of Thomson Delmar Learning.
Milady's Standard Cosmetology. (2004). Clifton Park, NY: Milady, an
   imprint of Thomson Delmar Learning.
Bickmore, H. (2003). *Milady's Hair Removal Techniques*. Clifton Park,
   NY: Milady, an imprint of Thomson Delmar Learning.
http://www.fda.gov

Waxing Protocols

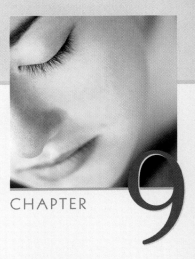

CHAPTER 9

KEY TERMS

blending	glabella	hood
effleurage	histamine	septum

LEARNING OBJECTIVES

After completing this chapter, you should be able to:

1. Know how to apply the appropriate precare for a waxing service.
2. Know how to correctly position the client for each waxing service.
3. Know the correct method of applying and removing soft wax.
4. Know the correct method of applying and removing hard wax.
5. Know how to provide appropriate aftercare.
6. Give appropriate home care advice.

INTRODUCTION

In the previous chapter we discussed the different types of waxes available and which type of wax is the preferred choice for which hair growth situation. Once the correct choice of wax is understood, how it is used is paramount in providing a successful procedure. Waxing incorrectly may not only mean an unsatisfactory outcome when hair is not properly removed, but may also cause injury to the client.

This chapter details the correct protocols for using both hard and soft wax to remove hair on all parts of the face and body, both for men and women. Understanding and applying the techniques will minimize the risk of injury or discomfort to the client.

CLIENT PREPARATION

The degree to which the client is received, treated, and prepped for a procedure is a testament to the professionalism of the technician. When the client is well received, appropriately draped, and carefully prepared, he or she will immediately feel relaxed and in capable hands. Client preparation also means bringing the client into a room that is clean, orderly, and prepared, and that has everything necessary readily available to avoid the technician having to "abandon" the client in search of the missing item. Below are further guidelines to consider when preparing the client.

Positioning

Correct positioning is important not only for the comfort of the clients during the service that they are to receive but also for the comfort of the technician while providing the service with ease, accuracy, and efficiency. The table should be at a suitable height to avoid fatigue or back discomfort. Correct posture should be employed to minimize the risk of back injury. The technician should stand close to the area to avoid leaning awkwardly. The treatment table should be centrally located in the room with easy access from all sides. When the table is too close to a wall, movement is restricted and the technician cannot follow through with pulls, which could result in snapping the hair or bruising the client.

Once the client is positioned for the service, the technician should begin by washing the hands in front of the client, drying the hands with a paper towel, and using the paper towel to turn off the faucet before discarding it. Now the technician is ready to prepare the area of the client's skin that is to be waxed.

Cleansing

Many of the manufacturers of hair removal wax offer an array of products for prewax and postwax care to complement their brand of wax. There are also a number of standard products available to prepare the skin. Prior to waxing the face, all makeup should be cleansed because oil on the skin and the oils in makeup prevent the wax from gripping the hair. The cleansing should be done as gently as possible to avoid overstimulating the skin in that area. A spray cleanser is faster and more economical for cleansing larger areas of the body, such as the arms, legs, and back.

After the cleansing, a manufacturer's numbing solution or spray may be applied to the area. The face should never be sprayed directly with a numbing product, but instead gently dabbed with a saturated cotton square. It usually takes two to three minutes for the numbing product to take effect. Excess numbing product may need to be removed if it contains an oil base that may prevent the wax from adhering to the hair.

Pretreatment

As mentioned previously, there are pretreatments that are available by the wax companies, but also available are suitable "generic" pretreatments like tea tree oil. Tea tree oil is an essential oil that has the ability to completely evaporate from the skin without leaving a greasy film to inhibit the grip of the wax. Tea tree oil that is 100 percent has antibacterial and soothing properties that quickly absorb into the skin. Many oils on the market may have as little as 5 percent with added carriers, so it is important to check the label to make sure that the tea tree oil is 100 percent. Only a trace amount of tea tree oil is necessary to be effective, just what is absorbed onto a cotton-tip applicator by sliding it around the lip of the bottle, rather than dipping the entire cotton tip into the oil.

After cleansing, the area should be lightly dusted with a talc-free, fragrance-free, cornstarch-based dusting powder using a piece of cotton. The powder serves to absorb any remaining moisture and oil. On larger body areas, if the hair is light and not easily visible, it also helps to mark where waxing has been done and still must be done.

WAXING FOR WOMEN

In this section, we will discuss those components of waxing that are most commonly unique to women, working from head to toe. While there is an increase in the popularity of waxing services for men, women still outnumber men for hair removal services. With any face waxing, it is helpful to ask new clients if the service is for a special occasion and to let them know of the associated risks of redness, irritation, and pimples, as well as the possibility on rare occasions of bruising and lifting of skin. Also important to discuss with the client are the other adverse reactions that can result from continuous waxing of the face (not including the eyebrows or upper lip).

The finer vellus hair, mostly associated with female facial hair, has shallower follicles closer to the epidermis, with less of a blood supply. With frequent waxing, particularly when removing the hair against the direction of growth, the follicle may gradually grow deeper into the dermis and closer to a richer blood supply, causing the hair to become thicker and longer. As the female client enters menopause, the hormonal balance changes. The effects of estrogen that "buffered" the male androgens diminish, causing the androgens to stimulate the hair growth in this area. In time, the hairs on the chin, with multiple wax treatments, may not be removed with wax, leaving the technician or the client to remove them with tweezers. The extensive regrowth can be unsightly, and ingrown hairs and folliculitis could result. As the client's skin matures, it becomes more fragile, and wax treatments could cause an adverse reaction.

The Forehead

Hairlines are often asymmetrical or otherwise undesirable to the client. Often women will wear bangs or style their hair to disguise these irregularities. A simple solution to even out the hairline is waxing. Even though the hair at the hairline is terminal, it is often finer than the rest of the scalp hair. If this is the case, it can be waxed in small sections. Because the skin in that area may be delicate, a cream wax or even a hard wax is recommended. Terminal hair that is of the same strength as the rest of the scalp hair, with a deep follicle, should not be waxed but eliminated with electrolysis.

To proceed with the waxing service, the client should be positioned in a semireclining position. She should be given a mirror, and, together with the technician, the desired hairline should be discussed. The hair to be removed should be isolated, and the hair that is to remain should be clipped back or covered with a disposable nurse's cap to protect the hair from any threads of wax. The hair that is to be removed should be trimmed to 1/4 inch with either scissors or a hair trimmer. Next the area should be cleansed, the pretreatment solution applied, and the area dusted with powder. At the same time the technician can be clearly ascertaining the direction of hair growth.

Forehead Hair Removal with Hard Wax

Hard wax should be applied in small sections of approximately 1 inch by 1-1/2 inches, initially against the direction of the hair, following immediately back over the top in the direction of hair growth. (See Figure 9–1.) The wax should continue to be applied to approximately 1/8 inch thick or until the hair and skin is not visible underneath. The wax should be ready to remove when it has set. It ought to be soft, pliable, and opaque, not wet and shiny looking. The edges ought to be clear with a slightly thicker edge where the pull is initiated. Holding the skin taut with one hand at the start of the pull, the edge is flicked up with the thumb and the wax quickly removed with the growth. Immediate pressure should be applied to the

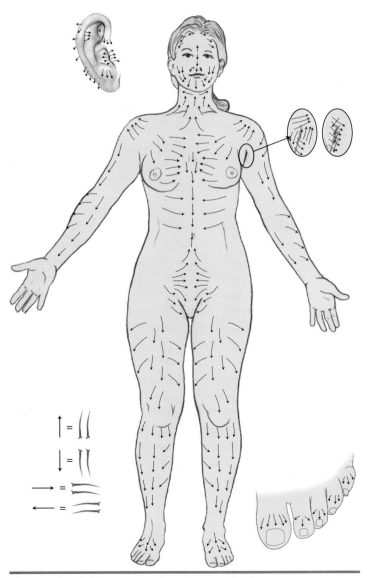

Figure 9–1 Hair growth directions, anterior

area. Adjacent areas are waxed until the unwanted hair is cleared and then the area soothed with an aftercare lotion.

Forehead Hair Removal with Soft Wax

Soft wax should be applied in small sections of approximately 1 inch by 1-1/2 inches, following the direction of growth to a point where it ends in a hair-free zone. The wax should be thinly applied with the edge of the spatula at a 45-degree angle. A 1 inch by 3 inch strip of muslin or Pellon is then placed over the wax, making sure there is plenty of free edge to grasp in the hair-free zone. Muslin works better than Pellon on small areas that have stronger hair as Pellon may have a tendency to separate, leaving a thin layer of Pellon and wax on the skin. Quickly give two firm but brisk rubs over the area, in the direction of hair growth, then with one hand, holding the skin taut at the free edge, grab the free end, and quickly pull back the strip, following as closely to the skin as possible. Immediately take the hand that was holding the skin taut and apply pressure to the area just waxed. The next adjacent area is treated, again ending in an area that is hair-free, and so on until the job is complete. At the end of the service apply a soothing aftercare lotion.

The Eyebrows

Waxing of the eyebrows is not simply about the removal of unwanted hair, as it is for most other parts of the body; it is also about aesthetics. Understanding shape, balance, and artistry are all important in shaping eyebrows. To create the perfect shape for a client takes a good eye. Knowledge of the basic rules of eyebrow and face shapes will benefit the client greatly. If the client is coming in to get her eyebrows waxed and shaped for the first time, the technician should take notice as she initially enters the room. Her appearance and image can define the kind of look she wants her eyebrows to reflect. Is she sophisticated or sporty? Well-groomed individuals generally appreciate more precise and defined eyebrows, whereas sporty or more casual individuals may be comfortable with a more natural look that just requires a little "clean up." The sophisticated client who comes in on a day off may be dressed down, so a few simple questions can be politely asked to hone in on the client's image as you wash your hands. Is the hair long or short? Women with short and/or fine hair are suited by a thinner, more defined brow; conversely women with thick and/or longer hair may be suited by a brow with more substance. The age of the client is also an important consideration. The sophisticated, thin eyebrow of a woman in her forties may not suit a teenage girl. A more mature woman may benefit from a more obvious arch, especially if her eyelids are starting to hood, because it gives the illusion of more lift and opens the eyes more. Generally speaking, the younger

hood
when the upper eyelid falls over the upper eye lashes

female should sport a more natural eyebrow shape. As a woman ages, the eyebrows can gradually become thinner and more defined, but she may have thick and unruly white or grey hairs that will need to be removed or trimmed. Another factor to consider is whether the client generally sports a full face makeup on a daily basis or typically does not wear makeup. The former may opt for a more defined brow that will complement or be complemented by the eye makeup, and the latter client may prefer keeping the look of the brow natural and not too thin. If it is the client's first eyebrow wax, clear communication is important to achieve the desired look.

Brow and Face Shape

In addition to the *image* factors listed above, there are other factors to be considered when assessing the shape of an eyebrow, so the client should be placed in a semireclined position for an eyebrow service and handed a mirror for viewing the desired shape and any irregularities. The client's hair should be secured off the face so that the face shape and eye placement can be assessed, as well as to prevent hair from getting in the way of the waxing procedure.

Clients with a round or broad face (see Figure 9–2) or wide-set eyes (see Figure 9–3) benefit by bringing the point of the arch to the inside of the pupil as the client looks straight ahead, creating the illusion that the face is narrower or that the eyes are closer together. Narrow faces (see Figure 9–4) or close-set eyes (Figure 9–5) benefit by placing the point of the arch to the outside of the pupil as the client looks straight ahead,

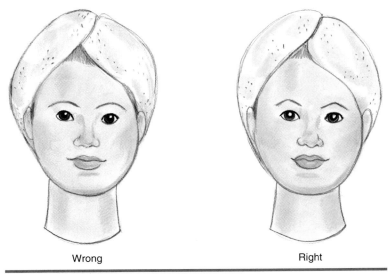

Wrong   Right

Figure 9–2 On a round face the eyebrow arch should be defined on the inside of the pupil

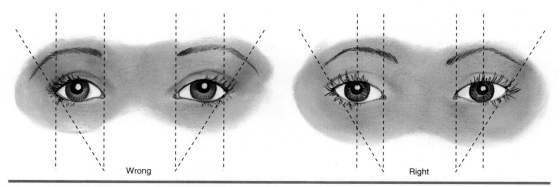

Wrong   Right

Figure 9–3 The arch position for wide-set eyes

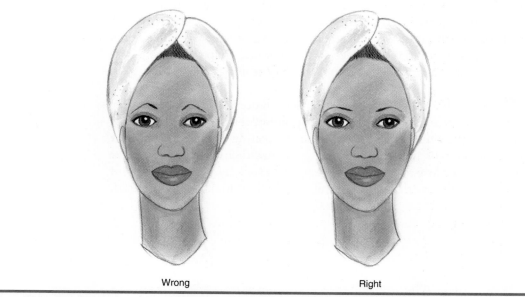

Wrong   Right

Figure 9–4 The correct and incorrect brow arches for a narrow face

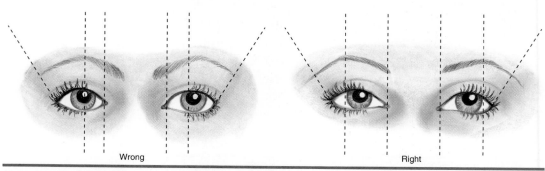

Wrong   Right

Figure 9–5 The arch position for close-set eyes

creating the illusion that the face is wider or the eyes are more in balance with the face.

When defining the eyebrow shape, the following guidelines should be used (see Figure 9–6), bearing in mind that these guidelines are applied to a perfect oval-shaped face with eyes that are positioned in perfect balance and proportion to that face shape. The start and point of the arch can be changed with subtle adjustments to create that desired illusion of balance and proportion.

When waxing the glabella, the area between the brows, a common mistake is to wax away the brow hair that grows straight up or turns inwards, resulting in the brow line starting farther in than it should. It would be better for the hairs to be trimmed around and the corner taken off. When hairs grow inward, they can be removed by tweezing in the direction of the desired new growth rather than being waxed away. This is accomplished by grasping the hair as close to the follicle opening as possible, turning the hair with the tweezers to the new desired direction of growth, then tweezing them out. Over time, with this repeated method, the hair can be retrained to grow in the desired direction.

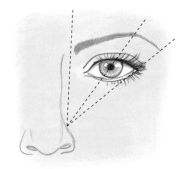

Figure 9–6 Use these guidelines when defining the eyebrow shape: 1. Start; 2. Point of arch; 3. End point of eyebrow

glabella
the area between the eyebrows that causes a frown

Brows with Hard Wax

Once the desired eyebrow shape has been ascertained, and after the aforementioned pretreatment, with a small spatula, apply the wax to the entire area under the brow, first against the direction of hair growth coating the underside of the hair, then immediately going back over the same area in the direction of growth, rather like frosting a cake. A thicker application is necessary so that neither hair nor skin is visible through the wax. The strip of wax should have a clean, even edge all the way around for clean removal and be somewhat thicker at the edge, where it will be lifted for the removal. Watch for the aforementioned signs that the wax is ready for removal.

Peel up a small edge of the wax on the outer edge of the eyebrow and, with a thumb, hold the skin taut. Grasp the wax, and pull quickly against the direction of growth as close to the skin as possible. Immediately apply pressure to the area. Once the use of hard wax has been mastered, the wax can be applied to the second eyebrow while waiting for the wax on the first eyebrow to set. When applying wax to the glabellar area, the same rule applies: Apply the wax first against the growth, then back on top in the direction of growth, and remove against the direction of growth. A point to remember is that hair grows upward between the brows but downward at the top of the nose. After the wax has been removed, tweeze any stray hairs that were not removed or any stubs that were too short to grip the wax. Waxing is mass tweezing, so to tweeze any remaining hairs puts those follicles in the same telogen stage as the waxed hair, offering a longer lasting result. After waxing and tweezing, a soothing antiseptic lotion may be gently massaged on both eyebrows simultaneously, finishing with gentle pressure at the temple. This service should be performed in approximately 20 minutes using hard wax, and 30 minutes for complete reshaping.

Use these guidelines when defining the eyebrow shape: 1. Start; 2. Point of arch; 3. End point of eyebrow.

1. **Start**—The first point of reference (see Figure 9–6), point 1, is the start point and is identified by resting a thin, wooden applicator orangewood stick or pencil along the side of the nose, just above the nostril, in the cleft of the nose and straight up to the inner corner of the eye. As some clients have wider nostrils than others, which could affect the start line, placing the stick just above the nostril gives a more accurate start point. The point above the inner corner of the eye where the stick passes will determine where the eyebrow should start. Any hair to the outside of the stick should be removed, unless the eyes are wide set, and any space on the inside should be filled with an eyebrow pencil unless the eyes are too close together.

2. **Point of arch**—The second point of reference, point 2, is to locate the arch, and it is the arch that can also be slightly adjusted to correct a misproportion. To find the correct point of the arch for a normal face shape and eye placement, the client should be looking straight ahead, the stick placed at the base of the nose and angled so that it crosses in front of the pupil. The point at which the stick touches the eyebrow is where the point of the arch should be. With broad-shaped faces, the arch can be brought in slightly to just above the pupil when looking straight ahead or just to the inside of it. Conversely, with narrow faces the arch can be adjusted farther to the outside of the pupil.

3. **End**—The final point of reference, point 3, allows us to locate the correct ending of the brow. To do this, the technician should slide the stick, still at the base of the nose, farther around so that it crosses over the outer corner of the eye. The point at which the stick meets the brow is where the brow should end. Any hair that goes beyond the stick should be removed, and any space on the inside of the stick should be penciled in. If the end is too short and not penciled in, the client, from her profile, may look like she does not have an eyebrow.

There should be a clear ascent from the start to the point of arch and a clear descent from the point of arch to the end. The line should be gradual and tapered without going from too thick on the ascent to too thin on the descent.

Brows with Soft Wax

Once the desired shape of the eyebrow has been ascertained, and the area prepared for waxing, a tiny amount of wax on a thin applicator is used to separate and pull down, away from the brow line, any hair that must be removed. While the actual waxing procedure is better done standing behind the client, this part of pulling down the hairs of the first brow only, can be done with the technician facing the client. After this is done, the technician moves behind and with the applicator applies a small amount of wax on it along the underside of the brow, from the start point, following the direction of growth to the end point. The wax should be thinly applied with the edge of the spatula at a 45-degree angle. A 1 inch by 3 inch strip is placed over the wax, leaving a free edge of muslin or Pellon at the end point to grasp. After two quick rubs, also in the direction of hair growth, the forefinger and middle finger are placed at the end point holding the skin taut, and the strip is pulled quickly backward, against the hair growth, parallel and as close to the skin as possible. Gentle pressure is then quickly applied with the fingers that held the skin taut. The process is repeated on the other eyebrow; then the glabellar area is waxed in an upward direction, rubbing on the strip twice and pulling down, and afterwards removing any hairs at the top of the nose growing downward.

Follow with any necessary tweezing, which should be done before any soothing lotion is applied because the lotion causes the tweezers to slide up the slick hair and not tweeze easily, causing additional discomfort to the client. A soothing lotion can then be gently massaged over the waxed area. Using both hands, massage the lotion into the area simultaneously, finishing with gentle pressure on the client's temples, before lifting. This ensures a pleasant finish to the service. This procedure should take 15 minutes for a regular eyebrow wax and 30 minutes for an eyebrow shape. Avoid waxing the eyebrows if there are signs of eye irritation or infection, such as conjunctivitis.

> If any wax falls onto the client's lashes, request that the client keep the eyes gently closed. Slide some damp cotton under the client's lashes, and then, using a cotton-tip applicator and petroleum jelly, stroke down the lashes until the wax slides off.

> Eyebrows frame the eyes and give the face expression. Well-shaped eyebrows can also create an illusion, by enhancing facial features, correcting the irregularities of eyes that appear too far apart or too close together, or changing the appearance of a face that is too thin or too broad.

Upper Lip

The upper lip under the nose can be divided into two equal sections for hair removal. The hair grows downward and outward at a slight angle, following the lip line.

Under the nose, however, it grows straight downward. As it is impossible, due to the position of the nose and the mouth, to pull the hair against its growth to remove those hairs, the hair, which is usually fine, is easily removed when pulling across the lip line against the growth with the rest of the hair on that half of the upper lip.

To prepare the client, cleanse the area, apply tea tree oil, and then dust the area with powder.

Upper Lip with Hard Wax

With a medium sized applicator, the hard wax is initially applied against the growth from the edge of the mouth upwards to the septum. Then, with a little more wax, glide back over in the direction of growth following the same guidelines of thickness and readiness mentioned for the forehead and eyebrows. (See Figure 9–7.) The wax can be removed in the direction of growth as soon as it becomes opaque, although the technician who is experienced in using hard wax can proceed in applying the wax to the opposite side of the upper lip while the first side is hardening. (See Figure 9–8.) On completion the area is soothed with an appropriate aftercare lotion.

Upper Lip with Soft Wax

Using a medium-sized applicator, apply a thin layer of wax, starting under the septum of the nose, in a downward, outward direction. It is important to make sure that the area under the nostril is covered and that no hairs are missed on the edge of the nostril and no wax enters the nostrils. This is an area that should not be immediately rewaxed. There are often noticeable hairs bordering the lip line and the outside corner of the lip line that stand up and bother clients, particularly visible in rear-view or magnifying mirrors. The tissue of the lips is fragile and can be easily lifted, so considerable care should be taken to avoid getting wax

septum
the part of the nose that divides the two nostrils

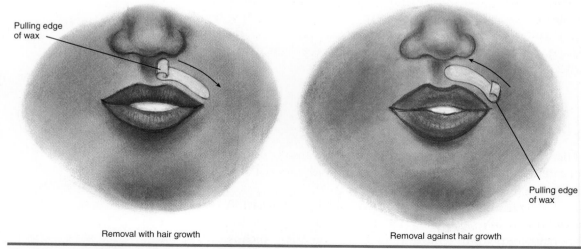

Pulling edge of wax

Pulling edge of wax

Removal with hair growth

Removal against hair growth

Figure 9–7 Applying hard wax to the upper lip

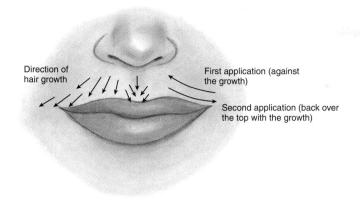

Direction of hair growth

First application (against the growth)

Second application (back over the top with the growth)

Figure 9–8 Two different techniques for removing hard wax from the lip

on the lips. If any wax gets on the lips, do not remove it with a strip but use either petroleum jelly or a wax-removing lotion for the skin. Immediately after the wax is applied, place the 1 inch by 3 inch strip over it, leaving enough of a free edge on the outside to grasp. With fingers holding that same outer edge of the lip taut and stable, grasp the strip and pull it quickly across the lip in the opposite direction of hair growth, as close to the skin as possible. Follow through with a quick, sweeping movement, beyond the waxed area.

Quickly apply pressure to the area with the hand that held the skin taut to ease the smarting sensation. Finish this service by applying appropriate aftercare, which can be massaged in by the technician using both hands simultaneously from the corners of the mouth inwards to the septum then back outwards and ending with gentle pressure on the outer corners of the lip.

The Chin

Chin waxing often includes not only the chin, but also the small area just under the jaw. While waxing this area offers a quick fix and a temporary solution to the unwanted hair, it can have a negative impact on the client later on, particularly if soft wax is used and is removed against the hair growth. As discussed above, soft wax causes the vellus hair on the chin to grow back in an irregular fashion, standing up, looking wispy. Also, the wax removes not only the hair that is unwanted but also the nonproblematic vellus hair, leading to more irregular regrowth. Continued waxing may aggravate the hair growth in this area, which is a secondary sexual characteristic of male hair growth, starting at puberty. Another downside is that the area that has been waxed clean makes the hair adjacent to it appear more obvious. As the chin area does not have the boundaries that the upper lip and eyebrows have, it is easy to continue to wax increasingly larger areas with the result being that the more it is waxed, the more it will need to be waxed, spreading the problem along the jaw and up the sides of the face. After multiple wax treatments, the client must deal with problems like excessive irregular hair growth that must grow in before it can be waxed again, ingrown hairs, folliculitis, and the risk of injury to the skin as it matures, becomes fragile, and develops liver spots. The client will be unable to use many antiacne or antiaging treatments.

Therefore waxing should *not* be considered the primary choice of hair removal for the chin, especially if the client has never removed the hair with wax before. It may be better to recommend other forms of hair removal, such as electrolysis or laser. If the client does not consider those methods options, then hard wax or sugaring should be considered, because both techniques remove the hair in the direction of hair growth without distorting the follicle and its regrowth.

Chin and Hard Wax

Hard wax would be the better choice of wax, as the wax is gentler, less stimulating to the skin, and removed in the direction of growth; therefore it will not cause the same distortion to the hair follicles that soft wax does. The area under the jaw should be dealt with first. Ask the client to tilt back the head, and then apply the wax to the underside from the jawbone down the throat in the direction of hair growth, which is usually straight downward. Farther down the neck, the hair starts to slightly change direction, growing away from the center of the neck. If there is a considerable span of growth, the area can be divided into two strips in the center. If three strips are warranted, the first strip will be in the center; the second and third will be on either side. The wax is applied in a manageable strip, following the guidelines mentioned above. While one strip is hardening, the wax can be applied to a second and even third area that is not immediately adjacent, depending on the speed of the technician applying the wax. The wax can quickly be removed one strip after the other until the area is cleared, quickly applying pressure after each pull. Waxing the top of the chin is usually done in two or three sections, depending on the amount of hair growth. Do not cross from one surface or plane to another, which means do not take the wax downward or across the jaw bone, but instead address one surface area at a time. Failing to do this and trying to wax across a plane ignoring the contours of the face makes achieving a successful, clean pull, close to the skin, impossible. Different planes should be dealt with separately. When pulling the strip backward, remember to hold the skin especially tight at the jawbone and to apply direct pressure right after. End the service with a mild antiseptic soothing lotion.

This service should be performed in 20 minutes.

Chin and Soft Wax

If there are a few unwanted hairs on the chin, and the client is not interested in electrolysis, another less aggravating method of removing those hairs is to use the wax on the strip left over from the client's lip wax, and, with a finger, press on each hair and quickly pull away, limiting the amount of vellus hair from being disturbed.

The Sides of the Face

Waxing the sides of the face can create problems for the client just as waxing the chin can. The client should be informed of all the adverse consequences. If the hair is visible but minimal in quantity and requires removal, electrolysis should be the first choice. If there is a significant amount of hair, and the client rates favorably in the Fitzpatrick Scale, then laser hair removal may be a good option to recommend. If neither are options, then hard wax is more desirable than strip wax to avoid distorting the follicles. Also, hard wax better grips the stronger hairs of the sideburn but without irritating the skin as much. Sugaring is an option, too, if the hair is not too strong.

Sides of Face with Hard Wax

Make sure the client's hair is well pinned back. Hand the client a mirror and ascertain exactly what hair is to be removed. If the sideburns must be shortened, begin by selecting the hair equally on both sides of the face that should be removed, pinning back the remaining hair well. A good rule of thumb is to use the middle knob of cartilage on the inside edge of the ear called the tragus. After isolating the hair to be removed, any hair that is more than 1/2 or 0.5 inch long should be buzzed or trimmed with scissors to 1/2 or 0.5 inch. Pretreat in the usual manner. With a medium sized applicator, apply the wax to the area in the usual manner for hard wax, making sure that the edge where the pull is to be initiated is in a hair-free zone so that the hairs are not going to be uncomfortably snagged as the edge is flicked up. As the first area is setting on one side, an application can be made to the other side. Removal is done with the growth.

This service should take between 20 and 30 minutes, depending on whether the hair must be trimmed. More time would be needed if it is the client's first face wax and other suggestions are going to be offered.

Sides of Face with Soft Wax

After isolating the hair and preparing the skin as listed above, apply the wax in the usual manner for soft wax. If the area to be waxed cannot be completed in one section, begin on the inside edge (toward the nose) first, followed by the area closer to the ear. Remove in the usual manner. Proceed with the second side in a like manner. Calm the area with a soothing antiseptic lotion. This service should take between 10 and 20 minutes, depending on whether the hair must be trimmed. More time would be needed if it is the client's first face wax and other suggestions are going to be offered.

Axilla

There is often asymmetry to the hair growth of the underarms. One side may have two different directions of growth while the other side may have three directions. While soft wax works well on this hair, it must be applied following the different sections of hair growth. If there are different directions in the same cluster, there could be breakage and some hairs left behind. Because the same area cannot be waxed over a second time with soft wax during that service, the remaining hair must be tweezed. Hard wax is very effective in this area, because it goes on against the hair growth, coating the hair in all directions. As the wax hardens, it grips the hair and lifts it away from the delicate skin of the underarms. A more thorough removal is achieved.

Whatever the choice of wax, the preparation of the client is the same. To prepare and position the client for this service, have the client first remove the clothing, and provide an appropriate drape for modesty. The client should lie face up and flat on the table. The area should be cleaned with a mild antiseptic cleanser, and all traces of antiperspirant or deodorant removed. If the hair is long so that it curls over, it should be buzzed or trimmed to 1/2 inch in length, making it easier to evaluate the different directions of hair growth as well as making it more comfortable. The axilla should be dusted with powder. The client raises the arm to be waxed above the shoulder, placing the hand behind the head. The other hand should then reach across the body and move the breast tissue down and away from the underarm. Do not wax the underarms if the client has had a mastectomy or suffers from mastitis.

Axilla and Hard Wax

Hard wax should be applied to the axillary area in small sections of approximately 1 inch by 2 inches, initially against hair growth, then back over the top with hair growth. A few hairs may grow in different directions in the same cluster and the hard wax, when applied correctly, can cover the entire hair shaft, including hairs growing in different directions. As the wax sets, it shrinks and grips the individual hairs tightly. The wax should be removed against the predominant hair growth in this area. Flick up the edge of the wax where the pull will begin, and hold the skin as taut as possible. Pull the wax away as fast as possible, as close to the skin as possible. Complete the waxing service and soothe the area.

Axilla and Soft Wax

The initial section should be along the outside edge. The technician should stand behind the head of the client. The wax should be thinly applied with the edge of the spatula at a 45-degree angle in the direction of growth. Before removal, if there is a chance of hitting the client in the face, have the client turn the face away. Firmly press the strip over the wax and rub in the direction of growth, allowing enough free edge to grasp at the end. Place the free hand firmly at that same end, holding the skin taut, and quickly pull against the hair growth and as close to the skin as possible. Follow the movement through, close to the skin. Starting to pull upward too soon will bruise the client and/or cause extreme redness. After removal, quickly apply pressure to the area. Proceed to the next section, repeating in the same manner until the hair has been removed. Apply a soothing lotion to the area. If the underarm is particularly tender, a cool cotton compress of cold water and baking soda can be applied to the area while the other side is being waxed.

To continue on the other side, have the client switch arms, placing this hand behind the head and using the free hand to pull the breast tissue down and away from the area. Wax the second axilla, being careful to observe the hair growth direction, as it could well differ. Reassure the client that any blood spots are due to the fact that the hair was removed at the dermal papilla or root and that the blood spots are a sign of successful epilation. Make sure the client has no residual stickiness in the axillas, because this can make the area feel tender if the skin sticks together. It is also annoying to find clusters of clothing fibers stuck to the wax in that area.

Arms

Strip wax is the fastest, most effective way to remove hair from the arms. However, because of the pulling direction against the growth of the hair, the hair may start to grow back in an unruly fashion, sticking up. Hard wax or sugaring will prevent unruly regrowth, particularly if it is a client's first time for an arm wax and the client is getting the service for a special occasion, but does not anticipate it being repeated in the near future. However, both hard wax and sugaring methods are slower methods.

For hair removal of the forearm, the client should be given a gown or apron to protect the clothing. The client should be sitting on the treatment table, legs dangling over, with the technician standing in front of the client. The forearm should be sprayed or wiped with an antiseptic solution, then dusted with powder.

Arms and Hard Wax

The client should hold the arm outstretched with the palm facing up. Begin by waxing any unsightly hair on the inside where there is less hair. Apply the hard wax following the general application rules or the manufacturer's directions. Do not apply hard wax to an immediately adjacent section where the two sides of the section touch, but place the second application with the space of a single application in-between. The in-between area is treated after the other two strips of wax have been removed. The forearm is completed all the way up to the elbow, paying attention to the direction of hair growth.

If the hair of the upper arm is more obvious and requires complete removal, then the client should relax the arm, allowing the forearm to rest on the lap. The wax should be applied initially against and then immediately in the direction of growth, which is downward, toward the elbow. The technician should remove the hair in the direction of growth in sections starting toward the elbow and working upward toward the shoulder, "blending" if necessary at the top.

Arms and Soft Wax

The hair grows downward toward the wrist, so the wax should be applied thinly and downward, following the growth. Continue up the lower half of the inside arm, toward the wrist. Apply the strip over the wax, leaving enough of a free edge to grab. Rub and remove in the usual manner. The next section to wax should be just above the previous section. After completing the inner arm, the client should turn the still-outstretched arm so the palm faces downward. Holding the arm firmly in place and starting down at the wrist, apply the wax across the top of the arm from the inside (thumb side) to the outside (little finger side), the width of the strip. Remove in the usual manner. Continue in strip size sections all the way up the forearm to the elbow. Next, have the client hold the arm straight upward, bent at the elbow, and apply the wax to the side that follows down from the little finger. This can be done in two sections.

The hair grows downward, toward the elbow. Apply the wax to the first section, starting near the wrist, working up, toward the elbow. Proceed in the usual manner.

Most often, the upper arm has just a few hairs right above the elbow. These can often be removed with the wax that is already on the strip if soft wax is being used. The strip will remove the more obvious hairs, leaving some shorter hairs behind. This technique is known as blending, because it produces a gradual link between complete hairlessness and more dense hair.

Hands

After completing the lower and upper arm, the technician should proceed to wax the knuckles and hands, if necessary. When waxing the hands and fingers, it is important to have the client make a fist, tucking the fingers underneath, thereby tightening the skin. Also, as the client's hand is "floating" without solid support, it is important to have a good grip of the hand when removing the wax, which means that pressure cannot be applied after the pull because both hands are occupied.

Hands and Hard Wax

To wax the hand, take the hand and apply the wax in the usual manner for hard wax. The hair growth is usually downward, toward the fingers, and angling out, toward the little finger. The entire top of the hand, not including the fingers, can be done at one time. On the fingers, the hair grows toward the middle knuckle, so take one finger at a time, starting at the thumb, and work toward the little finger. Apply the wax in the usual manner. Once the wax is applied to all fingers, it should have set enough to start removing, beginning again at the thumb and quickly pulling off with hair growth. After removing all the hair, take the hand in a handshake grasp and apply a soothing lotion along the topside, toward the elbow (and shoulder, if upper arm was waxed) and down the underside to the hand. If the hand was waxed, finish by massaging the lotion into the hand and fingers. Massage the thumb and little fingers simultaneously, followed by the ring and index fingers, and finishing with the middle finger and thumb a second time.

Hands and Soft Wax

Soft wax is the preferred wax for this area. To wax the hand, take the hand and apply the wax in the direction of the growth, which is usually downward, with soft wax, toward the fingers, and angling outward, toward the little finger. The entire top of the hand can be done at once, not including the fingers. Have the client form a fist by tucking the fingers under, because this tightens the skin. Apply the strip over the entire area, and rub in the direction of growth. As the client's hand is "floating" without

blending
waxing technique that transitions wanted hair into unwanted hair, preventing a line from occurring

solid support, it is important to have a good grip of the hand when pulling back quickly against the growth. If the fingers have hair that needs removing and it is only slight, it can often be removed with the wax that is already on the strip. The hair grows toward the middle knuckle, so by taking one finger at a time, pressing the wax onto the hair, rubbing in the direction of growth, and quickly pulling off against the growth the hair can be removed. If it cannot, complete the process by applying the wax. After removing all the hair, take the hand in a handshake grasp and apply a soothing lotion along the topside, toward the elbow (and shoulder, if the upper arm was waxed), and down the underside to the hand. If the hand was waxed, finish by massaging the lotion into the hand and fingers in the manner described above.

Bikini Wax

The standard bikini waxing was originally designed for removing the unwanted hair that poked out the sides of swimsuits. Once seasonal, now it is a desired service year-round regardless of swimsuit wear. Regrowth is often softer, lighter, and less dense when the area is waxed exclusively and regularly. Standard, professional conduct is extremely important in this waxing service, perhaps above all others. This is a time when most clients, especially first-time clients, feel the most vulnerable. A cheerful and confident professional manner helps to put clients at ease. Less anxiety means less discomfort. Show the client into the wax room and clarify what type of bikini wax is desired. Provide a drape and a pair of disposable underpants in the treatment room and inform the client that you will step outside the room at which time the client should remove all clothing from the waist down. She may leave on her underpants, if it is for a regular bikini wax, or change into the disposable pair. The client may also keep socks on and get onto the table and cover herself with the drape. Knock before reentering the room. Analyze the area, skin, and hair, and ascertain if you will need the client's help in stretching the skin. Bikini waxes can be classified in three ways, according to how much hair should be removed. They are American (or standard) bikini wax, French bikini wax, and Brazilian bikini wax. Communication is very important so that the client clearly understands what is removed and what is left with each type of bikini wax.

American Bikini Wax

This is the removal of hair exposed at the top of the thighs and just under the navel when wearing a regular bikini bottom. When doing a regular American bikini wax, strip wax is preferred.

The standard honey style wax works well, but, providing the hair is not too coarse or too short and stubbly, the cream wax also works well. If the client is wearing her swimsuit or her own briefs, they should be protected with a paper towel, with one corner placed down the crotch area, so that two corners can be folded into the sides and the remaining corner tucked over the top. Using a small applicator, pull out from under the panty line any hair that must be removed, leaving the remainder tucked in behind the panty and giving a clean, even line to both sides of the bikini area. If the hair is so long that it curls, it should be trimmed to 1/2 inch. This can be done quickly with scissors for a small amount. If there is a considerable amount, then an electric buzzer will be faster. Cleanse the area with an antiseptic cleaner and pat it dry. The area should then be dusted with powder. Have the client leave one leg straight and bring the sole of the other foot to the level of the knee. If working first on the right side of the client's bikini area, have the client place the *left* hand firmly on the paper, fingers straight downward. Ask the client to keep her hands on the paper at all times, to avoid getting wax on them. The free hand should be placed on the outer edge of the thigh to help pull the skin taut. Working on the bent leg, apply the wax with the edge of a large spatula in the direction of hair growth. The first application should be to the section farthest away and only up to the femoral ridge. The direction of hair growth is usually downward, following the panty line. However, toward the denser hair on the pubis bone, the hair grows more horizontally and inward, toward the center. Place the strip over the wax, leaving space to grab the free edge. Rub twice in the direction of growth, and then place that same hand firmly at the end of the strip with the free edge. The skin should be held especially taut in this area. Grab the strip and pull backward in a swift, continuous manner, as close to the skin as possible. Do not cut the movement short; make sure to follow through with the movement, even slightly beyond the placement of wax. Remember that lifting too soon will make the client uncomfortable and could cause bruising. Apply immediate, firm pressure to alleviate the discomfort.

Once all sections leading up to the panty line have been removed of hair, the hair that grows down from the femoral ridge can be removed. The client should bring the sole of the foot a little higher to just above the knee. Apply the wax just two-thirds of the way down in the downward direction of hair growth, leaving enough space at the bottom to place the hand to hold the skin taut. Place the wax strip over the area, again leaving enough of a free edge to grasp. Rub twice, vigorously, then, holding the skin as taut as possible, quickly pull the strip straight upward, as close to the skin as possible, and follow by quickly placing the hand firmly on the area for relief. Finally, to finish that side, have the client lift the leg to the chest, grasping the ankle with the opposite hand, drawing the leg across the body. This should expose the last remaining third of the hair that was too near the table to apply the wax. This position also ensures that the skin is nice and taut. The wax is applied as before, downward, with the pull upward.

If the client is going to have a full leg wax or an upper leg wax and she can maintain this grasp for a little longer, it is an excellent position from which to remove the hairs from the top/back of the thigh, while the skin is tight. Halfway down the back of the thigh, the hair changes direction and grows across from the outside in and should not be removed in this position. One side of the bikini area should always be completed before going to the other side.

French Bikini Wax

Named for the high cut French style thong, this is the removal of everything, including the hair of the anus and labia, leaving only a strip of hair in the front, on the pubis. Follow all directions for a standard/American bikini wax (see preceding section), paying special attention to the cleaning and powdering of the areas to be waxed. The technician must wear gloves for this service. For removing the hair on the labia, hard wax is the preferred wax, as it grips the strong hair in this area while reducing the risk of injury to the delicate skin of the area. Because the hair grows inward toward the vaginal opening, the rules of soft wax requiring removing against the growth cannot be applied. Hard wax can be effectively removed in this area. The hard wax is applied in strips of 1 by 2 inch strips.

To remove the hair between the buttocks, there are two positions. Technicians and clients develop their own preferences.

The first position is to have the client lie flat on the back and raise the knees to the chest and turn the soles of the feet in together (see Figure 9–9). The client can grasp the feet between the legs with one hand, leaving the other hand free to move the panties aside. Although hard wax may be preferred in this area, strip wax can be used successfully. The wax is applied downward to a small section on the lowest, inside part of the buttock. The strip is placed over the wax, given two firm rubs and removed in the usual manner. The wax is then applied to the next section above and so on until the area on that side of the inside buttock is cleared of hair. The client should then switch hands, moving the panties to the opposite side, and grasp the feet with the other hand. Remove the hair in the same manner as on the previous side.

The second position for French bikini waxing is to have the client turn over and kneel (see Figure 9–10). With one forearm resting on the table in front of her, the client has a free hand to move the panties to one side and to help separate the buttocks. The area is then waxed in the same

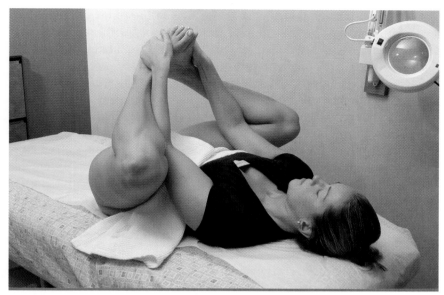

Figure 9–9 First position for the French bikini wax

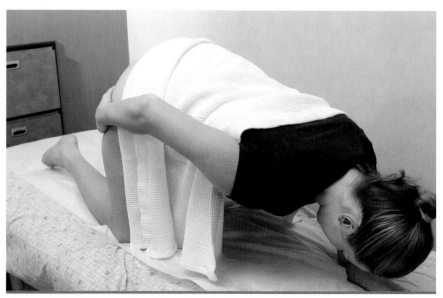

Figure 9–10 Second position for the French bikini wax

manner as the previous position (see above), except that the wax is applied from the side of the anus toward the vaginal opening. The client must switch hands when the technician is ready to switch to the other side of the inside of the buttocks.

The final part of the French bikini wax is the removal of the hair around the labia. This area should be waxed only with hard wax, and the application strips should be kept small, approximately 1 inch by 3 inches. There are experienced technicians who successfully use gentle soft waxes on the labia with small muslin strips, but training and experience on friends and colleagues is crucial before attempting it as a *paid for* service on the general public. Because the direction of hair growth on the labia is inward, the pull in this direction cannot be outward, against the growth, so the strip is pulled upward. A swift outward pull on the labia majorum *against* the hair growth could result in a laceration in the crevice between the labia majorum and labia minorum, which is distressing for the client and technician and could result in possible litigation. (See Figure 9–11.)

Brazilian Bikini Wax

The Brazilian bikini wax is the removal of absolutely everything. For the Brazilian bikini wax, the hair is removed as described for the French bikini wax (see preceding section), including the area between the buttocks and the labia. In addition, the hair on the pubis is removed. Because of the direction of hair growth, the coarseness of the hair, and the delicate skin of the labia, hard wax should be used for this area. Explain to the client that blood spots may appear and are to be expected. With any first-time bikini wax, advise the client to return within three weeks for a follow-up wax. After that the client should space waxing service every 4 to 6 weeks.

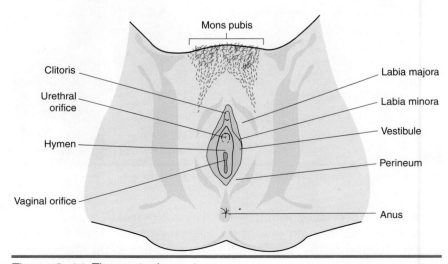

Figure 9–11 The vaginal opening

All traces of wax should be removed at the end of the service using plenty of soothing antiseptic lotion. Salicylic acid can be applied with cotton to the front aspects, but it may sting uncomfortably if applied to the labia, and can be applied the next day. This helps remove any redness and bumps and reduces the risk of ingrown hairs.

Legs

In this area soft wax is the preferred wax for its speed and effectiveness and the fact that the skin of the extremities is usually not as delicate as the face. Also, the hair is already a terminal type of hair and not likely to be made worse by waxing with soft wax, and the client may indeed experience slow and softer regrowth. There is considerable difference between half leg waxes that include a half upper leg or a half lower leg. The hair of the upper leg may be less dense when compared to the lower leg, but a larger surface area still must be covered, taking more time and using more wax than the lower leg. This should be reflected in the cost of the service and the time allowed for the hair removal. Additionally an upper leg wax or a whole leg wax does not include the bikini area, which usually involves an additional cost.

If the whole leg is to be waxed, the legs should be prepared by having the client lie supine (flat on the back) with the legs flat on the table. If the client has poor mobility in the hips and cannot turn the legs inward or outward very easily while lying on the back, it may be easier to first position the client lying prone (face downward), with the feet off the end of the table. This position supports the hip and offers a better range of motion to the client. Mist or spritz the top area with an antiseptic lotion, then dust the entire area with powder. Have the client bend the knees and place the soles of the feet on the table, and then apply the lotion and powder as far underneath as possible. To prepare the limbs, it is faster and more enjoyable for the client if the technician works simultaneously by spraying the cleaner on both limbs and wiping in sequence up the limbs with both hands, finishing at the fingers or toes. Wipe any excess moisture off with two tissues, one in each hand, and dust the legs with powder. The client can now straighten the legs. If the feet and toes are to be waxed with the leg wax, this is a good time to wax them. Make sure the area to be waxed is warm. If the feet are cold, the wax will remain behind and not lift off with the strip. Apply the wax to the top of the nearest foot, applying it downward, toward the toes. Quickly apply the strip, before the wax cools, and quickly pull it off, as close to the skin as possible. Muslin works better in this area as the Pellon may pull apart and leave the wax behind. End the pull with immediate pressure to the area. If there is very little hair on the toes, the wax on the strip may be sufficient to remove those hairs simply by pressing the wax onto the hair and quickly pulling away, making sure that the pressure is in the direction of growth and the pull is in the opposite direction. Once the foot has been cleared of the hair, start on the inside lower leg at the bottom, by the ankle. Dip the spatula well into the wax so that approximately 3 inches of the spatula are coated in wax. Scrape excess wax off the underside of the spatula, then hold it at a 45-degree angle, and start at approximately 7 inches up from the ankle. Glide the spatula downward with the hair growth for the same 7 inches using the edge of the spatula, allowing a thin layer of wax to slide off it and onto the leg. Apply the strip, leaving enough of a free edge to grab and rub twice in the direction of growth and remove in the usual manner, against the hair growth and close to the skin. Apply immediate and firm pressure. The next application should be directly above the previous one, proceeding in the same manner until the knee is reached. Return to the bottom of the leg and begin the process again, this time applying the first strip of wax to the area just to the inside of the shinbone. Continue removing the hair in the usual manner, in sections moving up the leg, again stopping at the knee. Rotate the foot as necessary to work on each side of the leg.

To wax the knees, have the client bend the leg, putting the foot flat on the table. This area has coarse patches of dry, dead skin cells as well as folds of skin on some clients. This position ensures that the skin is tight. Apply the wax in downward, outward sections, from the middle of the knee to the lower half. Apply the strip, rub downward, and remove quickly upward, working around the knee. Next, apply the wax to the top part of the knee in a downward direction to the middle. Apply the strip, rub, and remove it against the growth.

After the knee is completed, move to the upper leg. If the upper leg is not going to be waxed, move to the other side. It helps to move the wax around to the opposite side on a cart if unable to reach over. To wax the upper leg, the technician stays at the original side and has the client lower the leg back downward. When waxing this area, it is very important that the skin is held taut with every pull. The skin on the thigh is often looser than the lower leg, and there are often more folds of skin around the knee, behind the knee, and on the back of the thigh. The direction of hair growth on the upper leg is downward in the middle and outward on either side. Begin by waxing the middle, applying the wax in a downward direction, toward the knee. When the middle section is cleared of hair, the outer thigh should then be waxed in sections starting downward, toward the knee. The wax is applied starting at the middle, going outward. Apply the strip and rub over it in an outward motion. Holding the skin very taut is especially important in the outer thigh area, for the client's comfort, as well as to minimize bruising. The strip is then pulled in the opposite direction, back toward the center. This procedure is continued up the outside of the thigh to the point where there is no hair growth at the top.

At this point, the client should bend the leg, bringing the knee outwards to the same position used for a bikini wax. Starting down near the knee, the wax is applied from the middle outward. Be careful not to go too far down toward the table, because enough room must be left to hold the skin taut for the pull back upward. Another reason is that the hair at the back of the thigh changes direction, growing up, toward the buttocks, and the flesh from the back of the thigh may be pushed forward when the client is lying on the back. Before pulling the strip upward, make doubly sure that the skin is held as taut as possible. This is an area that can bruise easily if the pull is not swift and clean. Complete the sections of the inner thigh up to the bikini, but not the bikini area, unless that is part of this service.

At this time, ask the client to bring the knee to the chest, if able, grabbing the leg behind the knee. This tightens the skin on the back of the thigh, allowing the removal of the hair back there with less discomfort. This works well for clients who may be overweight or have loose skin. Only the hair growing straight toward the buttocks should be removed in this manner. Any hair growing across the back of the thigh should be removed with the client lying prone. After completing the inner thigh, move to the opposite side and continue removing the hair in the same manner as the first side. When the hair removal of the front and sides of both legs is completed, lotion should be applied to the waxed areas, removing any remaining wax, so that the client does not stick to the paper when turning over. More powder should also be applied at this time, especially if the client has been perspiring.

The hair generally grows across the calf from the outside inward with the growth pattern changing behind the knee. Start at the bottom of the lower leg, applying the wax from the outside inwards in the direction of growth and removing against the growth, and continue up the calf in the same manner to the back of the knee. Generally, the hair also crosses from the outside of the thigh growing toward the inner thigh for the first one-half to two-thirds of the thigh. At the top, it often changes direction, growing straight upward, toward the buttocks. Some clients may have a spiraling hair growth pattern on the back of the thigh. Clearly evaluate the hair growth directions, and wax following the standard rule for soft wax application and removal. When all hair has been removed from both legs, pamper the client by applying plenty of lotion and using gentle effleurage movements. Massage and soothe the legs using upward movements up the middle and a little lighter stroking down the outside. The half-leg treatment should take approximately 30 minutes.

effleurage
a rhythmic, gentle stroking of the skin, often just using the fingertips, which does not attempt to move the muscle underneath

■ WAXING FOR MEN

The areas male clients most commonly choose to have waxed are the back, the shoulders, between the eyebrows, and the outer ear. Some, especially swimmers or body builders, have the chest and legs waxed, too. Occasionally, male clients enter the salon dressed as women and request more extensive waxing. Men requesting sex-change operations are often required to go through psychiatric testing and are asked, before succumbing to major surgery, to live and dress as women for a period of time. Eventually, these clients may opt for hormone therapy, laser treatments, and/or electrolysis prior to male to female transgender surgery. Until then, however, they may choose to have much of the torso hair waxed away, along with the arm and leg hair. These situations may be awkward for the technician, but they are also awkward for those requesting the services. Confidence, compassion, and professionalism from the technician are paramount. Clearly ascertain from clients which hair they would like to have removed, and clearly explain to the clients what can and cannot be done as well as what the clients can expect.

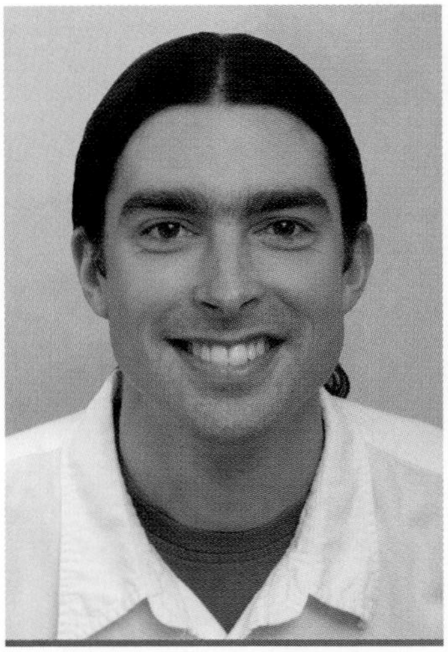

Eyebrows

Most of the time, with men, it is just the glabellar area, often called the "unibrow," that needs waxing (see Figure 9–12). Occasionally, a little tweezing under the brow is warranted. Often, the brow hairs are long and unruly, and trimming them with scissors can make a big difference in their appearance. Men's eyebrows should not be waxed in the same way women's eyebrows are waxed. Men often do not want a sophisticated look but a more natural look that is simply well groomed. Men do not expect high arches.

To wax and groom men's eyebrows, cleanse, pretreat, and powder the client's eyebrows in the usual manner. Offer the client a handheld mirror and discuss the shape, what should be removed, and what should stay. Using a small amount of wax on the end of a thin, wooden applicator, isolate the hairs under the brow that should be waxed off. Apply the wax in the direction of growth. Apply the strip, also rubbing in the direction of growth, and quickly pull away, against the growth. After completing both eyebrows, move to the center. For men, the eyebrow should always start just to the inside of the corner of the eye; everything else in the glabellar area can be waxed away. Most of the hair in the glabellar area grows upwards, but there may also be a significant amount of hair at the top of the nose that grows downwards, and should also be removed following the appropriate guidelines. (See Figure 9–13.)

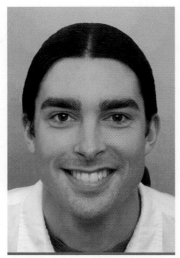

Figure 9–12 Before waxing eyebrows

Figure 9–13 After waxing eyebrows; note the masculinity is maintained

Backs

When men book back waxes, they generally want all the hair removed from just below the waistband upward. If the client is wearing a business suit and will be returning to work, suggest that he remove his pants and upper clothing. Provide a hanger on which to hang the clothes and a towel or drape to place around the waist. Leave the room while the client changes. If the client does not need to remove his pants, have him at least remove the belt from his pants for comfort, then have him lie prone on the table. His arms should be upward, with the elbows sticking outward. The client should rest the side of the face on the tops of the hands. Place two paper towels along the top edge of the client's pants. If the hair is longer than 1/2 inch, it should be trimmed (see Figure 9–14). If using an electric trimmer, cover the wax pot or trim the hair well away from the wax to prevent "fly aways" from entering the pot. Stand on the same side on which the wax is going to be applied, changing sides after that half is completed. Gloves should be worn for this service, because blood spots are inevitable. Warn the client that he will feel a cold spray, then spray the area with a mild antiseptic solution. Wipe off any excess moisture with a paper towel, and dust with powder.

Begin the hair removal at the area just above the waistband of the pants. Soft wax is the preferred wax for this area due to its speed and effectiveness. The first application of wax should begin from the outside edge of the torso where the hair growth starts (see Figure 9–15). Using a large spatula, dip into a full pot of wax until one-half to two-thirds of the spatula is covered. Remove the spatula, scraping the underside of the

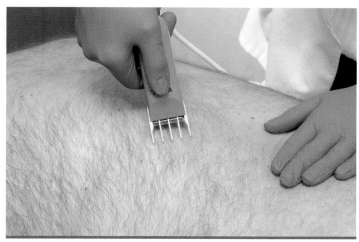

Figure 9–14 Position, placement, and preparation of a client for back waxing

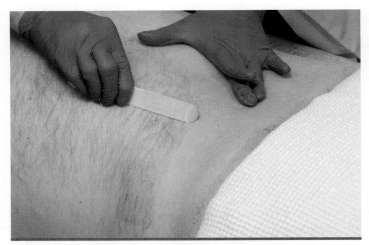

Figure 9–15 Initial wax application to back

spatula on the side of the pot or on the scraping rim that is provided. Using the edge of the spatula, glide inward, following the direction of hair growth toward the base of the spine, allowing a thin layer of wax to cover the area. Apply the strip, leaving a 1 inch free edge at the farthest end. Rub the strip twice in the direction of growth, and then, with the free hand placed over the base of the spine holding the skin taut, quickly pull backward and downward against the growth and as close to the skin as possible. It is important to follow the movement through, in a downward motion, to where the hair growth started. Quickly apply firm pressure with the free hand. The next application should be right next to the preceding one. If the length of the strip will be too long to do in one try, remove the strip on the outside first. The second strip should be toward the middle, the third strip to the side of the first, and the fourth strip above the third, going to the middle. Continue on in this manner until reaching the top. At the top, the hair starts to grow downward in the center, along the spine. Complete the removal on that side by following the waxing rules and directional changes.

At this time, include the back of the shoulder if it is requested. When that side is complete, move to the other side of the table and repeat the process. With the gloves still on, apply plenty of soothing antiseptic lotion to the area that was waxed. Be careful not to extend beyond that, because there may be a few more strips to do with the client sitting up. A cool compress soaked in a baking-powder solution can also be applied for a few minutes. It is not unusual for hives to develop in this area, though they will subside in an hour or so. Applying an over-the-counter salicylic acid product to the area will help reduce the redness and bumps. Because the client cannot see the back, the technician must let the client know when the blood spots have diminished and when it is safe to get dressed. Do not let the client risk getting blood spots all over his clothing.

The client should now sit on the edge of the table, facing the technician. At this time, with the arms at his side, the rest of the shoulder area can be waxed and any blending toward the front can be done, making sure both sides are balanced and even. The shoulders are waxed in a similar manner to the knees, one surface area or plane at a time, without attempts to round a curve with the strip. The hair on the shoulder usually grows inward to the center of the shoulder from the back, and inward toward the center from the front. Waxing the front is considered a separate service (part of the chest wax), but blending a little with wax already on the strip is acceptable.

Chest

Before waxing a man's chest, have the client sit on the side of the table and discuss which areas he would like cleared of hair. Some men book this service wanting abdominal hair or hair in front of the shoulders removed right up to the chest area but leaving the hair on the chest (i.e., above and between the breasts) intact. Make sure the task is clearly understood. Gloves should be worn for this service because blood spotting is likely. For this service, the client should be lying supine. Stand at the side of the table for the side that is being worked on, changing sides after that half is completed.

When waxing a man's chest, the hair must be approximately 1/2 inch long. If it is longer than that and curly, it should be trimmed to 1/2 inch long. When trimming the hair with an electric trimmer, trim it well away from the wax, or cover the pot, because the hair will "fly" into the wax pot. After trimming the hair, warn the client that he will feel a cold spray. Spritz or wipe the entire area with a mild antiseptic solution. Wipe away any excess with a paper towel, and dust the area with powder. Soft wax is the preferred wax for this due to its speed and effectiveness. The first application of wax should begin on an outer edge, working upward and inward, toward a denser area. The wax should always be applied in the direction of hair growth, rubbed in the direction of the hair growth, and removed against hair growth. A large strip should be used. As the area becomes dense, the wax applications should be in smaller strips, applying immediate pressure after each pull. On completion, soothe the entire area with aftercare lotion.

Ears

The hair on the outer rim and lobes of the ear can be waxed but not hair inside the ears. Men often trim ear-lobe hair with scissors, leaving it bristly. Waxing the hair will result in much softer regrowth. To wax the earlobes and ear rim, have the client lie supine or assume a semireclined position. Cleanse and dry the area. Both hard and soft waxes are effective in this area. With hard wax the applications are small, following the usual guidelines for hard wax, or the manufacturer's recommendations, starting at the top of the rim. Hold the top of the rim for the removal downward. With soft wax the wax is applied to the lobe in a downward direction with a narrow stick; then a small strip is placed over the area. The *earlobe* must then be held taut with the free hand, and the strip pulled quickly upward. Proceed to the area above. Apply the wax in a downward motion along the rim. Apply the strip, again rubbing downward. Holding the top portion of the lobe taut, pull quickly upward, against the growth. After completing the second ear, soothe the area with lotion, massaging both earlobes simultaneously for a more pleasurable end to the service.

When mastered, 10 minutes should be more than enough time for this service.

■ POSTTREATMENT CARE

After the hair removal, any residual stickiness should be removed with a soothing wax-removal lotion, which most wax companies manufacture and distribute. Massage the area very gently to avoid further stimulation.

Swelling may result due to the trauma of waxing, mainly on the upper lip, more so with strip wax than with hard wax. Swelling can be treated with ice in a bag or with cold stones immediately following the service.

Hives can also occur, which is a histamine reaction. Hives can be avoided the next time if the client takes Benedryl® or a similar product before the service. Many wax companies sell complementing aftercare soothing products. Another form of aftercare that can be used is salicylic acid, which can sting on initial contact with the skin but then takes away redness in 15 to 20 minutes. For areas that look particularly tender, a cool compress can be made by soaking a clean towel or cotton in a solution made of a tablespoon of baking soda and a pint of water with ice. The compress can be applied to the area for 10 minutes and then removed with any residue. For clients who are prone to breakouts after facial waxing, high-frequency treatments can be applied by a licensed aesthetician. If the equipment is readily available, applying a cataphoresis treatment will help soothe the skin, reduce the redness, and close the pores.

Clients should not take hot baths or use hot tubs the remainder of the day after the service.

Avoid tanning (sun or booths) for at least 24 hours postwaxing or until all erythema has subsided.

histamine
a normal substance found in the body that is released from injured cells

Posttreatment Care

Remove stickiness with a soothing wax removal lotion, massage in gently without causing further stimulation.

Treat erythema and bumps with salicylic acid.

Treat swelling with ice bag or cold stones.

Apply cataphoresis if available to close the pores and soothe the skin.

Give client posttreatment guidelines: Avoid tanning and hot tubs for 24 hours. Avoid makeup and perfumes until signs of trauma or irritation have passed.

Book the client's next appointment.

Sunless tanning products should not be applied to the skin for 24 hours or until signs of waxing have disappeared.

Clients should not apply perfumed products to the area that was waxed for at least 24 hours.

Conclusion

Waxing continues to be a popular and affordable method of temporary hair removal, even with the growing popularity of laser. Manufacturers continue to try to improve the wax by making waxes that are gentler to use on more delicate areas in response to the needs and wants of clients who use skin care that compromises the delicate epidermal tissue or who use the increasingly popular Brazilian bikini waxes. While strides have been made in this regard, and strip waxes are promoted as kinder and safer for the most delicate skin, hard waxes may be the better option. Protocol as laid out in this chapter should continue to be followed to avoid unnecessary trauma with either type of wax. The rules for hard and soft wax application and removal are generally accepted worldwide; however, the technician should also consider the manufacturer's guidelines listed on packaging or included separately. It is also important to know all the regulations required by the state board for waxing and to adhere to those regulations. There is nothing more unnerving for a technician than causing trauma or injury to a client during a waxing service. It is distressing for the client, who must live with scabbing and/or bruising for a number of days, and if the service was booked before an important occasion, it causes further distress and embarrassment at that event. The technician can apologize profusely, offer remedies, and provide the service without charge. While these are appropriate gestures, they will not undo the damage.

Certainly, some clients may be unaware of their skin care product ingredients and are willing to assume the risk; others may fail to accurately report certain factors that may contraindicate the service, but this is out of the technician's control. As long as a full initial consultation has been given to every client, follow-up questions asked at *every* return visit, and a release signed at every visit, the technician is somewhat assured that a correctly applied service will be without adverse effects, other than short-term redness. When protocol and procedures are followed, negative incidences and reactions are considerably reduced, and the waxing services will be satisfying.

▶ ▷ ▷ TOP 10 TIPS TO TAKE TO THE CLINIC

1. Correct positioning and posture prevents injury to both client and technician.

2. Eyebrow waxing is not just about hair removal but also about creating an illusion and balance.

3. While waxing eyebrows and the upper lip is acceptable, waxing the chin is not advisable.

4. The safest and most suitable wax for a French or Brazilian bikini wax is hard wax.

5. Hard wax is applied initially against and then immediately with the direction of hair growth, and is removed with the growth.

6. Soft wax is applied with the growth and removed against the growth.

7. Technicians should wash hands before and after each client.

8. Gloves should be worn for waxing services and discarded at the end of the service.

9. Appropriate draping is an important part of the service.

10. Communication is vital to avoid waxing away more than is desired.

BIBLIOGRAPHY

Milady's Standard Comprehensive Training for Estheticians. (2003). Clifton Park, NY: Milady, an imprint of Thomson Delmar Learning.

Milady's Standard Cosmetology. (2004). Clifton Park, NY: Milady, an imprint of Thomson Delmar Learning.

Bickmore, H. (2003). *Milady's Hair Removal Techniques.* Clifton Park, NY: Milady, an imprint of Thomson Delmar Learning.

http://www.fda.gov

Threading and Sugaring

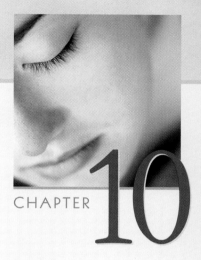

CHAPTER 10

KEY TERMS

epilepsy	khite	threading
fatlah	phlebitis	thrombosis
hemophilia	psoriasis	

LEARNING OBJECTIVES

After completing this chapter, you should be able to:

1. Discuss the history of threading.

2. Define the benefits of providing threading.

3. Prepare sugaring formulations.

4. Know how sugaring is applied and removed.

5. Discuss how sugaring has evolved in the United States to meet our demands for speed, efficiency, and economics.

INTRODUCTION

threading
method of hair removal using strands of thread

khite
Arabic word for threading

fatlah
Egyptian word for threading

Threading, also known as "banding," is a method of hair removal that uses a looped and twisted cotton thread maneuvered by the technician's fingers. The most common area for using threading is the face. Although not as common as other means of hair removal, threading is worthy of mention in this book because it is a fast, inexpensive method of mass tweezing that does not cause trauma to the skin. It is a method of hair removal worth considering for individuals who have skin care treatments or use products that prohibit waxing. Threading is a technique that is difficult to self-teach, and thus should be learned from an experienced threader.

■ HISTORY OF THREADING

Threading is a hair removal technique that has been used for centuries in Middle Eastern countries such as Iran, Turkey, India, and Pakistan. In Arabic, threading is known as khite, and in Egyptian, fatlah. It is an inexpensive method of hair removal that is usually passed on from generation to generation. The technique is predominantly found in Asian, Indian, and Arabic neighborhoods, but is gaining popularity in many parts of the United States. For many clients, finding an experienced and skilled "threader" is like "finding gold."

Benefits of Threading

The benefits of threading, in the hands of a master threading practitioner, are multiple. Threading is mass tweezing, but is accomplished at a much faster rate. The results can also be compared to waxing, but without trauma to the skin. Because threading does not affect the skin, it is an effective method of hair removal for individuals who are unable to tolerate waxing on the face due to prescription and other product use (for example, Retin-A®, Differin®, alpha hydroxy acids) or facial treatments that cause negative reactions when waxing is used. The level of discomfort during threading treatment is usually less than electrolysis, but is similar to tweezing. Because the hairs are snagged faster than tweezing, the plucking sensation is more tolerable.

Threading is an inexpensive service to provide, requiring only the use of strong household cotton thread, an antiseptic pretreatment, and soothing aftercare. The speed of an experienced and skilled technician with the minimal product overhead equates to a good profit margin.

Preparation of Equipment and Treatment Area

The technician must use a new, clean, and sterile thread for each client. The thread loops can be preformed and placed in a UV sterilizer and then placed in a covered box. The client should be placed in the treatment chair lined with a fresh sheet, towel, or paper.

Preparation of Client

The technician should protect the client's hair by wrapping it to avoid snagging hairs on his or her head. After the hair is wrapped, the technician should thoroughly wash his or her hands. The area of the client's skin to be treated should be cleansed of makeup, wiped with a mild liquid antiseptic, and allowed to dry. Avoid using creams, as they will remain on the hair and reduce the gripping effectiveness of the threading.

Application of Threading Technique

The most popular areas for the threading technique are the eyebrows, the area above the eyebrow (up to the hairline), sideburns, sides of face, upper lip, chin, and the area under the jaw.

The thread used should be a strong cotton household thread, clean and sterilized. Thread length should range from 24 to 30 inches. Shorter lengths are easier to control when learning and developing the skill, and are also better for technicians with smaller hands. As the practitioner becomes more skilled, a larger loop of thread is more manageable. The two ends of the thread are knotted together forming a loop. The forefingers, middle fingers, and thumbs are placed through each end of the loop in a "cat's cradle" fashion. The loop should be twisted at one end approximately a dozen times. The twists are then coaxed into the center of the loop, making sure the knot is at one end near the fingers so it does not interfere with the twisting. Threading is done by placing the upper end of the twist under the unwanted hairs so that they hang over the twist, then quickly manipulating the twist upwards by spreading the lower fingers, thus entrapping or snagging the unwanted hairs and plucking them out. (See Figures 10–1 and 10–2.) This is followed by quickly spreading the upper fingers, thus moving the twist towards the lower fingers, dropping some of the plucked hairs. The technician then moves quickly to another area of unwanted hairs. The fingers must move rapidly across the area at a rate of one movement approximately every one-fourth of a second.

As the twist gets congested with hair, it inhibits the rapid movement of the twisting, so a new part of the loop should be twisted or a new thread used. After the service is complete, a soothing lotion should be applied to the skin.

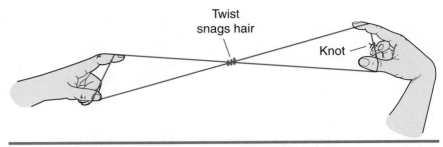

Figure 10–1 Two-handed threading

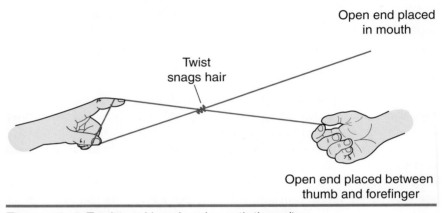

Figure 10–2 Traditional hand and mouth threading

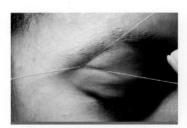

Figure 10–3 An example of threading

A second more traditional technique that many threading practitioners use is to put one end of the loop of thread in the practitioner's mouth gripped between the teeth and to maneuver the loop from just one end. This method is usually applied by threading practitioners when working on themselves. While the *idea* of this method may seem unhygienic to many, there have been no data to suggest that it is harmful to a client; however, one should check with the state's cosmetology or aesthetic regulatory board. (See Figure 10–3.)

Indications and Contraindications to Threading

An indication in the case of hair removal, as discussed previously in the text, is the sign, signal, or symptom that a problem exists and warrants treatment. Conversely, a contraindication points to signs, signals, or symptoms that alert us not to treat with a particular method or in a certain manner.

Table 10–1 Time Needed to Thread Specific Areas

Eyebrows	up to 15 min
Upper lip	10 min
Chin	10 min
Sides of face	20 min

The cost of the service should be approximately one-third less expensive than waxing.

The effect of regrowth with threading closely resembles that of waxing and tweezing.

Indications

The most popular areas for threading are on the face, including eyebrows, hairline, and upper lip, as well as between the eyebrows, along the jaw, under the chin, and on the sides of the face. (See Table 10–1.)

Contraindications

The foremost reason for not using a threading service is broken, irritated skin. Although no wax is applied to the skin with threading, the thread drags along the surface of the skin. Sunburned skin can also be aggravated by threading treatments. Clients with active eczema and psoriasis should not be treated unless the condition is dormant. Also, clients with an active

- Threading is a good alternative for clients who do not tolerate waxing on the face due to prescription and other product use (for example, Retin-A®, Differin®, AHA's) or wax treatments that cause a negative reaction.
- It is an inexpensive method of hair removal, requiring only the use of strong household cotton thread, an antiseptic pretreatment, and soothing aftercare lotion.
- Threading is a minimal product service, and when administered by an experienced practitioner, the service is achieved quickly (faster than tweezing) for a high profit.
- The discomfort level is usually less than electrolysis and waxing and is similar to tweezing, but the plucking sensation is faster and therefore more tolerable than tweezing.

herpes outbreak and visible lesions should not be treated unless the condition is dormant.

Downside to Threading

Threading is not an effective method of hair removal for large parts of the body. However, women in countries where threading is the predominant method of hair removal use the technique on their own legs and use the single-handed with mouth method for the arms.

Threading can be uncomfortable because the hairs are snagged out of the skin faster than tweezing, but slower than waxing. Depending on an individual's discomfort threshold or tolerance, threading may not be his or her preferred choice.

Another downside to threading is that, if not done with care and accuracy, the technician may also unwittingly remove vellus hair that was not problematic. Removing vellus hair may encourage it to grow back in an irregular fashion or become terminal hair, thus aggravating the hair growth situation. This is more of a concern when treating the upper lip, chin, sides of the face, and area under the jaw, but is generally not a concern for the eyebrows. One of the reasons the vellus hairs may transition is because of the way threading pulls the hair out (i.e., not in the direction of growth, but randomly and straight up), which means some of the follicles become distorted. The regrowth hair may stand up in a wispy fashion where it once was flat on the skin.

Last, as the hair grows back, there may be an increase of folliculitis, pustules, and inflammation that can cause pigmentation problems.

Conclusion to Threading

When performed by an experienced technician, the results of threading are very effective. A threading practitioner who knows what he or she is doing can beautifully shape eyebrows. Threading is a skill that takes practice to master, but is well worth the effort once learned. It is definitely a viable option for clients who are unable to tolerate waxing.

▪ SUGARING

Like threading, sugaring is an ancient method of hair removal that found its way to North America and is an increasingly popular method of hair removal. Customers like the idea of an ancient, well-utilized technique, as well as the fact that the sugar paste is 100 percent natural. As ancient as the sugaring method is, it is still employed in its original form around the world. However, the technique has evolved in the Western world with different aspects and consequences, which will be discussed in this section.

History of Sugaring

Sugaring is a method of hair removal used for centuries in the Middle East, North Africa, and the Mediterranean. Sugaring is believed to have been discovered as a form of hair removal in ancient times, possibly quite by chance, when sugar paste was used to treat a wound, to dress a burn, to prevent infections from developing, and to aid in healing. The removal of the paste would also remove the hair while leaving the skin with very little irritation. Ancient Egyptians believed body hair to be unacceptable and unclean and used shaving or tools like tweezers to remove the hair. Sugaring was a faster, less painful, and more effective method that also exfoliated the skin, leaving it smoother and without stubble. Because sugaring epilates the hair, the regrowth is softer and finer, so it is understandable that it has become a lasting and preferred method of hair removal around the region.

While sugaring techniques have remained basically unchanged in many regions, when the technique arrived in the United States, it started to evolve dramatically. Now there are two very different types of sugaring, just as with waxing: the applicator-applied/strip removal method and the hand-applied/nonstrip method. It is important to recognize the differences between these techniques as they have different effects on the skin and hair.

Manufacturers who have jumped on the sugaring bandwagon, due to its low production costs, have begun to distinguish themselves by "improving" the product with additives and promoting the faster method of using strips to remove the sugar paste and hair. The features of sugaring have now changed. With these "improvements" what was once a somewhat slow method that caused little distortion to the hair follicle by the way it was applied and removed is now applied in the same way as the strip method of soft waxing (applied with a spatula, covered with a strip, and removed by pulling in the opposite direction of growth). What was once, and still is, marketed as a gentler method of hair removal that causes little irritation to the skin is now sold in jars and cans along with a multiple array of soothing lotions and gels for aftercare relief, while the original method required only a warm, moist cotton or cloth for aftercare. People using Retin-A® or AHA's may require more soothing agents because they are more prone to irritation.

Benefits of Sugaring

While sugaring has many benefits, those benefits are determined by the method of sugaring employed, mainly whether it is the hand-applied method or the spatula-applied method. These two application methods will be discussed individually and separately to illustrate the benefits of each method.

Benefits for Hand-Applied Method

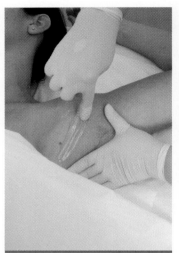

Figure 10–4 A client having sugaring

The foremost benefit of the hand-applied method of sugaring (see Figure 10–4) is that there is no risk of burning because it is applied at body temperature. Trauma is also reduced because no rosins are added to the natural hand-applied sugar paste, and consequently the paste does not adhere to the skin. The lack of adhesion to the skin means there is a minimal risk of bruising during the removal process. Because sugar paste does not adhere to live skin cells, it will only remove the hair and exfoliate the loose skin cells of the stratum corneum with minimal discomfort and trauma to the skin. The hand-applied sugaring method can be used safely on dry psoriasis and dry itch eczema. Because of the application temperature and the fact that it does not adhere to the skin like waxes containing resins, this treatment is considered to be safe to use on areas with varicose veins or spider veins. However, caution, common sense, and good judgment should be used with regard to these conditions. Because of the temperature and adhesion qualities, the same area can be treated more than once without risk of irritation or trauma. As there is no risk of burning or tearing the skin, this method is considered safe to use on individuals with diabetes, but a physician's approval should still be obtained and a medical release signed.

Because the sugar paste is applied by hand, the paste goes underneath and over the top of the hair gripping it from all sides, close to the follicular opening, so the hair length need be only 1/16 inch in length for the removal of virginal (previously untreated) hair. Because the hair is removed in the direction of growth, there is no distorting of the hair follicle or breakage of the hair at the follicle opening. The regrowth hair is often lighter, softer, and less dense. Another benefit to the client is that the sugar paste has natural antiseptic properties, which inhibit bacterial growth, causes less irritation, and reduces possible breakouts in the days following the service. Because the sugar paste is not reused on other clients, it is an extremely hygienic method of hair removal. The final treatment-related benefit is that the sugar paste is water soluble, therefore making the clean-up for the client easy and gentle.

The easy clean-up of sugar paste is also beneficial to the technician. Equipment, walls, floors, and treatment tables can be easily wiped down with hot water, following with the usual disinfectant and sanitizer. Another benefit for the technician is that the sugar paste is relatively inexpensive, especially if "homemade."

Downside for Hand-Applied Method

While there are many benefits to the hand-applied sugaring method, there are a few significant downsides. The primary downside is that the method is slow and time consuming to perform, especially on larger areas. It is not a preferred method for larger body areas like the legs and back. There is some minimal discomfort similar to, but not as uncomfortable as, waxing. Folliculitis and ingrown hairs may result. However, the risk of these conditions is considerably less with the nonstrip sugaring method than with both the spatula-applied sugaring method and waxing methods.

Benefits for Spatula-Applied Method

The most important benefit to the spatula-applied method is that there is no risk of burning (provided it has been tested) because it is applied at a cooler temperature than hot wax. Unlike the hand-applied method, the spatula method is much faster to accomplish, therefore making it more practical for treating larger areas. As with the sugar paste used in the hand-applied method, the paste will not adhere to live skin cells and will only remove the hair and exfoliate loose skin cells of the stratum corneum with minimal discomfort and trauma to the skin. This means it can be used safely on dry psoriasis and dry itch eczema. However, this is *only* the case if the sugar paste is resin free and 100 percent natural. Some manufacturers add resins to "improve" the product, but in doing so take away many of the advantages of sugaring. Because of the temperature and adhesion qualities of sugar paste (providing it is resin-free), the same area can be treated more than once without the risk of causing irritation and trauma. Regrowth hair is lighter, softer, and less dense. As with the hand-applied sugar paste, clean-up of the equipment, walls, floors, and treatment table is easy because the sugar paste, if resin-free, is water soluble. This also means easy clean-up for the client. Like the hand-applied method, the sugar paste has natural antiseptic properties, inhibiting bacterial growth, and is hygienic because the sugar paste is not reused on other clients.

Downside to Spatula-Applied Method

The first and most important downside to the spatula-applied method is the risk of burning, because it is applied with a spatula and not by hand. The sugar paste must be tested for appropriate temperature prior to the application. There is some discomfort with this method, similar to waxing in sensation. As the sugar paste is removed against the hair growth,

The Differing Benefits of Sugaring Techniques

- There is a minimal risk of bruising because the sugar paste does not adhere to live skin cells and pull at the skin during removal.
- Because of the application temperature and the fact that it does not adhere to the skin like waxes containing resins, sugaring is considered safe to use on areas with varicose veins or spider veins. However, caution, common sense, and good judgment should be used with regard to these conditions.
- Because the sugar paste does not adhere to live skin cells, the paste will only remove the hair and exfoliate the loose skin cells of the stratum corneum with minimal discomfort and trauma to the skin, and can be used safely on dry psoriasis and dry itch eczema.
- Because of the temperature and adhesion qualities, the same area can be treated more than once without the risk of causing irritation and trauma.
- As there is no risk of burning or tearing the skin, sugaring is considered safe to use on individuals with diabetes. However, a physician's approval should be obtained and a medical release signed.
- The hair length need be only 1/16 inch in length for removal for previously untreated hair.
- Regrowth hair is lighter, softer, and less dense.
- Easy clean-up of the equipment, walls, floors, and treatment table is possible because the sugar paste is water soluble.
- Clean-up is easy for the client.
- Natural antiseptic properties, which inhibit bacterial growth, are present.
- This method is hygienic because the sugar paste is not reused on other clients.
- This method of hair removal is inexpensive if the sugar paste is homemade.

hair may grow back in a more unruly fashion, not lying close to the skin, also causing folliculitis and ingrown hairs.

Sugaring Paste

The sugar paste is formed by mixing sugar, water, lemon juice, gum (Arabic or ovaline from the acacia tree), and heating it until a syrup is formed.

Table 10–2 Recipe for Sugaring Paste

Recipe for Sugar Paste

Ingredients:

2 cups sugar

1/4 cup lemon juice

1/4 cup of water

All ingredients should be combined and slowly cooked over a low heat. The mixture should not be heated above 250°F. Use a candy thermometer to read the temperature accurately. The mixture should cool in a glass jar. It should be used at body temperature when applied by hand, or can be warmed in a microwave or in a bowl standing in hot water when applied with a spatula.

This is a home kitchen recipe. The results from this recipe are not guaranteed by this publication.

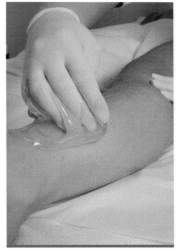

Figure 10–5 The hand application of sugar paste

The gum is beneficial to the consistency, if readily available; if not it is often omitted in home recipes. (See Table 10–2.) For hand-applied methods the sugar paste mixture should not be too runny; one should be able to manipulate it into a ball. For sugaring using a spatula or strip, the paste can be thin, but still not too runny, and should have a consistency similar to molasses. Most sugar paste made and used in the Middle East is 100 percent natural. However, companies are now manufacturing what they call sugaring paste, but they add resins to their product, which causes confusion as it is not true sugar paste if resin is added. When 100 percent natural, the sugar paste is considered hypoallergenic and is not irritating to the skin. However, some sugar paste brands may have added gums and resins along with fragrances, which may make it more irritating to the skin. It is important to read the product labels to check the ingredients listed.

APPLICATION TECHNIQUES OF SUGARING

There are two distinctly different sugaring methods: (1) application and removal by hand (see Figure 10–5), and (2) application by spatula (see Figure 10–6) and removal with a strip. While the techniques for spatula-applied sugaring are similar to those of spatula-applied waxing, the hand-applied sugaring method is unique.

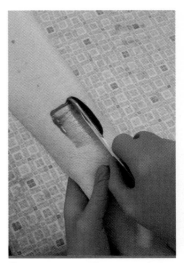

Figure 10–6 The spatula application of sugar paste

When hair removal is to take place on the face and the client has not had the service done in this area before, it is important to do a patch test first. This tests the client's reaction to the service and indicates whether the client should have the treatment within a day or two of an important engagement. Any reaction, particularly a histamine reaction, will appear almost immediately, and if microorganisms have been introduced to the vulnerable area, pustules may appear up to 48 hours after the treatment. The patch test is important mainly for clients with a known skin sensitivity or for those who have an important function coming up, especially if any resins have been added to the sugar paste used with the spatula method. The test should be done on the face but in an area less noticeable (for example, toward the front of the ear).

Application by Hand

Before the treatment begins, the technician should wash hands and apply latex or vinyl gloves. Some technicians doing the nonstrip method apply only one glove to the hand doing the stretching, not to the one handling the sugar paste because gloves make the paste awkward to handle. The gloved hand applies gentle pressure to the skin after each "flick," which may affect some people choosing sugaring as a service. The area to be treated should be cleansed with an antibacterial cleanser and should be free from dirt, makeup, and lotions in a manner similar to the preparation for waxing. The skin should feel warm to the touch for a more effective and comfortable treatment. If the skin is cool and goose bumps are causing the hair to stand upright, discomfort may be increased and some of the hairs may snap.

The area should be lightly dusted with a gentle powder that is free from chemicals, perfumes, and aluminum that could irritate the skin posttreatment. The powder will absorb any residual moisture, which will help make the treatment more effective.

The sugar paste is then manipulated into a ball. It should be pliable and easy to manage. The paste is pressed and pushed against the hair growth and back over the top followed by a quick flicking motion that is parallel to the skin, pulling the sugar paste off *in* the direction of hair growth. (See Figures 10–7 and 10–8.) If any hair remains behind, the sugar paste can be reapplied to the same area.

When the area is cleared, the same ball of sugar can be used to remove hair on the adjacent area, and so on, until the service is complete. The sugar ball can be used on the same client throughout the duration of the service or until it becomes so congested with hair that it is rendered ineffective, in which case a new ball of sugar paste is put into use. The sugar paste can be used on the face and later on the body but not vice versa at the

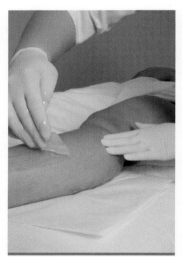

Figure 10–7 The manual removal of sugar paste

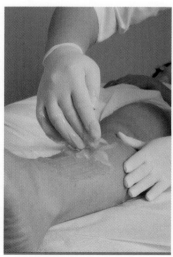

Figure 10–8 The manual removal of sugar paste

risk of cross contamination and the potential risk of an outbreak of pustules on the face. For obvious hygiene reasons, the sugar paste should be disposed of after the service and not reused on another client.

Application by Spatula with Strip Removal

Application by spatula is done in the same fashion as hot wax: apply in the direction of hair growth, apply the muslin or Pellon strip over the top, rub in the direction of growth, and quickly pull away against the growth close and parallel to the skin (see Figure 10–9). For a more detailed description of this technique, see Chapter 8. Some cans of sugar paste, especially those with added resins, require the temperature to be hotter than that of the ancient hand-applied method, and are therefore more like hot wax, and subject to the same guidelines, concerns, and contraindications of soft wax.

Posttreatment Care

Any remaining sugar paste (that is resin-free) can be removed from the client's skin with a warm moist washcloth on larger areas or moist cotton rounds on small areas. The client should not have to leave feeling sticky.

Clients who develop histamine bumps can take an antihistamine if they choose, but the technician must not supply antihistamine. Clients should be advised by the technician to refrain from using fragrances or deodorants on the treated areas and to avoid the sun or tanning booths for 48 hours after the service.

Clients can usually go 6 to 12 weeks between treatments, although this will vary between individuals and depending on the parts of the face

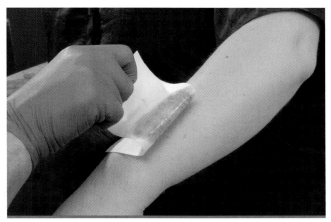

Figure 10–9 Removal of sugar paste using a muslin strip

and body treated. The more frequently clients are sugared as a method of hair removal, without using any other method in-between, the longer they will be able to go between services. Sugaring technicians regularly make the assertion that the time between each treatment may increase the more they use sugaring as their only method of hair removal.

Indications

Any area may be treated by sugaring (excluding nostrils, inner ears, genitals, and men's beards). Hair length with virgin hair growth of 1/16 inch can be sugared, and any area of previously shaved hair or coarser hair of 1/8 inch may be treated.

Contraindications for Hand-Applied Method

The contraindications for the hand-applied method include chapped or broken skin. Sunburned skin should not be sugared until the sunburned areas have healed completely. Pimples, pustules, moles, skin tags, and warts should be avoided. Certain conditions warrant physician approval, including phlebitis, diabetes, and hemophilia. Herpes and herpes simplex (aka cold sore) should not be sugared during an active outbreak. Clients who are frequently prone to herpes outbreaks can take prophylactic medication prior to their appointments. Pregnancy, particularly during the third trimester, can be contraindicated if the areas requiring sugaring take more than 20 minutes of the client lying flat on her back, in which case the client should wait until after the birth of the baby.

Contraindications for Spatula-Applied Method with Higher Temperature Wax

Because the removal process of the spatula-applied method of sugaring is performed against the direction of hair growth, it is not a good method of hair removal for the chin and sides of the face. Removing hair in this manner, over time, causes irregular regrowth. The hair grows back sticking up, and the vellus hair that once was perpendicular to the skin with a shallow follicle begins to grow at a deeper angle where it gets an increased blood supply. When this happens, the hairs regrow as terminal hairs, stronger, coarser, and with pigment. This condition becomes problematic because the hairs are required to be 1/8 inch in length before they can be removed again. When this happens, clients get into a frustrating cycle of hair growth, removal with possible erythema, and a possible rash. This is followed by a week or so clear of hair that is then followed by regrowth of previous hair removal treatments.

phlebitis
inflammation of the wall of a vein

hemophilia
recessive genetic disorder occurring almost exclusively in men and boys in which the blood clots much more slowly than normal, resulting in extensive bleeding from even minor injuries

Sugaring should not be performed over moles, skin tags, warts, pimples, pustules, or any broken or excoriated skin at the risk of injury or introduction of microorganisms. Herpes and cold sores should not be sugared during an active outbreak because of the risk of spreading the virus and also causing further injury. Prophylactic medication should be taken prior to service. If the skin shows signs of sunburn, it should not be sugared until the sunburned areas have healed completely. Likewise, inflamed, irritated, damaged, and compromised skin should not be treated.

Certain topical skin care treatments like glycolic peels, AHA's, Retin-A®, Accutane®, and Differin® compromise and affect changes to the epidermal tissue, so clients using any of these products should not be treated with the higher temperature sugar paste. Skin disorders such as eczema, seborrhea, and psoriasis may be treated with sugaring depending on the severity. Minimal flakiness of dead skin cells can be sugared, but not if the skin is broken. In mild cases, the skin may benefit from the exfoliating effects of sugaring, but in more advanced stages, broken skin could result. Therefore, it is imperative that technicians receive signed releases from clients prior to the service.

Scar tissue, including keloids, should not be sugared with this applicator method. While individuals prone to keloid scarring should not be sugared, clients who have a healed scar can receive sugaring in an adjacent area. Likewise, one should not sugar over varicose veins with this method of sugaring, especially if it is a higher temperature sugar paste and has added resins, at the risk of causing further injury to the vein, but the surrounding areas may be treated. Fractures and sprains should not be sugared until the area is completely healed. A technician should also avoid using this method for clients with other medical conditions such as phlebitis, thrombosis, and any circulatory disorder, as well as those prone to easy bruising, hemophilia, and diabetes. However, clients with diabetes may be able to be treated depending on the severity and the degree of healing, and should consult with their physicians, get written approval given, and sign a release. Regardless, a technician should never treat the lower extremities of a client with diabetes with this sugaring method. In addition, clients who experience a lack of skin sensation should not receive sugaring treatment. Likewise, clients with epilepsy can receive the service, but only with caution and physician approval and only if the epilepsy is controlled for a long period of time with medication. Because some epilepsy drugs cause a tendency for easy bruising, physician approval must be attained prior to the sugaring service. Technicians should receive a physician's note, and should have the client sign a release. Finally, clients who are pregnant should not receive this type of treatment if the areas requiring sugaring take more than 20 minutes of lying flat on her back.

psoriasis
skin disease marked by red scaly patches

thrombosis
formation or presence of one or more blood clots that may partially or completely block an artery, for example, flowing to the heart or brain or a vein

epilepsy
medical disorder involving episodes of abnormal electrical discharge in the brain characterized by seizures, convulsions, and loss of consciousness

Conclusion

Sugaring is an effective method for hair removal, and probably a better choice over hot strip wax for the face when using the hand application and removal method. The downside to hand-applied sugaring is that it takes more time than using either the spatula application method or waxing, making it more time consuming on larger areas and therefore not very cost effective. However, the product is cheaper to purchase or make, and, providing it is a 100 percent natural sugar paste, there is less need for costly cleaning agents and aftercare lotions. Care should be taken to read labels and choose the most suitable sugaring product.

▶ ▷ ▷ TOP 10 TIPS TO TAKE TO THE CLINIC

1. Threading is also known as banding.
2. There are two methods of threading: two-handed combination, or one-hand and mouth combination.
3. Threading is an excellent method of hair removal for clients using Retin-A®.
4. Threading offers a good profit margin with low product cost.
5. Hand-applied sugar paste is removed in the direction of hair growth.
6. Spatula-applied sugar paste may not be 100 percent natural, and may have resins added.
7. Spatula-applied sugaring shares many of the same contraindications as hot wax.
8. The contraindications for the spatula-applied method of sugar are different from the hand-applied method.
9. Specific conditions like diabetes and epilepsy require physician approval prior to the service.
10. Neither threading nor sugaring should be performed on clients with a herpes outbreak.

CHAPTER QUESTIONS

1. Name two benefits of threading.
2. Name two contraindications of threading.
3. Why is threading viable for people who cannot tolerate waxing?

4. In which direction is nonstrip sugar paste applied?

5. In which direction is spatula-applied sugar paste removed?

BIBLIOGRAPHY

Bickmore, H. (2003). *Milady's Hair Removal Techniques*. Clifton Park, NY: Milady, an imprint of Thomson Delmar Learning.

Milady's Standard Comprehensive Training for Estheticians. (2003). Clifton Park, NY: Milady, an imprint of Thomson Delmar Learning.

Alexandria Sugaring Company. Available at http://www.alexandriasugaring.com

Electrolysis

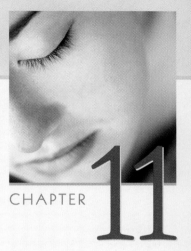

CHAPTER 11

KEY TERMS

acne vulgaris

alternating current

ampere

anaphoresis

anions

anode pole

blend method

cataphoresis

cathode pole

cations

circuit

circuit breaker

conductor

converter

cortisone

diathermy

direct current

electrologist

electrology

electrolysis

electrolysist

electrons

ethyl alcohol

fuse

galvanic electrolysis

grand mal

hydrochloric acid

hyperpigment

insulator

ionization

iontophoresis

isopropyl alcohol

milliampere meter

milliamperes

ohm

Ohm's law

petit mal

phoresis

point effect

rectifier

rheostat

steroid dependent dermatoses

thermolysis

transformer

volt

watt

LEARNING OBJECTIVES

After completing this chapter, you should be able to:

1. Understand the evolution of electrolysis.

2. Know the indications and contraindications for electrolysis.

3. Name the three modalities of electrolysis and explain how they work.

4. List the basic differences of various needles.

5. Understand theoretic electrolysis techniques.

6. Know how to provide appropriate pretreatment and aftercare, including advising clients on home care.

243

INTRODUCTION

This chapter covers the history and development of electrolysis and how it has evolved over the years into a widely used and accepted method of hair removal. Electrolysis is the only permanent method of hair removal recognized by the FDA and AMA. This chapter also deals with the three modalities of thermolysis, galvanic electrolysis, and the blend, and how those modalities work.

■ HISTORY OF ELECTROLYSIS

In 1869, ophthalmologist Dr. Charles E. Michel began to research a method of safely and permanently removing ingrown eyelashes from his patients' eyelids. Michel devised a method of inserting a surgical needle into the hair follicle that was connected to a dry cell battery by a conducting wire. After applying a measured amount of direct current, he observed that the hair did not regrow. In 1875, he documented and published his findings, and electrolysis was born as a method of permanent hair removal.

It was then quickly adopted as a method of treating not only ingrown eyelashes but unwanted facial hair. The process, while effective for one ingrown eyelash, was slow and laborious for facial hair. By 1916, Professor Paul Kree developed a more efficient method by using multiple needles at once. Galvanic electrolysis, which uses multiple needles, became the most popular method for decades following and was a major catalyst in the development of electrolysis as a profession for hair removal. A number of years later, in 1923, an article about the use of high-frequency current for hair removal was published by Dr. Henri Bordier of France. This application of high-frequency current became known as thermolysis due to the heat produced to destroy cells. High-frequency thermolysis was introduced as a much faster method of treating unwanted hair. However, with this method there seemed to be a higher percentage of regrowth, and its effectiveness greatly depended on straight, undistorted hair follicles as well as an accurate probe and insertion depth to ensure the destruction of the dermal papilla.

By 1938, Henri St. Pierre and Arthur Hinkle had introduced a methodology combining the best of galvanic and thermolysis modalities, which they called the "blend" technique. Galvanic and high-frequency electrolysis could be combined both alternately and simultaneously. The resulting technique was faster than the galvanic modality, not quite as fast as thermolysis, but more effectively destroyed the dermal papilla,

electrolysis
the use of an electric current to remove moles, warts, or hair roots

galvanic electrolysis
a modality of electrolysis using direct current with positive and negative poles that causes the production of caustic lye in the hair follicle, which in turn causes the hair's destruction

thermolysis
the breakdown of a substance by heat; as it pertains to electrolysis, used synonymously with diathermy

especially on distorted follicles. While thermolysis or diathermy is still the most popular modality used in other parts of the world, the blend method or technique has become the most accepted and popular method in the United States.

diathermy
a treatment accomplished by passing high-frequency electric currents to generate heat; as it pertains to electrolysis, used synonymously with thermolysis

Electrolysis, Is It Still a Valid Technique?

Electrolysis is as valid today as it ever was. There is a growing desire for a permanent solution to unwanted hair, as evidenced by the increasing popularity of laser hair removal. Individuals who find that their hair or skin color is unsuitable for laser hair removal or who have contraindications to the service can still achieve permanent results with electrolysis. While laser hair removal continues to improve, it offers permanent *reduction* but not necessarily permanent *removal*. For the remaining hairs that were not permanently removed, electrolysis provides the means for permanent removal.

Benefits of Electrolysis

Electrolysis is currently the only proven method of permanent hair removal recognized by the FDA, although it now recognizes that laser hair removal offers permanent *reduction*. Unlike laser hair removal, electrolysis can be performed successfully on all types of hair: blonde, dark, gray, straight, curly, vellus, or terminal. It can also be used effectively with all races and on all skin types: dry, oily, or mature.

Electrolysis can also be performed on all parts of the face and body, except for the inside of the nose or the inside of the ear, and is even used to treat the penile shaft prior to male-to-female transgender surgery.

Electrolysis is a method that can remove hairs with great precision, one at a time, making it a great choice for shaping eyebrows or softening a hairline. It can remove single offensive hairs on the chin, leaving the vellus hair intact, unlike waxing that strips everything in its path.

Downsides of Electrolysis

The most frustrating downside of electrolysis to many clients is that electrolysis requires the client to stop other forms of hair removal other than trimming or shaving on the areas to be treated, so the hairs will be long enough and visible enough to be treated. It is difficult for some people to allow hair to grow in before treatment. Electrolysis is seen as costly to some who consider tweezing as free. Many people do not appreciate the negative, long-term impact of tweezing, which is that when an offensive hair is tweezed often finer vellus hairs are caught up in the tweezers. Over a period of time with multiple tweezing, the vellus hairs begin to grow deeper as the follicles become distorted, and on reaching the richer blood supply the well nourished hairs begin to grow in as terminal hairs with pigment, exacerbating the problem. Clients believe that the hair they tweezed on their chin last week is the same one they are seeing this week, not realizing that the telogen stage of the hair in that area is 12 weeks; therefore the tweezed hair, removed at the root, will not reappear for three months. This also means that the client probably has a much greater hair growth problem than he or she realized.

Electrolysis can cause discomfort for some people. We all have different thresholds and tolerances for discomfort. As has already been discussed, there are products to minimize the discomfort, but for some individuals it is not enough.

When undertaking electrolysis for treating the unwanted hair, one needs to recognize that a protocol of regularly scheduled appointments has to be adhered to, so that the technician can recognize and treat the anagen hairs. Regularly scheduled appointments can be difficult for busy people. To succeed, electrolysis requires a commitment to the program of treatments and a temporary reorganization of time and priorities.

Electrolysis treatments can, like most methods of hair removal, cause redness (erythema), bumps, and swelling. This may influence when the client will schedule appointments. It may be difficult, for instance, for the client having to return to work, as makeup should not be worn for 24 hours after the treatment, which may be difficult for some women. The client should know that there are treatments like cataphoresis and products available to help soothe and camouflage the face. Extensive electrolysis work may take months, even years, to complete, not because of the skill of the technician, although this may be the case if the technician is not trained or is poorly trained. Rather, the work takes so long due to the stages of hair growth and the length of those stages, and other contributing factors like polycystic ovarian syndrome or medication that continually stimulates the follicle and causes excessive hair growth.

ELECTRICITY, ELECTROLYSIS, AND SAFETY

Electrolysis is a safe and effective method of hair removal when administered correctly. There have been tremendous strides and improvements made to electrolysis equipment in the past two decades, incorporating a more ergonomic design with new and improved safety features. For example, timing and intensity can be preset to cease the current flow

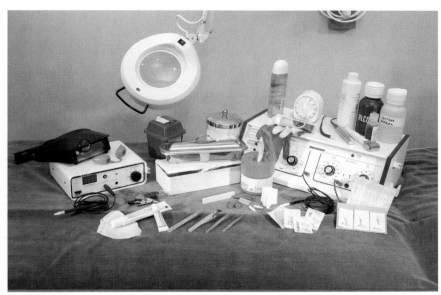

Figure 11–1 Electrolysis machines and supplies

after the set time, allowing for consistency. Of course, no matter how much improved the equipment has become, it is to no avail if the user does not follow the manufacturer's guidelines for placement, usage, and maintenance. It must be thought of first and foremost as a piece of electrical equipment. (See Figure 11–1.)

Basics of Electricity

To understand electrolysis one must first understand the basics of electricity, or electrology. Electrical energy, whether it is direct current (DC) used for galvanic electrolysis or alternating current (AC) used for thermolysis, destroys the dermal papilla in the hair follicle, resulting in permanent hair removal. A clear understanding of electricity ensures a better understanding of electrolysis equipment.

Electric energy can be produced through five main sources: friction, magnetism, heat, chemical reaction, and atomic reaction. The result of these five sources is the flowing of negatively charged particles called electrons along a pathway called a circuit, by means of a conductor. A conductor is a substance that allows the free, easy, unrestricted flow of electrons. Examples of good conductors are most metals, especially copper; steel electrolysis probes; saline (water and salt mixture); and the human body. An insulator inhibits or causes resistance to the flow of electrons. Examples of insulators are rubber, plastic, wood (dry), and glass. Hair is also a very poor conductor of electricity and does not

electrology
the general study of electricity and its properties

electrons
stable, negatively charged elementary particles that orbit the nucleus of an atom

circuit
route around which an electrical current can flow, beginning and ending at the same point

conductor
a substance that allows electricity to pass through it

insulator
a material or device that prevents or reduces the passage of electricity

withstand heat well, which is why electric tweezers are completely ineffectual as a method of permanent hair removal.

The flow rate of electrons can be measured by a unit called an ampere. In electrolysis, flow is measured in milliamperes. A milliampere is 1/1,000 of an ampere. The milliampere meter measures current in 1/1,000s of an ampere. The quantity of current flowing through a circuit is controlled by a rheostat, which is the intensity control dial on the epilator unit.

Other common electrical terms worth understanding when using electrical equipment include ohm, Ohm's law, volt, watt, rectifier, and converter. All of these terms are used when dealing with electricity.

An ohm is a unit that measures the amount of resistance, indicating whether a higher voltage is required to push a current through a conductor. Ohm's law is the requirement of 1 volt to push the current of 1 ampere through the resistance of 1 ohm; voltage = current × resistance. Volt refers to the force needed to send 1 ampere of electric current through 1 ohm of resistance. A watt is the unit measure of electrical power involving the flow of current along a conductor and the voltage; 1 kilowatt = 1,000 watts. A rectifier converts AC to DC, while a converter changes DC to AC. (See Figure 11–2.)

A transformer increases or decreases the voltage of AC. There are two types of electricity, based on electron flow: direct current and alternating current. Direct current (DC) is the flow of electrons in one direction, even and constant. Alternating current (AC) is the rapid flow of electrons, first in one direction, then in the opposite direction. An

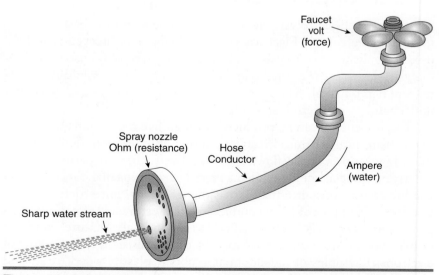

Figure 11–2 A diagram of watt including volt, ampere, and ohm

oscillating current is similar to AC except that oscillation has a higher frequency.

Safety Features

Certain safety features prevent electrical damage or injury. The first is a fuse. A fuse is a thin wire designed to hold a specific amount of electricity. If more than the desired amount of electricity flows through the fuse, which happens when too many appliances are plugged into the same outlet, the fuse wire overheats and breaks, discontinuing the flow of electricity along the circuit. When the fuse breaks, it must be replaced. Care should always be taken to make sure the correctly sized fuse is used and that the corresponding outlets are not overloaded with appliances generating more electricity than the outlet should handle.

The second safety device is the circuit breaker, which is used instead of a fuse. The circuit breaker works by throwing a switch when there is an overload of electricity, thereby discontinuing the flow of current. To restore the flow of current, one simply needs to flick the switch back on. However, one must first make sure that the elements that caused the circuit breaker to throw the switch are eliminated or sufficiently reduced.

Electrolysis equipment should always be plugged into its own socket with a grounded, three-pronged plug and surge protector. It should never be "stacked" into an adaptor with other electrical appliances, especially large appliances like refrigerators or air conditioners, or even microwave ovens. To do so could affect the even flow of current. If another appliance requires a surge of current, the result could be a reduction of electricity to the electrolysis equipment, requiring the operator to boost the current flow. As the surge ends, excessive current from the epilator could significantly damage the skin. The analogy is to being in the shower and having another water source (for example, another shower, dishwasher, or washing machine) divert hot water. The person in the shower turns up the hot water. When the other source cuts its hot water, there is a sudden burst of hotter water back in the shower, which can be startling and extremely uncomfortable.

Care of the Equipment

Safety for a technician means knowing your equipment, taking proper care of it and following manufacturer's directions for setup, use, and maintenance. As with all electrical equipment, the electrolysis unit should be properly grounded and plugged into an outlet designated for its use only and with no adjustments made to the plug. The unit should be kept away from direct heat (for example, sun or heaters) and should be kept well away from water. If a unit comes into contact with water, it

converter
a device used to change alternating current to direct current

transformer
a device that transfers electrical energy from one alternating circuit to another with a change in voltage, current, phase, or impedance

direct current
electric current that flows constantly in one direction

alternating current
electric current that regularly reverses direction

fuse
an electrical safety device that contains a piece of metal that will melt if the current running through it exceeds a certain level

circuit breaker
an automatic switch used in electricity to prevent the flow of electricity in an overload of electricity

should be turned off and checked for damage by a licensed electrician recommended by the unit's manufacturer. The unit should never be opened by an untrained or unlicensed electrician; to do so will invalidate any existing warranty.

The unit should be kept free of dust and have adequate ventilation. The cords should be kept untangled and away from items and edges that might weaken them or cause them to fray. Do not clean the unit with volatile chemical substances or water. Chemical substances can remove important markings, and water can enter the unit, damaging it internally. Instead the unit should be dusted each day and regularly wiped down with a *damp* cloth and mild disinfectant.

Bulb Test

A test bulb can be purchased from any electrolysis supply company. It works by clipping one clip to any metal portion of the electrolysis unit and the second clip to the metal portion at the end of the probe (with the plastic cap removed). The current is applied by depressing the foot switch. If the light bulb illuminates, the needle cord is working well.

If the bulb does not light up, there could be a rupture in the needle cord that is preventing the current from flowing freely to the tip of the needle. The needle cord needs replacing.

A busy electrolysis business should have a supply of replacement cords and even a backup epilator should a significant problem with the main epilator require shipping it across country for repairs.

■ TYPES OF PERMANENT HAIR REMOVAL

There are three modalities of permanent hair removal based on the type(s) of electric current that they use: thermolysis, which uses alternat-

---

Troubleshooting Problems with Electrolysis Equipment

If the unit does not appear to be working, there are certain steps that should be taken before a call is made to the manufacturer or an electrician. (See Table 11–1.) Going through the checklist first will save time, as the electrician or manufacturer will probably ask the same questions, and the problem may get resolved before the call needs to be made.

Table 11–1 Troubleshooting Electrolysis Equipment

No current is being produced at the probe.

- Is the epilator plugged in and turned on?
- Is the epilator receiving power from the outlet? If not, check the outlet with another appliance.
- Does a fuse need replacing, or has a switch flipped at the circuit breaker?

The power indicator light is on, but no current is producing at the tip.

- Are all dials (rheostat) where they should be?
- Is the foot switch connected properly to the epilator?
- Is the needle holder cord properly connected to the epilator?

There is still no current.

- Does the indicator light come on when depressing the foot switch? If the light fails to come on, the problem is with the foot switch or the foot switch cord or adaptor that plugs into the epilator. If the light does come on, the foot switch is working and the problem lies elsewhere, possibly in the needle holder or the handheld electrode or their respective cords and adaptors. Further isolate the problem by eliminating the handheld electrode, unplugging it, and switching it to thermolysis mode.
- Does the probe produce current in thermolysis mode? If yes, the problem was with the handheld electrode and most probably the cord, which should be replaced. If no current is produced at the probe in thermolysis mode, then there is a very good chance that the problem lies with the needle holder or the cord. The needle holder and cord should be replaced and retested. It is always worth having spare cords to prevent having to cancel clients, which inconveniences those clients and sacrifices revenue. If there is still no current at the probe in thermolysis mode, then an additional test can be done with a small light bulb.

ing current, galvanic electrolysis, which uses direct current, and the blend method, which combines alternating and direct currents simultaneously or sequentially.

Thermolysis

Thermolysis, also called diathermy, shortwave, and radio wave (the same waves as in microwave ovens), is a method that uses AC to produce oscillating radio high-frequency waves. The high-frequency current oscillates in a range of 3 to 30 megahertz, or 3,000,000 to 30,000,000 cycles per second. The Federal Communications Commission (FCC) has assigned three frequencies for use: 13.56 megahertz, 27.12 megahertz, and 40.68 megahertz.

The 13.56 megahertz frequency is used most commonly in electrolysis today. Clinics with equipment using an alternative frequency are subject to federal prosecution.

The high-frequency (Figure 11–3) waves travel down the probe and, when the probe is placed in the follicle and surrounded by the moisture of the soft tissue cells, the water molecules of the soft tissue start to vibrate, producing heat. This heat causes tissue damage called electrocoagulation and can destroy the dermal papilla. The probe itself does not become hot, but the high-frequency electromagnetic field generates heat through vibration in the water molecules. The moister the tissue is, the more heat that can be generated. As there is generally more moisture at the base of the hair follicle, more heat is often generated there. The heat is even more directly targeted to the dermal papilla at the base of the hair follicle if an insulated probe is used, because heat is first produced at the

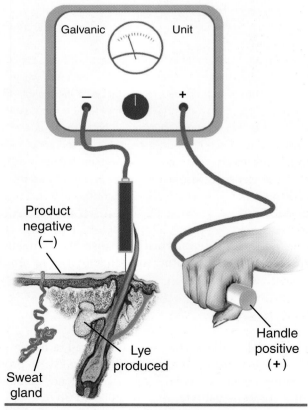

Figure 11–3 Galvanic current on a client

tip, known as the point effect. It then rises in a droplet shape toward the upper portion of the hair follicle.

Benefits and Downsides of Thermolysis

When a technician understands the benefits and downsides of each of the three modalities, the most appropriate choice can be made for the particular hair growth situation, dependent on the level of training, understanding, and skill with that modality. Thermolysis has multiple benefits and downsides, listed below, with regards to training and mastery of it.

Benefits of Thermolysis

Thermolysis is the most straightforward method of electrolysis to learn. There is no calculating that needs to be done, as there is for galvanic electrolysis. The two variables that form the treatment energy are the strength of the current applied and the length of time of the application of the current. This produces variable treatment energies for different types of hair and body parts. Thermolysis is fast and can treat a number of hairs very quickly. A skilled technician can treat a new hair every few seconds. Finer vellus hairs and hairs with straight follicles, like the upper lip, can be treated quickly and successfully with thermolysis with very little regrowth. With this method, there is no risk of "tattooing," a complication that can occur with galvanic electrolysis, and is further described below.

Downsides of Thermolysis

While thermolysis is relatively easy to learn, compared to other modalities, it is much harder to master the perfect insertion required for the destruction of the dermal papilla that is necessary for permanent hair removal. Thermolysis requires thorough teaching and a development of the practical skills necessary for an accurate insertion.

Thermolysis is not as effective on coarse hair because the required amount of heat, sufficient to destroy the dermal papilla, could cause a negative reaction in the skin. A lower current means that there will be some regrowth, which can be eliminated on a lower current with a subsequent visit, but the better option would be to use the blend method. Thermolysis is not as effective on distorted follicles, but multiple treatments to a once distorted follicle do eventually straighten it, making thermolysis still possible for permanent removal, although the time for permanency is greatly extended. Thermolysis equipment does not provide for the opportunity to deliver an aftercare treatment of cataphoresis to soothe the skin the way that galvanic electrolysis or the blend method can.

point effect
the concentration of high frequency current at the tip of the probe

Thermolysis takes its name from the Greek word *thermo*, meaning heat, and *ysis*, meaning to dissolve. It is also commonly called diathermy, a more outdated term; "high frequency," for the alternating current (AC) it uses; and "shortwave," again for the high-frequency shortwaves that produce heat-inducing action via a probe to destroy the dermal papilla. The high frequency shortwaves that are emitted off the probe react with moisture in the cells at the dermal papilla, shaking them up and creating a turbulence that creates heat, and it is the heat that destroys the dermal papilla desiccating and destroying it. The facts that it is fast, effective, and relatively (compared to other methods of electrolysis) easy to learn make it a popular method, and it is still the most common method of electrolysis around the world.

GALVANIC ELECTROLYSIS

Galvanic electrolysis is *true* electrolysis. Although electrolysis has become the general term for permanent hair removal, including thermolysis and the blend, *galvanism* is true electrolysis. Galvanic modality uses DC (see Figure 11–3), which flows in one direction, from the negative pole to the positive pole. The galvanic modality is a product of electrochemistry using electrical energy to bring about a chemical change. This change happens when an electrode (for example, a handheld metal rod), carrying a positive charge of electricity, is conducted by the metals (electrolytes) in the body and the negatively charged electrode (for example, the probe) is inserted into the follicle. The result is that the current flows from negative to positive and, as the negatively charged probe lies in the follicle surrounded by soft tissue, an electrolytic chemical action, called ionization occurs in which ions, released from atoms in the tissue, rearrange themselves, forming new substances. Two molecules of salt ($NaCl$) and two molecules of water (H_2O) in the tissue cells separate and regroup to form one molecule of hydrogen gas, one molecule of chlorine gas, and two molecules of sodium hydroxide ($NaOH$), also known as lye. Lye formation interests the technician, because it is the lye that effectively decomposes the soft tissue.

ionization
a process in which an atom or a molecule loses or gains electrons, acquiring an electrical charge

Benefits and Downsides of Galvanic Electrolysis

Like thermolysis, the galvanic modality offers a permanent solution to unwanted hair, and yet the benefits and downsides to galvanic electrolysis differ in many ways from its sister modality.

Benefits of Galvanic Electrolysis

Galvanic electrolysis does not work with the speed of thermolysis, but what it lacks in speed can be made up with accuracy: the chemical reaction caused by the galvanic current is able to "bleed" down distorted follicles to destroy the dermal papilla. The accuracy of insertion is not as crucial for galvanic electrolysis as it is with thermolysis, making it a good modality to learn with. Galvanic electrolysis offers the highest success rate in lack of regrowth. An accurate insertion is less important with galvanic electrolysis than it is for thermolysis, because the caustic *lye* that is produced "bleeds" down to the dermal papilla, causing its damage or destruction. As a result, galvanic electrolysis is a good choice of modality for the newly trained, less experienced technician. Because of its ability to "bleed" in the follicle, distorted and wavy hair follicles can be successfully treated; although the probe may not bend and go all the way down to the dermal papilla, the lye will continue to bleed down to the base and effect the necessary change. The lye produced in the hair follicles continues destroying the hair follicle even after the treatment session is over.

Downsides of Galvanic Electrolysis

Galvanic electrolysis is the slowest method of permanent hair removal. The chemical action needed to produce sufficient lye to destroy the dermal papilla can take a number of minutes on each hair.

The extended application of the current can cause an irritating sensation for the client. A client with a high-strung or nervous disposition may be unable to tolerate the slowness or discomfort; therefore, it may be harder for the client to remain still throughout the current application. With this method the client's full cooperation is necessary for successful treatment, which includes remaining still for extended periods and keeping the electrolysis circuit flowing by continuously holding the electrode. After the session, the lye can continue to treat follicles and can continue to be a source of discomfort and irritation to the client.

Another significant downside to the galvanic method is the risk, especially with older equipment lacking in safety features, of tattooing. Tattooing occurs with an incorrect cord setup that can result in permanent black marks on the skin. This happens when the positive pole is connected to the probe, causing hydrochloric acid in the metal of the probe, which creates a permanent tattoo in the skin that is very difficult to remove.

Ionization Principles

To understand galvanic current with regard to electrolysis, one must first understand the science of *ionization* and the use of positive (+) and negative (−) poles to separate substances into ions. An ion is an atom or a

Galvanic electrolysis, sometimes referred to as "true electrolysis," is the original modality used for permanent hair removal. Galvanic current is DC, that is, current that moves continuously in one direction. DC in a saline (salt-water) solution causes the separation and rearrangement of the chemical components, that is, water (H_2O) and sodium chloride (NaCL) into new substances including sodium hydroxide, also called lye (NaOH), and hydrogen gas. This process, called electrolysis, occurs in similar fashion on the soft tissue in the hair follicle.

hydrochloric acid
a colorless acid that is highly acidic

cathode pole
pole used to negatively charge ions

anions
negatively charged ions

anaphoresis
process whereby ions are negatively charged

anode pole
pole used to positively charge ions

cations
positively charged ions

cataphoresis
the process whereby ions are positively charged

blend method
method of electrolysis that combines thermolysis and galvanic electrolysis

group of atoms carrying an electric charge. When negatively charged using the cathode pole, the ions are called anions, and the process is called anaphoresis. When positively charged using the anode pole, the ions are called cations and the process is called cataphoresis. The anode cord for an electrolysis epilator is usually red, and the cathode cord is usually black.

BLEND METHOD

The blend method uses the slower but effective method of galvanic (DC) electrolysis with the fast-acting benefits of thermolysis (AC). These two modalities can be applied simultaneously or sequentially, leading with either method. The AC and DC pass down the same needle. The DC causes the production of sodium hydroxide (lye) at the base of the follicle, and the AC action heats up the lye, improving permeability and bringing about a faster and more effective destruction of the dermal papilla and tissue of the hair follicle. Conversely, the AC generates heat in the follicle causing increased permeability of the lye produced by the DC. Therefore the blend method is the combination of two types of current, rather than a machine, although units are sold that offer both thermolysis and galvanic electrolysis within the epilator, making the blend method possible. The blend method reduces the treatment time to one-quarter of that of conventional galvanic current alone. The thermolysis modality is the easiest to learn but requires greater skill to master, because it requires an accurate probe for successful destruction of the dermal papilla. The galvanic method is the next easiest to learn and understand; the blend method is considered the most difficult to learn and apply, but it is well worth the effort for its superior results when applied successfully.

Benefits and Downsides of the Blend Method

The blend method incorporates the benefits of both thermolysis and galvanic modalities, and also the downsides of the two methods. (See Figure 11–4.) Whether or not a technician chooses to use this method will undoubtedly be determined by the benefits of the blend method on the hair follicle weighed against his or her ability to learn and master it.

Benefits of the Blend Method

The main benefit of the blend method is that it works for a significant number of hairs, especially curly and kinky hairs that have curved

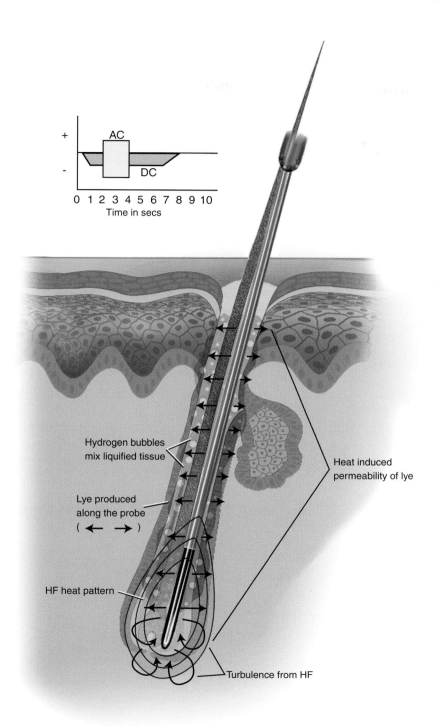

Figure 11—4 Effect of the blend method on the hair follicle

follicles, incorporating the accuracy of the galvanic action with the speed of thermolysis. The blend method is an effective and versatile method of treating a wide range of hairs on all parts of the body at a wider range in their hair growth cycle. Using high frequency for a longer time on a lower-intensity setting and following it with the galvanic is effective for treating hairs from their early anagen stage right up to their high telogen stage.

Downsides of the Blend Method

The blend method is the most difficult to learn and master. The planning and calculating of accurate, effective treatments is complex, and while those tasks might be made easier by an automatic epilator, the complexities of computerization may remain a challenge for some. Not knowing how to accurately calculate and apply the blend method could cause damage to the skin from overtreatment. The damage is visible as eschars, blanching, pitting, or dimpling of the skin.

■ PRINCIPLES OF PHORESIS

Phoresis is the scientific term for the process in which chemical solutions can be forced into the unbroken skin using the galvanic current. In electrology and esthetics, phoresis is used in two main forms that are called iontophoresis: (1) anaphoresis and (2) cataphoresis. (See Table 11–2.)

phoresis
process in which chemical solutions can be forced into unbroken skin using galvanic current

iontophoresis
a method by which drugs or solutions are introduced into the body via electrical current

> Phoresis is the process in which chemical solutions can be forced into unbroken skin using galvanic current.

Table 11–2 Side-by-Side Comparison of the Different Types of Phoresis	
Cataphoresis (Anode)	**Anaphoresis (Cathode)**
Produces acidic reactions	Produces alkaline reactions
Closes the pores	Opens the pores
Soothes nerves	Stimulates and irritates nerves
Decreases the blood supply	Increases the blood supply
Constricts blood vessels	Dilates blood vessels
Hardens and firms tissue	Softens tissue
Has antibacterial qualities	

Iontophoresis

Iontophoresis is the use of galvanic current to introduce water soluble products into the skin using the anode (+ pole) and cathode (– pole) with DC. Iontophoresis is the aesthetic term used for ionization.

Dual-Roller Iontophoresis

Iontophoresis uses two ionto rollers for the ionization treatment. One roller is attached to the negative (cathode) pole, the other to the positive (anode) pole. The client need not hold an electrode. Lotions or a piece of gauze soaked in a water soluble solution are applied to the skin, and the rollers are passed over the skin, causing ionization.

Anaphoresis

Anaphoresis is the process of using the negative (cathode) pole to force substances into unbroken skin. The current flows from the negative to the positive pole and produces alkaline reactions. This reaction is stimulating, increasing the blood supply and visibly dilating blood vessels, as well as opening the pores, improving the skin's ability to absorb substances.

Cataphoresis

Also known as "positive surface galvanism," cataphoresis is the process of using the positive (anode) pole, in the form of a roller that acts as the electrode, to distribute galvanic current to the surface of the skin. The client holds the negative (cathode) pole in the hands. The current forces water soluble acidic pH substances into the unbroken skin. There are two ways of applying the gauze, which can be premoistened with witch hazel. The gauze can be wrapped around the roller or applied directly to the skin and the roller moved across the gauze.

   In this method, the current flows from the positive to the negative pole. In electrolysis, it is used to stop the chemical reaction, soothe the skin, and provide antibacterial protection after treatment. It can also be used after waxing to soothe irritated or inflamed areas and as a treatment with a facial. It is not applied after thermolysis.

Indications for Electrolysis

Indications for electrolysis would be a desired removal of unwanted hair, regardless of texture (coarse terminal or fine vellus) or pigment (gray, blonde, red, or black) on any part of the face and body, including genitalia, with exceptions being inside of the nose and inside of the ear.

Contraindications for Electrolysis

Besides the conditions, diseases, or medications that may temporarily or permanently preclude a client from receiving electrolysis, some situations may allow the technician to proceed with caution, with the approval of, or under the direction of, the client's physician.

A contraindication may be temporary like a sunburn, long lasting like a pregnancy (the service can be given postpartum), or permanent like diabetes mellitus (a chronic disorder).

Individuals with acne vulgaris should receive no electrolysis in the vicinity of the affected area due to the high presence of bacteria and the possibility of cross contamination. In addition, acne vulgaris is a painful condition, and electrolysis only adds discomfort to the already traumatized area. Certainly, electrolysis helps control acne outbreaks by eliminating hairs that get trapped in the infected follicles and by providing galvanic current, which destroys sebaceous glands in the hair follicles. However, treatments should be held off until the active outbreak has passed and there is little sign of infection. The client should be referred to a dermatologist and receive a course of facials to control the condition as soon as possible.

While asthma does not preclude electrolysis, caution should be exercised. This illness is nervous in origin, and those with it may be prone to attacks when feeling anxious about the procedure. The frequency and severity of attacks should be documented and may help determine if electrolysis can be given. Every step should be made to relieve any apprehension and anxiety the client may experience. Treatments should start at a low current level and progress cautiously.

Clients with blood-pressure problems may be treated with electrolysis, but caution should be used when treating those with high blood pressure problems, particularly when those clients show anxiety.

Heart conditions are contraindicated unless it is with the knowledge, approval, and supervision of the clients' physicians. Physician approvals must be in writing. Clients wearing pacemakers should not receive galvanic electrolysis or the blend method unless the positive electrode is placed so the flow of current does not pass through or near the pacemaker, for example, work on the toes. If the client is to receive thermolysis, the clinician should be sure that the high frequency of the epilator will not interfere with the pacemaker, which can happen if the pacemaker is "synchronous"; that is, it stimulates the heart on demand, as opposed to asyn-

acne vulgaris
the "common acne" characterized by blackheads and pimples; found most commonly in teenagers and young adults

chronous, which delivers a constant rate of electrical stimuli to the heart. Also people with heart conditions often present with poor circulation and bruise more easily.

In December 2002, the FDA put out a warning to all medical workers to be on the alert for patients with deep brain stimulator (DBS) implants and to avoid treating those patients with diathermy. The risk of exposing a patient who has this implant to a diathermy treatment is serious injury and possibly death. The DBS acts as a regulator for the brain to stabilize the tremors associated with diseases like Parkinson's disease, Tourette's syndrome, and dystonia. Patients are asked to avoid shortwave diathermy treatments, which may heat the metal implants and associated leads. The FDA has listed certain equipment it considers a threat, and diathermy epilation units are not listed. However, as studies in this area are still inconclusive, it is prudent to treat no individuals with these implants until research is complete and there is conclusive evidence that it is safe to treat these individuals.

Considerable care should be taken in treating a client with diabetes, also known as diabetes mellitus. The severity of this illness, including the kind of treatment the client receives for it, should be well documented. Include whether the disease is controlled by diet and exercise, with an insulin pump, or regular insulin injections. The lower extremities should never be treated with electrolysis, because the loss of some sensation to the skin makes it difficult to judge appropriate levels of intensity. Also, the skin has diminished ability to heal. While these problems are more severe in the lower extremities, they also affect other parts of the body, including the face. The need for meticulous hygiene, sanitation, and sterilization cannot be overemphasized. The client should be advised of the importance of following home-care procedures to promote faster healing in a condition that otherwise inhibits healing. Guidance or a referral from the client's physician is necessary.

Electrolysis should not be performed over varicose veins, due to the risk of puncture and bleeding.

Attacks of both types of epilepsy, grand mal and petit mal, can be triggered by electrolysis current. If the seizures are infrequent and controlled by medication, it is possible to perform electrolysis on these clients, particularly if the unwanted hair is emotionally stressful for the client and there is a real need for the service. However, clients with epilepsy *must* be evaluated by their physicians before receiving electrolysis treatment. The physicians will determine if the treatments would be safe. Receive the physicians' approvals in writing.

Most skin disorders like sunburn or acne are temporary, and only the area affected need be avoided. Other skin disorders, like herpes, may be

grand mal
a serious form of epilepsy in which there is loss of consciousness and severe convulsions

petit mal
a form of epilepsy marked by episodes of brief loss of consciousness without convulsions or falling

contagious, and the client should not be treated even in areas where the skin is not affected. Other skin disorders may be indicative of a serious chronic disease like lupus, which contraindicates electrolysis.

When using galvanic current on clients that have metal implants, which include pacemakers, pins, rods, plates, and intrauterine devices (IUDs), the client may feel discomfort, so the pathway for the handheld electrode should be positioned such that the current does not pass near any metal implants. Thermolysis may be a better choice.

Doctors' Consent

Any time there is a condition that may be contraindicated or questionable for treatment, clients must always receive consent in writing from their physicians. There could be serious legal ramifications were something to happen, even if it was not triggered or affected by the electrolysis. Technicians must follow protocol to avoid a damaging lawsuit. If there is any question of a client's well-being, the service should not be provided. The client should be advised of other options.

The technician should always use vigilance with clients' health and well-being, and not try and make a diagnosis beyond expertise. Instead, the technician should know when to refer to a physician for further evaluation.

ELECTROLYSIS FOR DIFFERENT TYPES OF HAIR

The choice of modality is not as important as ensuring that whatever choice is made is carried out with skill, accuracy, and the proper training. The technician's goal is always to destroy the dermal papilla of as many offending hairs as possible, in the shortest time with no lasting adverse effects to the skin. With that in mind, there is enough experience and documentation in the three modalities of electrolysis to appreciate the benefits of one modality over another, given certain variables (for example, the type and quantity of hair to be removed). Different types of hair require or benefit from the use of different modalities. Being educated and accomplished in the use of all three modalities affords the technician the choice of selecting the most effective modality for the type of hair that needs removing.

Electrolysis for Vellus Hair

With an extensive amount of vellus, thermolysis is the most effective modality of electrolysis.

A lower-density current at a shorter duration minimizes adverse skin effects while effectively and quickly destroying the dermal papilla. However, when using thermolysis in shallow follicles like those on the upper lip, a higher intensity current and shorter duration, like the flash method, will help prevent high-frequency blowout, visible as blistering surface damage from excessive steam created in the follicle.

Electrolysis for Coarse Hair

Thick, coarse hair benefits more from galvanic electrolysis when there are only a few hairs, because this method is slower and the client will want all offending hairs removed in one session, if possible. The blend method would be the sensible choice if there were too many hairs to remove in one session using galvanic electrolysis exclusively. The amount of thermolysis current required to destroy the dermal papilla on strong, coarse hair could be significant enough to cause discomfort to the client and possible damage to the skin from overtreating. Coarse hair, in large quantities like that on the leg, benefits from the blend method of electrolysis.

Electrolysis for Curly Hair

Hair that is wavy, curly, or kinky generally has a crooked follicle. Because getting to the dermal papilla with a straight probe is not possible by sliding it down the hair follicle, the galvanic method should be the first choice if there are just a few hairs. This is because the destructive, galvanically produced chemical reaction of sodium hydroxide (lye) is able to "bleed" down to the dermal papilla to effectively damage or destroy it. The blend method is preferred if there are multiple hairs that need removing in one session, because it includes the destructive benefits of the lye "bleeding" down to the dermal papilla with the additional boost of speed from the thermolysis modality. Curly hair should have the curl trimmed off it, which will help determine the angle and direction of growth.

Distorted Follicles

Distorted hair follicles usually are formed by long-term tweezing or waxing against the hair growth and tweezing combined. Thermolysis in distorted follicles is a challenge; to succeed at it requires considerable experience and skill. It often means using that "sixth sense" that experienced technicians develop to figure out the angle of distortion. Distorted hairs can be treated successfully with thermolysis, especially in the early anagen phase when the follicle is shallow and less distorted. The better choice for distorted hair follicles is galvanic electrolysis, especially if the hairs are few and not too coarse, or the blend, if there is a significant number of coarse hairs with probable distortions for the same reasons described with curly, wavy hair. Although it is difficult to ascertain at the outset which hairs and how many are distorted, it is safe to assume that if a client has been tweezing a significant number of hairs daily or even a few times a week for a number of months or even years, most will be distorted.

■ THE TREATMENT PROCESS

After completing the consultation, considering all the variables, and formulating a treatment plan, the treatment session can begin. The room should be clean and orderly, with all necessary supplies on hand. Sterilized items should be ready in their closed containers, and the lamp and equipment should be wiped down and turned on.

Hands should be thoroughly washed and gloves donned. The client should be positioned on the table and draped. Draping is important to avoid skin-on-skin contact and thereby reduce the risk of cross contamination. Draping protects the technician and the client. Draping also inspires confidence in the client that the technician is a professional allied health worker. Washable goggles or damp cotton pads help when working on clients' faces to shield those clients from the glare of lamps. However, sanitize goggles between clients, and discard cotton rounds after each client. During a long, gray winter, clients may prefer the "therapy" of bright lights. Allow them that choice.

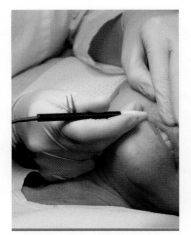

Figure 11–5 The one handed technique

One Handed Technique

The probe is held like a writing implement, in the right hand if right handed, and in the left hand if left handed. The forceps are also held point up in the same hand by the three fingers tucked underneath. When it is time to use the forceps, the probe is slipped back between the forefinger and second finger and the forceps are slipped forward in the same grip the probe was in. After the epilation, the forceps are taken back by the middle, index, and little fingers with the top upward, toward the thumb, and the probe is swung back to its original position, gripped by the thumb and forefinger. With this technique, the free hand can maintain an effective stretch, along with the little finger and underedge of the dominant hand. The shorter 23.4 cm forceps fit more comfortably in the hand, with the one handed technique. (See Figure 11–5.)

Two Handed Technique

The probe is held in the same manner as in the one handed technique, but the forceps are held in the opposite hand. There are two variables to epilating the hair using this method. The first is to epilate the hair with the hand that is holding the tweezers. (See Figure 11–6.)

This is considered faster, because there is no time wasted switching the forceps, but one may question the flexibility, steadiness, and sensitivity of using the less-dominant hand for this purpose. It may be harder to determine the resistance on the tug of a hair and whether it is truly released due to the destruction of the dermal papilla, or whether it just has a thick hair sheath. Sometimes, the more-dominant hand can make a better determination. However, with practice there is no reason that kind of sensitivity cannot be developed in the less-dominant hand.

The other two handed method is to hold the forceps in the opposite hand to the probe but to then switch the forceps to the dominant hand for the epilation. Some technicians consider this to be less time effective, because the forceps are still switched. Switching the forceps to the other hand also disrupts the effective stretch. However, it does ensure an accurate epilation, using the sensitivity of the dominant hand. Another consideration is the angle of the epilation. When epilating with the less-dominant hand, there is a risk of pulling the hair upward instead of outward, in the angle and direction of growth. If the dermal papilla was not destroyed, the hair may be tweezed, and in a direction that will distort the follicle. Therefore, when using the less-dominant hand to epilate, take care to ensure that the hair is epilated in the same direction and angle of the probe. This is easier to do with the one handed method.

Stretching the Skin

The stretch of the skin, when done correctly, is vital in achieving a perfect insertion. It helps to open the follicle and lift the hair, allowing the probe to slide down the underside of the hair shaft. The stretch is always accomplished with both hands. Some fleshy areas, like the areola or a double chin, require considerably more stretching than other areas, where the skin may lay tightly over a bony protrusion, like the shinbone. The stretching will be determined by whichever hand is holding the forceps. If the probe and forceps are in the same hand, then the less-dominant hand is free to use as many fingers as necessary to accomplish the most optimal stretch. If the less-dominant hand is using the forceps to epilate, the stretching must be assumed by the little finger and the edge of the hand that follows down from it. When the less-dominant hand holding

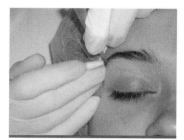

Figure 11–6 The two handed technique

Stretching the skin correctly is vital for an accurate insertion. It opens the follicle and lifts the hair so that the probe can be more readily inserted down the underside of the hair shaft for more accuracy. Stretching may require the full use of both hands, using the side of the hand that follows from the little finger, on larger fleshy body areas, or just a few fingers on a small area like the upper lip.

the forceps has to pass them to the probing hand, the stretch is often lost and must be reestablished. Stretching should not be heavy or forceful. It should not depress the skin, and it should not feel uncomfortable to the client. Overstretching or stretching incorrectly at bad angles will cause an inaccurate insertion. The stretch should be light and sufficient to open the follicle and lift the hair slightly for an easy and accurate insertion.

■ INSERTION TECHNIQUES

The focus should always be on accuracy, rather than speed, in hair removal. Accurate probing and correct application of treatment energy make electrolysis permanent. It is not a race to remove as many hairs as possible in a session.

Hairs immediately adjacent to one another should not be epilated at the risk of overtreating the area and damaging the skin, particularly in sensitive areas like the upper lip or eyebrow.

If working two sides of an area, the use of a timer is helpful to divide the session time equally and avoid running out of time before moving to the opposite area, giving an unbalanced treatment.

The coarsest most obvious hairs should be removed first, progressing to the next most obvious.

Avoid working in one area, which creates an obvious bald patch surrounded by more dense hair.

Gauging Follicle Depth

The first couple of probes should be to gauge follicle depth and to establish an effective working point, which is the treatment energy required to destroy the dermal papilla, combining the current density and duration of the current. Treat one hair with minimal treatment energy going to the learned and assumed depth. Grasp the hair at the follicular opening, and slide the hair outward. If it is an intact anagen hair, hold it next to the probe tip to ascertain its length. Observing where it ends on the probe will determine the depth of the follicle. There will be some variation, but doing this to a few random hairs will approximate average depth.

Shallow insertions create a more intense heating pattern, so reduce the treatment energy if moving to shallow or early anagen hairs after treating hairs in deeper follicles, otherwise the skin could sustain damage at the opening to the follicle.

Begin on an initial follicle with the lowest treatment energy recommended for the area. If the hair does not release, increase the treatment energy a second time. If the hair still does not release, try a second follicle and so on, increasing the energy until the hair releases. Do not treat the same follicle more than three times. Although it is permissible to apply the treatment energy more than once, it should be the exception, not the rule. It is far better to establish an effective working point using the minimal amount of treatment energy to effectively destroy the dermal papilla and release the hair, because doing so avoids the multiple double insertions that are time consuming and could cause damage from overtreating follicles.

PEET, PERT, PEST

The PEET, PERT, and PEST techniques were developed and based on the theory that as the hair, combined with the external and internal root sheaths, takes up so much of the follicle, it often impedes direct access to the dermal papilla by the probe. Through the PEET, PERT, and PEST techniques, technicians have experienced good results in the destruction of the dermal papilla.

Preelectrolysis Epilation Technique (PEET)

The hair is plucked from the untreated follicle, the needle is inserted into the empty follicle, current is applied, and the needle is removed from the follicle. This technique is worth utilizing if the hair was inadvertently tweezed, or perhaps a hair got caught in the tweezer during the epilation of the previous hair. It is worth entering the empty follicle with the probe and applying the treatment energy in the hopes of destroying the dermal papilla.

Postepilation Reentry Technique (PERT)

With the PERT technique, the standard electrolysis treatment is performed first with the hair in the hair follicle, then again to the empty follicle once the hair has been epilated. This is the equivalent of "double dosing" if it is thought, on observing the epilated hair, that a complete destruction has not taken place. Care must be taken with this technique, not to overtreat the follicle and damage the skin.

Postepilation Sustained Entry Technique (PEST)

The PEST technique is accomplished using the two handed method. The technique is to first perform the standard electrolysis treatment to the hair follicle, and then, while leaving the needle in place with one hand, epilate the hair with the other, repeating the current application to the empty follicle and then removing the needle. PEST is like PERT (see preceding section), but by leaving the probe in the follicle, it ensures that the correct empty follicle is being retreated.

Incorrect Insertions

Incorrect insertions not only reduce the effectiveness of the current application but they can be damaging to the skin by puncturing the follicle walls or causing surface damage (see Figure 11–7). Probing too deeply often draws blood, which is visible at the follicle opening. This occurs with technicians who are not yet experienced nor adept at feeling the base of the follicle or who have selected a probe that was too long for the follicles in the area being treated.

Other causes are when an accurate depth of the follicles was not ascertained at the start of the treatment or when an early anagen hair was treated because it was believed to be a full-grown anagen hair after shaving. Providing the insertion was not too deep, the dermal papilla can still be destroyed, but not without creating the unnecessary nuisance of drawing blood. A too-shallow insertion is more of a problem with thermolysis

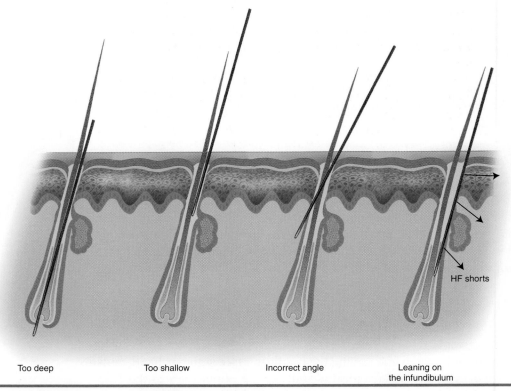

Too deep	Too shallow	Incorrect angle	Leaning on the infundibulum

HF shorts

Figure 11–7 Diagram of incorrect probe positions

because it simply means that the dermal papilla will remain untreated. This is not as serious a problem with the galvanic modality or the blend method because the lye, if enough is produced, will bleed downward to the dermal papilla. It will be a far more effective treatment, however, if the insertion is made to the correct depth. A shallow insertion also increases the risk of surface damage.

Insertion at an incorrect angle, a common cause of drawing blood, happens when the angle of the follicle is not correctly determined. If the probe comes into direct contact with the hair shaft, it may disintegrate the hair at the point at which it comes into contact with the probe, causing the top half to break away but leaving the lower portion attached. This is again an area in which a skilled and experienced technician may be more adept at feeling the sides of the follicle wall, particularly with a fine, two-piece probe, but even a newly trained technician with a sensitive touch can make the correct determination. The angle can be affected by nearby scar tissue or a nearby mole. An incorrect insertion can also be affected by overstretching or stretching the skin incorrectly.

If the skin is not adequately stretched and the angle of insertion is incorrect, the probe may come in contact with the side of the follicle. This could cause tissue damage, especially with thermolysis and the use of a noninsulated probe.

Once the probe has slid into the follicle, it should not be moved. Focus and a steady hand are vital while applying the treatment energy to ensure there is no movement. Movement during insertion causes tissue damage. An accurate count will ensure that the probe is not being withdrawn from the follicle while the treatment energy is being applied.

Precare

If the electrolysis treatment was performed accurately, but the precare or postcare was poor or lacking, an adverse reaction will occur in the following days, leaving the client reluctant to continue the course of treatments. Conversely, a thorough and appropriate pretreatment will minimize the possibility of any negative reaction to an appropriately performed treatment. The technician's hands should be washed and gloves donned. The treatment area should be thoroughly cleansed to remove all traces of dirt, grime, makeup, deodorants, and so on. This can be done with a gentle, all-purpose cleanser in a light, gentle manner so as not to overstimulate the circulatory system in that area. Next, the area should be prepped with an antiseptic. Ethyl alcohol 70 percent is effective and not as harsh smelling as isopropyl alcohol.

While either may be effective in high bacterial areas like the groin, underarms, fingers, and toes, they may be unsuitable for the faces of

ethyl alcohol
a colorless liquid with a fruity smell produced by fermentation; often used as a solvent; synonymous with ethanol

isopropyl alcohol
a colorless, flammable alcohol often used as a solvent

some clients because they are too drying and stimulating. Mild antiseptic lotions like witch hazel can be substituted in more sensitive areas.

After cleansing, a topical anesthetic can be applied if the client did not apply one before coming in for treatment.

While the anesthetic is taking effect, wipe the needle holder with alcohol and place a clean, sterilized needle cap on it. Next, select the appropriate sterilized probe, open it in front of the client, and, using sterilized forceps, place it in the needle holder.

In the case of galvanic electrolysis and the blend method, prepare the positive handheld electrode with the conductive gel or the moistened pad and hand it to the client.

To collect the epilated hair, either place a cotton square in the vicinity or wrap some clear tape in reverse around the opposite wrist to the hand that slides the hair out. Discard the tape after each client.

Make all appropriate settings and proceed with the treatment.

Posttreatment

The most suitable aftercare treatment for the client is often a question of trial and error. Just as people have differing reactions to the multitude of skin care lines, so they have differing reactions with aftercare products and techniques. Electrolysis supply companies have a wide range of recommended aftercare products to use on clients. Whatever one chooses, it is important to remember that the follicle itself is free of bacteria, after being treated with electrolysis current. While it is important to keep the vulnerable surface area of the skin free of bacteria, the area should not be

---

Postcare Treatment for Electrolysis

Posttreatment soothing can be accomplished by the use of witch hazel lotion or gel, aloe vera gel, or Caladryl/Calamine lotion.

Ice bags can be used to reduce swelling and puffiness.

Cataphoresis can be used to close pores, as well as to soothe and calm the skin.

Erythema on the face can be camouflaged by professional products.

Clients should be advised to avoid hot tubs, saunas, sun, and tanning booths for 24 hours, or until signs of the erythema and irritation have passed.

Clients should be advised to use clean, uncontaminated makeup and skin care.

"flooded" with any liquid, particularly water, that may transport micro-organisms too readily into an otherwise bacteria-free follicle. Clients who have had work done on the hairline or on the face should avoid shampoo-ing the hair for 24 hours. They should also avoid applying hair-grooming products to the hair if the hairline has been treated and avoid getting hair-spray on any treated area until the area has completely healed. Using a damp, but not saturated, washcloth or cotton with the product is key. Witch hazel lotion or gel is cooling and soothing to many people and has mild antiseptic properties. Others prefer aloe vera gel. Caladryl/Calamine lotions are effective if there are histamine-type bumps or inflammation on the skin, but they leave a chalky residue. If the area shows signs of puffiness or swelling, a few ice cubes placed in clean plastic is effective for clients to use. There are cold packs that can be prechilled and given to clients to use, but ice is more economical unless clients choose to rest in the facility with cold packs for awhile. Whatever product is used should be kept sterile by using a spatula if it is in a jar or by pour-ing it onto cotton if it is a liquid, without the cotton touching the lip of the bottle. If the client must return to work or has another engagement and would like the treated area camouflaged, waxing manufacturers have aftercare products that soothe and camouflage.

Major electrolysis probe manufacturing companies also have lines of aftercare products, some that are also tinted in different shades and can be applied after the treatment or purchased by the client for home use. These products are inexpensive and soothe, camouflage, and promote healing to the skin. They are preferred over makeup.

When the aftercare is completed, the technician should remove the probe cap and place it and the forceps in the holding tray containing a disinfection solution, before removing the gloves.

Aftercare/Home Care

Meticulous aftercare is essential to speeding the healing process and to avoiding pimples.

Clients' hands should be washed thoroughly before touching the treated area.

Clients should be informed that the current, when applied to the fol-licle, destroys bacteria in the follicle. Antiseptics applied before and after the treatment temporarily remove bacteria from the skin's surface. If little pustules become apparent in the days after the treatment, microorgan-isms may have been introduced in the day or two after the treatment, when the skin was still vulnerable and healing. These microorganisms may have been introduced through touching the skin with unclean hands, which is easy to do if it was a habit to feel for the hairs (for example, while driving), saturating the skin with water, thereby transporting microorganisms down into the follicle, or using face creams that have been contaminated by dipping fingers directly into the pot rather than using a spatula. Makeup that has been contaminated by touching fingers to the lip of the bottle or using dirty sponges can also become contaminated, and pose problems to the electrolysis client after treatment. If the client uses sticky hair products, changing the pillowcase more frequently will also help.

Skin Cleansing

Cleansers should be fragrance-free and designed for sensitive skin. Masks and rich creams should be avoided for 48 hours.

Avoid saturating the face with water for 24 hours after the electrolysis session. Body areas can generally be washed after 12 to 18 hours. Water too readily transports microorganisms down into an already vulnerable area. The face can be cleansed with appropriate lotions and removed with damp cotton or tissues. For the body, a perfume-free body wash or a gentle germicidal soap like Safeguard™ can be used. If the client has been in the habit of sticking fingers into the jar of face cream, recommend a fresh face cream jar and spatula, especially for the few days following the treatment when the skin is most vulnerable to infection.

Medicated Creams

Mild first-aid or antibiotic creams, such as Neosporin™ or Bacitracin™, can be applied, but not steroid creams like cortisone. Cortisone creams should not be used or recommended for aftercare for any client requiring their use for two weeks or more.

Long-term use of cortisone creams could cause the skin to develop steroid dependent dermatoses, meaning that the irritation could return, necessitating further use of the cream. It is lengthy and bothersome to "wean" the skin of cortisone dependence.

Makeup Removal

Avoid makeup for at least a day. Instruct the client to apply clean and sterile makeup. If the makeup may have been compromised with fingers or a well-used sponge, it may be worth purchasing new, "clean" makeup for the duration of the treatment. Avoid putting fingers to the bottle opening and contaminating the whole bottle. Also, avoid makeup sponges unless they are washed thoroughly after each use or are replaced regularly.

These are good hygiene habits to develop regardless of the reason. Cake makeup that uses sponges is generally more clogging and tougher to clean, so avoid it, if possible.

---

cortisone
a hormone secreted by the adrenal gland used to treat rheumatoid arthritis and allergies

steroid dependent dermatoses
a condition in which the long-term overuse of topical steroid creams causes the skin to require continued usage to keep the offending condition away

Makeup removal should be gentle and done with products that are perfume-free and designed for sensitive skin.

Hair

If the client is prone to breakouts on the face or neck after electrolysis, and all previous steps are being used to prevent the breakouts, another consideration may be the hair. If the client wears product in the hair, the product will pick up dirt and pollutants from the environment.

The dirt and grime often get transferred to the client's pillowcase and in turn to the client's skin. Because it is not recommended to saturate the face after the treatment, the client should not shower and wash the hair. Instead, the client can put a sleeping cap over the hair and use a clean, fresh pillowcase for the 2 or 3 nights following the treatment, until the skin has healed.

Ultraviolet Exposure

Tanning in a tanning booth or natural sunlight should be avoided while undergoing regular electrolysis treatments, meaning treatments once every two weeks. If there is any erythema to the skin, tanning may cause the skin to **hyperpigment** and produce brown spots. Advise clients to protect their skin from any ultraviolet rays with a sunscreen of at least SPF 15. SPF 30 can be used on the body, but it is generally too clogging for the face. Using an SPF 15 and reapplying it after a few hours is as effective as the SPF 30, but less clogging.

Bleaching Creams

Hair can be bleached, carefully following manufacturer's instructions, but not for at least 48 hours after the treatment or in areas still showing signs of irritation. As the bleached hairs grow out, it is clearly visible to ascertain the pigmented new anagen hairs.

hyperpigment
overstimulation of tyrosine in the melanocytes

electrologist
someone skilled in the use of electricity to remove moles, warts, or hair roots; synonymous with electrolysist

electrolysist
someone skilled in the use of electricity to remove moles, warts, or hair roots; synonymous with electrologist

Conclusion

You may have already decided to become an electrologist or electrolysist, or you may be a technician working in another hair removal field and are considering the benefits of adding electrolysis to your skill as an aesthetician or hair removal specialist. Electrolysis is a valued service that can only complement and enhance other hair removal and aesthetic services. Theoretical study, when paired with formal classroom training, provides an opportunity to establish a lucrative and rewarding career as an electrologist *and* a hair removal specialist.

>>> TOP 10 TIPS TO TAKE TO THE CLINIC

1. Electrolysis is currently the only proven method of permanent hair *removal* recognized by the FDA.

2. Electrolysis equipment should always be plugged into its own socket with a grounded, three-pronged plug and surge protector.

3. Thermolysis modality uses AC to produce oscillating radio high-frequency waves in the follicle to destroy the dermal papilla.

4. The Federal Communications Commission (FCC) regulating agency has assigned the 13.56 megahertz frequency for electrolysis.

5. Galvanic modality uses DC, which flows in one direction, from the negative pole to the positive pole to produce sodium hydroxide in the follicle to destroy the dermal papilla.

6. The blend method uses galvanic (DC) electrolysis with thermolysis (AC) applied simultaneously or sequentially, leading with either method to effectively destroy the dermal papilla.

7. Clients must receive a physician's consent in writing for any condition that may be contraindicated or questionable for treatment.

8. Stretching the skin correctly is vital for an accurate insertion.

9. Appropriate pretreatment and posttreatment care minimizes adverse reactions.

10. Clients should be given instructions for taking care of the treated area at home.

CHAPTER QUESTIONS

1. Name three of the five sources that can produce electric energy.

2. What is Ohm's law?

3. Name a good conductor and a poor conductor.

4. What is a milliampere?

5. What is the difference between AC and DC?

6. What is cataphoresis?

7. List three benefits of electrolysis.

8. List three downsides of electrolysis.

9. List five contraindications of electrolysis.

10. What are three things clients should avoid immediately after receiving electrolysis treatments?

11. Discuss how to gauge the depth of a hair follicle.

12. What is PEET?

BIBLIOGRAPHY

Bickmore, H. (2003). *Milady's Hair Removal Techniques.* Clifton Park, NY: Milady, an imprint of Thomson Delmar Learning.

Bono, M. (1994). *The Blend Method.* Santa Barbara, CA: Tortoise Press.

Gallant, A. (1994). *Principles and Techniques for the Electrologist.* Cheltenham, U.K.: Stanley Thornes (Publishers) Ltd.

Glor, F. (1987). *Modern Electrology.* Great Neck, NY: Hair Publishing, Inc.

Hinkle, A. R., and Lind, R. W. (1968). *Electrolysis, Thermolysis, and the Blend.* Los Angeles, CA: Arroway.

Meharg, G. E., RN, and Richards, R. N., MD. (1997). *Cosmetic and Medical Electrolysis and Temporary Hair Removal,* 2nd ed. Toronto, Ontario: Medric Ltd.

Building a Hair Removal Business

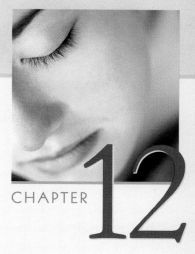

CHAPTER 12

KEY TERMS

accounts payable

accounts receivable

annual business plan

balance sheet

cost of goods sold

cost to acquire

cross-selling

database

deferred revenue

direct costs

economy pricing

fixed price

hot-sheets

income statement

indicators

indirect costs

inventory

marketing strategies

marketplace

overhead costs

penetration pricing

powering the patient
database

premium pricing

pricing strategies

product bundling pricing

purchase order system

referral programs

standard pricing policy

yearly business objectives

LEARNING OBJECTIVES

After completing this chapter, you should be able to:

1. Devise a business plan for your hair removal business.

2. Understand how to analyze your competition.

3. Create a price structure.

INTRODUCTION

Hair removal is an essential component of many skin care programs and is, from a business perspective, an essential service of medical and luxury spas. The treatment establishes repeat appointments and as such builds a clientele for the clinician and the spa. The financial success of providing hair removal services depends on several crucial business concepts, beginning with the development plan.

Writing a development plan (see Table 12–1) may appear to be a simple process, but is actually filled with details and decisions that may not have occurred to you otherwise. That is the beauty of a development plan—it makes you think, and then plan accordingly. During the process of thinking about how to develop your hair removal business, you will have to answer questions and solve initial problems. This process helps to make your development plan solid and void of holes that could potentially cause problems. The sections of a hair removal development plan are simple: getting your business started, and sustaining it.

■ GETTING YOUR BUSINESS STARTED

Getting your hair removal business started can be both exciting and challenging. Offering hair removal services can provide the opportunity to take a business to the next level or to be a stand-alone business that is exciting and financially rewarding. The start-up process involves evaluating the laser devices or processes, learning how to use a device, understanding the cost/price relationship, and creating marketing strategies to generate new clients. Adding a service to your menu will be hard work that needs to "bear fruit" as quickly as possible, and the best way to

marketing strategies
planned use of marketing elements and media pathways to create a strategy to introduce new clients or reactivate former clients

Table 12–1	The Development Plan
Equipment	Evaluate different devices, prices, and features to decide which are best suited for your business.
Pricing	Research demographic information, cost analysis, and competition to set a fair market price for hair removal services, while allowing for profit.
Marketing Strategies	Develop a marketing strategy that is both cost-effective and capable of generating new clientele.

accomplish this is through a strict and methodical process. The development plan for getting started with hair removal should address three issues: equipment/services, pricing, and marketing.

In the equipment category, you investigate hair removal lasers and decide which devices, components, and accessories best fit the need. An effective approach to accomplishing this goal is to make a list of the features you are looking for and why they are important. Addressing these questions before you meet with vendors will help you decipher the information about the devices available and help you select the most appropriate one for your business.

Pricing is the next category in the development plan. Your plan should begin with market research to find out how much the competitors are charging for particular services. This does not necessarily involve asking clients. Rather it is an investigative approach into other facilities, which entails calling or visiting other clinics to evaluate price and service. In addition, you should know your own costs and how to create a wide margin for profits. A certified public accountant (CPA) can help with this process.

The last category, marketing, is usually everyone's favorite part of the development plan. Marketing can involve promotions, advertising, gift with purchase, or other types of incentives to get clients through the door and entice them to buy services and products. It is great to watch new clients come through the door and leave satisfied with the services they received. However, without proper planning, marketing strategies can be ineffective.

An effective and comprehensive development plan is the launch pad for the success you will later enjoy.

Buying Devices

The success of a hair removal business begins with the proper selection of equipment and materials to provide the services. This includes items such as a laser hair removal machine, waxing pots and associated tools, and electrolysis equipment. Also, miscellaneous supplies needed to complete the job must be considered at some point.

Whether you are a business owner on the threshold of a new opportunity in hair removal or part of a well-established clinic looking to upgrade, purchasing the right equipment is key to success. But, shopping for new devices can be a hassle. While price is obviously important, it should not be the primary consideration. To ensure you get a device that fits your budget and needs, begin by evaluating the features you are looking for, rather than just the price. The cost of the hair removal systems will vary quite a bit, depending on the features. This is especially true if you want the machine to provide a variety of treatments such as IPL or vein treatments. Know exactly what you are getting for the price. A good consumer should know what the equipment includes and other important details, such as warranties and broken machine replacements. The old adage "you get what you pay for" is very true when it comes to purchasing this type of equipment.

There are now device catalogs that give information on a variety of machines, and this is usually a good place to start your research. Another reliable place to start is with the device manufacturers themselves. Conventions are a great way to "shop" around, be exposed to the latest state-of-the-art equipment, and see it in action. Association conferences that you attend for continuing education credits often have manufacturers showcasing their devices with representatives readily available to demonstrate and answer questions. When considering a manufacturer, research to find out if the company is well established. Does it have reliable safety and performance records? Do current customers believe the manufacturer has a reputation for quality and service? Will the company be "here today and gone tomorrow?" Has the device been stamped to verify it has been tested and listed? If the company is new to producing hair removal devices, has it made other devices with a solid reputation? Is the company the primary manufacturer or a reseller? Will it stand behind the device and provide service and support? Is the device FDA approved for achieving the results it is claiming, or is it just approved as a device that turns on and off? What type and duration of warranty comes with the device? Is the manufacturer registered with the FDA? If so, will the company be required by law to continue providing parts and service for seven years after the discontinuation of the device production?[1] In determining the general quality of a device, you should consider its physical stability, quality of component parts, ergonomics of the headrest, and ease of reading the dials. If you know a technician who has used a certain type of device, ask his or her opinion about its performance. This will help get an unbiased assessment separate from the manufacturer's statements about quality and performance.

Next, consider the features available. Have these features been examined and documented in peer-review studies that validate their advertised results? If so, who sponsored the study? If the manufacturer sponsored the study, the results may be skewed to show positive outcomes. Keep in mind warranties for repairs and maintenance. Your warranty should be for no less than one year with options for renewal. Be sure to get in writing the company's procedure for "down devices," which are those broken or otherwise inoperable. In these cases, will the manufacturer or reseller provide a comparable loaner? Will the loan be free or a rental with a cost you have to cover? A broken device without prompt service or replacement can be a revenue disaster. If a device breaks and you have to either wait for service or send the device back to the manufacturer without a replacement, you will be canceling patients or scrambling to offer other treatment choices. This could have catastrophic consequences on revenue, patient retention, and employee moral. If the manufacturer does not have a replacement device offer to bridge the repair gap, you will most certainly need to have a contingency plan to avert the aforementioned consequences. Contingency plans should include an arrangement with the manufacturer for a short-term lease or a loaner for the duration of the repair. Other options would include a backup unit or a day lease with companies that provide such a service.

By evaluating the features, you will begin to hone in on the price of the equipment. The next step in your development plan is to evaluate all related costs and set the retail price for the treatment. So if you are going to buy a more expensive device, make sure you can translate that into a higher retail price and, subsequently, better treatment.

Now that you know the fixed price of the various devices, you should examine the "variable costs" needed to perform services. Are there any disposable items that need to be factored into the cost? What are other variable expenses? A thorough understanding of related costs will help calculate the retail price point for the procedure per area and per patient.

Hiring and Training

Knowing whom to train can be straightforward in small clinics that have few available or qualified staff members. But in larger clinics, where there are several qualified technicians, selecting how many and which staff to train will be part business savvy and part intuition. You might think having many staff members trained will allow more procedures to be performed. However, unless the volume of hair removal business allows all qualified technicians to remain busy, you will have many people performing few procedures.

As we have mentioned, hair removal is highly technique sensitive, which means the more you do, the better you get.[2] Until client volume warrants training additional staff, limit the training to a few individuals who are the hair removal "experts." If these individuals are trained in laser hair removal, waxing, tweezing, and other forms of hair removal, they will become the experts. This allows them to provide full service hair removal, and will make your clients feel they are getting this treatment from the most qualified staff. Remember, because hair removal is technique sensitive, those with superior eye-hand coordination, as well as knowledge of who the best candidates are for which treatment, will excel.

fixed price
a price that remains the same, usually for a set time period

Sales representatives will often tell you, "this is the very best price." But, they often have the ability to make deals to drive business. Buying this equipment is somewhat like buying a car—prices are negotiable. Be sure to get all the extras you can, for example, an extension on the warranty. However, do not get duped into buying something you do not want or need.

Improvements in technology, "wear and tear" on equipment, and flexibility are all considerations when evaluating the financing options of hair removal devices. Once you have all the information in place for the purchase, talk with your accountant to be sure you are making the best choice for your business. A professional opinion on this can keep you out of financial trouble.

Training a hair removal specialist will be cost-effective for the business and financially beneficial for both the clinic and the specialist. But during the delicate introductory period, it is not without potential disadvantages. Concentrating hair removal training to a limited few risks the possibility of client defection in the event the staff member leaves the facility. While noncompete clauses, penalties, and threat of legal action can discourage departing staff from pilfering the client list, the fact is that clients have a right to transfer care. They will be less likely to do so, however, if they receive various services from other staff members, thus spreading the loyalty. So make sure your clients get a variety of services from different technicians.

There is never any way to know if a staff member is going to leave—sometimes it just happens abruptly. One way to plan ahead to recover training costs is by inserting a training fee into the employee contract. At the same time, training is a necessary expense for doing business, and spa owners should develop their ability to make good employee choices. As a business owner, you will strive to create customer loyalty to the business rather than just loyalty to the technician. Of course, you should also strive to make the working environment and benefits of employment create employee loyalty as well.

Cost Analysis

Conducting a comprehensive cost analysis is important for the technician and business owner alike. In order to make money, you have to understand how much it will cost to provide the procedure to clients. Cost analysis has two separate components: direct costs and indirect costs. Direct costs are all expenses that are directly related to implementing a hair removal procedure. These costs are offset only by payments of patients who receive this treatment. Most of our discussion will be related to direct costs. It can be confusing, so let us try to make it simple with some examples.

Direct Costs

With hair removal procedures, the direct costs (see Table 12–2) will include expenses related to items purchased—gel, gauze, linens, maintenance expenses, marketing hair removal services—and costs associated with training, insuring, and compensating employees. In other words, direct costs are those incurred solely due to hair removal.

Because costs usually are increasing, you need to evaluate expenses at least every six months. For example, hidden increases may occur; for example, did you give your employee a raise, or did the benefit structure change? Expenses like these should eventually be accounted for in the cost

direct costs
costs that are directly and exclusively attributable to a specific product or service

indirect costs
costs necessary for the functioning of the organization as a whole, but that cannot be directly assigned to one service or product

Table 12–2 Direct Costs
Example of a Single Hair Removal Treatment

Item	Cost	Percent of Revenue
Revenue per procedure	$210.00	
Time per procedure	30 minutes	
Direct cost of sales		
Lease[1]	21.76	10%
Maintenance contract	5.67	2.7%
Clinical supplies (gauze, gel, razor, tongue depressors, etc.)	2.00	0.09%
Linens	2.80	1.3%
Marketing campaign[2]	2.83	1.3%
Clinical employee wage	63.00	30%
Clinical employee benefits	16.38	7.8%
Total direct costs	**114.44**	**54%**

1. Based on 18 patient hours per week, the number of patient hours per year is 882. If the average time is 30 minutes, multiply the number of patient hours by 2 to get the number of 30-minute visits.

2. Marketing campaign is based on $5,000 annually and 1,764 hair removal visits per year. To find the annualized cost of any item divide the number of visits (1,764) into the cost of the marketing campaign ($5,000).

of the procedure. Although you should have accounted for much of the cost information when you were researching your devices and putting together your contracts, you need to continue to figure out changes to appropriately adjust profitability.

With your direct costs analyzed, add your standardized indirect cost formula (total overhead costs divided by the number of procedures performed). This calculation will give you an idea of how much you need to make for hair removal treatments to be profitable. The trickiest part is deciding to price your products to make it enticing enough to achieve profitability and sustainability.

Price Strategies

Although pricing strategies may seem a part of the marketing plan, pricing is quite different and should be evaluated independent of marketing. The theories and implementation of pricing can be very sophisticated.

overhead costs
indirect costs

pricing strategies
process by which a business determines the best way to price its product or service in order to entice customers while allowing for profit

Indirect costs are sometimes referred to as overhead costs and are applied to all procedures based on treatment time. Most clinics have a standardized overhead cost per hour.

Common indirect costs include rent, telephone, business telephone book advertising, and other generalized marketing.

inventory
an itemized list of merchandise or
supplies on hand

premium pricing
pricing strategy in which the price is
set high to compensate for a high
quality product, usually with a high
production cost as well

penetration pricing
pricing strategy in which the price is
set low, to allow for introduction into an
existing market

economy pricing
the low pricing of a product or service
as a means to entice costumers to buy

product bundling pricing
pricing strategy in which one or more
products or services are offered at a
discount

For the purpose of this text, we will focus on four distinct pricing strategies: (1) price and costs, (2) price and competitors, (3) price and customers, and (4) price and business objectives. These pricing strategies drive business objectives, compared to promotional pricing, which is an occasional "price break" that may be used to move overstock inventory, for example.

Pricing and Costs A business that offers hair removal must ensure the revenue it generates will yield a profit. Several different pricing tactics will help ensure that costs are covered, and should be evaluated based on different business models. The number of price tactics will depend on how many hair removal procedures you choose to offer and what the market will support. In the medical spa and day spa sector, one usually thinks of premium pricing, which uses high prices to communicate the uniqueness of the product or service.

The next type of price strategy that might be used in the spa is penetration pricing. With this strategy, the price is set low, to allow access into the market by gaining market share. The costs in this strategy are at a break-even or a loss of profit.

Next is economy pricing, which is a strategy that keeps costs low in order to provide the lowest cost to the customer. This is a very popular strategy and was made famous by Wal-Mart.

Product bundling pricing is a tactic commonly used in spas including the medical spa. This strategy is similar to the concept of *packages*, but is a bit more sophisticated because it combines multiple services (e.g., hair removal and facials bundled together). With product bundling, you look at the costs of each service and determine how much discount can be taken in exchange for collecting the fee in advance. Product bundling can also help the clinic: (1) be efficient in scheduling, (2) increase utilization by knowing the number of clients who have packages, (3) predict the number of patients that should be scheduling, and (4) introduce the clients to services that they may not experience otherwise.

While there are many other different types of pricing strategies (for example, product packages), these four are the most commonly used in the spa industry.

Evaluate your business objectives for the year before choosing a pricing strategy. Your objectives might include maximizing profits, attracting new clients, achieving a revenue goal, preventing further competition, or maintaining your market share. A business could use each of these pricing models at different times in the year to execute its plan.

Pricing and Competitors Entrepreneurship and competitiveness are often synonymous terms. In order for competition to translate into success, a hair removal business owner needs to walk the fine line between active interest and "nosy neighbor." By collecting small amounts of information, you can catch a glimpse of what the competition is doing with pricing, menu offerings, and employee compensation. The ability to collect and accurately translate this information into useful operational techniques for your own practice is a valuable skill for sizing up your own practice. The processes by which you choose to "get the goods" do not need to be extreme or invasive; you can draw conclusions simply by being watchful of advertising, listening to others, or attending public presentations.

Pricing and Customers   In retail business, it is said that the price of an item is the price the customer will pay,[3] meaning that the price of a product is consumer driven. This trend is also true in the spa or medical spa business. An important first step in setting your hair removal price is to understand your customer. Because hair removal services are competitive, customers may have already had the treatment at another clinic. For this reason, sometimes a brief customer survey is warranted. This is especially recommended if the service is being integrated into a larger facility to expand the menu. The survey should ask questions about the services that are planned and the products that will be used. Remember, perceived value tracks closely with the price a client is willing to pay. In a larger environment the survey should include a range of price such as $25–$50 and a choice of "yes" or "no" to answer this question on the survey. This will give the facility a good idea of a current client's perceived value of the newly added service. This price, of course, will not be the only marker used to set a price. In a smaller environment or as a single practitioner the process of surveying can be delicate because the technician has a personal relationship with the client. In this situation the question of pricing can be difficult and may be better avoided.

Although surveys can provide valuable information, they can be tricky to prepare. For example, framing questions so they do not influence the answer can sometimes be difficult. Therefore, a professional should prepare surveys that impact significant decisions, such as pricing. Otherwise, the information could be skewed or biased. Bear in mind that you cannot use the survey alone to create a price. Pricing is set based on several components: client surveys, competition pricing, and, last but not least, your costs and desired profits.

Pricing and Business Objectives   Pricing hair removal to facilitate the growth and profitability of your business is a smart industry tactic. However, when companies drastically cut prices in an effort to attract customers, the end result can be disastrous. To avoid using desperate, last option

Some simple survey questions might include:
- Have you ever received hair removal services?
- What method? Laser, electrolysis, waxing, other?
- If not, would you consider having the treatment?
- If appropriate for your environment, a question about pricing should appear. Survey the clients regarding what would be an appropriate price range for the various types of hair removal.

Example of a Three-Month Development Plan for Hair Removal Services

January

Objectives
1. Begin training programs.
2. Evaluate clinic database.

Tactics
1. Schedule training with clinic educator. Discuss with the manufacturer times for clinic meetings and educational presentations.
2. Create a criteria selection form for clinic database evaluation.

Goals
1. Complete training by February 25.
2. Have a list of potential clients from the database, ready for a marketing campaign by the end of January.

Costs
1. Training wages for all participating employees.

February

Objectives
1. Develop multipronged marketing campaign.
2. Evaluate progress of training to ensure we are on target.
3. Develop clinic goals.

Tactics
1. Develop email, in-house, and radio marketing strategies. Develop and print literature for hair removal, including informational brochures, "what to expect" literature, and pricing lists.
2. Evaluate testing of training sessions. Observe classroom and clinical training.
3. Analyze potential number of available clients.

Goals
1. Have literature ready by February 20. Have marketing campaigns ready to launch by February 20.
2. Ensure there are no glitches in the training process. Evaluate the model "reviews" of procedures.
3. Determine client and revenue goals.

Cost
1. Budget for printing literature.
2. Budget for first three months of hair removal marketing.

March

Objectives
1. Discuss goals with the staff.
2. Evaluate progress and schedule.
3. Understand the immediate success and opportunities of clinic performance.

Tactics
1. Meet with the staff and introduce the goals and bonus program for the hair removal launch.
2. Create a daily "hot-sheet."
3. Review feedback surveys from clients about the new treatment.

Goals
1. Get the staff excited and willing to participate in the growth of the new treatment.
2. Use the daily hot-sheet to ensure goals are being met.
3. Evaluate surveys for opportunities.

Cost
1. Bonus for staff members.

pricing decisions (and suffering the subsequent consequences), consider implementing a standard pricing policy. After using the tactics mentioned above to set the initial price, a standard pricing policy helps to guide the ongoing pricing process. The policy is a document controlled by the clinic manager or spa director that lists all the prices. The initial prices are calculated through a mathematical formula based on cost and a specific markup percentage. When prices are increased, the standard price is subsequently used based on the formula. This standard pricing method is far more effective than arbitrarily picking prices as in: "What is spa ABC charging? Oh, let us charge 50 cents less."

Standard pricing policies help the company meet its yearly business objectives. Yearly objectives are part of the annual business plan, which is a complex document that includes a budget, a marketing plan, and a growth plan. A comprehensive business plan updated on a yearly basis gives focus and depth to the business growth.

When a spa adds a service, such as hair removal, creating an isolated development plan for the growth of the procedure helps ensure its success. When you use a model such as the one depicted, you will want to make sure the information is sufficiently detailed and that it is tailored to your individual situation.

■ KEEPING YOUR BUSINESS MOVING

In order for your new hair removal service to thrive, you will need to keep up with the latest trends, regulations, and competition, which are collectively referred to as your business landscape. The business landscape will be the deciding factor in many areas, especially accurately and effectively marketing your hair removal program.

Three intertwined aspects of evaluating your business landscape are the marketplace, clients, and competition. Independently and consequentially, these three components are constantly changing. By identifying the present conditions of each component, you can evaluate the current landscape. The marketplace is different in every city, and it is sometimes even more localized than the city in which your business is located—it may be your local community. Therefore, in order to have a firm grasp on the marketplace, you must understand your city and local community.

With a comprehensive understanding of local dynamics, narrowing the area population down to your client base is the second and most misunderstood component of the business landscape. Understanding client base will have a domino effect on marketing, pricing, and many other components that are critical to the success of your business.

standard pricing policy
business document that outlines the specific price range of a given product or service, preferred pricing strategy, and circumstances during which each might change

yearly business objectives
part of the annual business plan that identifies the goals a business would like to attain during a given fiscal year

annual business plan
growth plan that outlines business objectives, marketing plans, and budgets for the period of one fiscal year

marketplace
any environment where two or more people buy or sell a product or service

Making a profit is the number one reason for being in business; otherwise, you are a nonprofit organization or out of business. Figuring out how to minimize costs, meet goals, pay bills, keep employees happy, and provide outstanding customer service can sometimes feel overwhelming. One particular strategy that ranks at the top to keep a business moving forward is revenue strategies or *how you price*. Understanding pricing strategies, how the competition determines price, and what the market will support in your client demographic requires insight, skill, and sometimes even intuition.

database
an electronic compilation of extensive categorical information relevant to business processes such as marketing or inventory

Finally, while knowing your marketplace and your clients will have a significant role in daily operations, understanding the competition does not. Therefore, it should not have an equal share of consideration. Worrying about your competition could become a distraction (or an obsession) that will only harm your practice. You should limit your understanding of similar businesses to the few bits of information you compile while assessing your competition (i.e., prices, menu, and promotions).

In addition to keeping current with your business landscape, moving forward includes accurate and regular monitoring, and daily tracking of operations and business risks. Establishing indicators and goals and understanding your financial statements plays a pivotal role. Reviewing indicators and goals weekly will help evaluate the performance of the technicians and the overall clinic. This review will pave the road to your success. In the following sections, we discuss the issues of your business landscape in more detail.

Understanding the Client

Understanding your client is helpful when designing your marketing plan. Most marketing principles are considered "the norm" because they have been proven to change or modify consumer behavior. However, a well-thought interpretation of your potential clients will help tailor your marketing campaigns to your client base rather than to broader populations. Enhanced collection and analysis will help refine marketing campaigns from conception to implementation.

An analysis of the existing client base will give you a composite sketch of your target demographic. The information to seek includes service preferences, price sensitivity, age, household income, knowledge of the industry, referral sources, and preconceived notions of the spa facilities and services.

Evaluate existing clients in the current database to identify those who might be interested in hair removal, based upon your composite sketch criteria. This can be done two ways: (1) through a survey, or (2) by a mathematical analysis based on growth. Using a survey is very simple if you create a brief questionnaire that clients fill out while waiting for treatments. To compensate clients for filling out the survey, you can offer them a hair removal treatment at an "introductory promotional price." Those not in the clinic during the time you are collecting surveys can be called or emailed with the survey.

Although using a mathematical approach may seem like "a stab in the dark," it is a useful and effective method. If you know the number of clients currently in your database, you can realistically project the potential number of clients that will eventually seek hair removal services. To accurately estimate the potential number, you should keep the number moderate, such as 2 to 5 percent of clients in the database.

With this information in hand, create an in-house campaign to capture patients. Current clients will be the first to experience and enjoy the hair removal treatment. To further increase the number of hair removal clients, create a referral offer for those who experience the treatment and refer a friend.

Understanding the Competition

Your competition is everywhere, even outside your business sector. Like it or not, the ideal is the marker against which the commonplace is compared. Your waiting area will be compared to the most exquisite furnishing fits for royalty. Your customer service will be held up to virtually unattainable standards. And yes, your treatment programs will be expected to surpass the abilities of the leading plastic surgeons. This is just what clients expect. This does not suggest your hair removal business should settle for mediocrity; rather it should ground you against putting emphasis on "keeping up with the Jones family" or overreaching your own business goals. Your hair removal business success will be served best by an internal motivation to satisfy your clients. Although other hair removal clinics in town and the Fortune 500 conglomerates across the globe are all competing for the same clients, you must shrink your description of competition to a short list of information that can facilitate your individual business goals.

Analyzing the competition can be distracting at times because you may want to know what they are doing, who their patients are, and what their treatments are. While it is important to know your competition's landscape, you should not become obsessed with them. The few key points to keep informed about your competition are pricing, common procedures, demographic target, and promotions. Once you know these few elements or have an idea of the direction of their business, stay informed but leave it alone. Use your time efficiently, by growing your own business rather than paying attention to someone else's business.

Researching competition across the country is important because it gives you an idea of the direction of the industry. Look for a few very progressive businesses on each coast and in the middle of the country. Stay current with what they are doing, including their pricing, procedures, promotions, literature, written materials, and Web site promotions. This will help you to know the trends and fads that develop in the industry and adjust your business if you wish.

Marketing

Developing marketing strategies (see Table 12–3) and watching them "bring in clients" can be very rewarding at times, but can be equally disconcerting at other times. Business growth followed by success is dependent on innovative and effective marketing. The marketing plan you create should utilize as many tactics as possible. Each tactic will have a different reach, appeal, and anticipated impact on the business. Your marketing tactics should remain varied and should include direct mail, email, newspaper, radio, television (if your budget allows), in-house strategies, and literature, to name a few.

Direct Mail

Direct mail is a commonly used tactic to introduce new services. The clinic or spa usually sends out a card or letter with an offer attached. Direct mail usually has a success rate of less than 1.5 percent. Although the average clinic believes direct mail to be a terrific way to introduce new services or products, it can be very expensive. Let us take a look.

Assuming a 1.5 percent success rate, sending out 1,000 cards will yield in 15 clients through the door. If the direct mail piece cost is $2.00 per card plus postage, the total per card is $2.39, which means the total cost for the mailer is $2,390. That means each of the 15 patients that come through the door must spend $158 each to cover just the cost of the mailer (not including overhead or profit. As you can see, an unexpectedly low yield in clients responding to a direct mail campaign could end up being very costly.

While direct mail can be successful, business owners should do the math to make sure the end justifies the means. Keep in mind that direct

Table 12–3 Marketing Strategies

Marketing Strategy	Breadth of Market Reach	Cost	Cost to Acquire Risk
Direct mail	Low	High	High
Email	Low	Low	Low
Newspaper	Moderate	High	High
Billboard	Moderate	Moderate	Moderate
Radio commercial	Moderate	Low	Low
Regional magazine	High	High	Moderate
Local affiliate television commercials	High	Moderate	Moderate

mailings are not a sure thing, and consider taking proactive steps to decrease the risk by "trimming the fat" from your mailing pool. For example, send direct mail pieces to only those clients who have responded positively to an in-house survey or who have visited the clinic in the past six months. A well-planned database should be able to do as much with little time. Also, consider a "cross-selling" direct mail campaign that combines one treatment (for example, a facial) with a promotional hair removal treatment. Because of the unpredictable nature of direct mail campaigns, you should consider mailing offers to a selected number of qualified patients rather than to your entire database.

Email

It is to your advantage to make it easy and rewarding for existing clients to volunteer their email addresses for in-house marketing and promotional use. By far, email is the most cost-effective means of communicating with clients. You can develop regular email specials and introduce new promotions with little effort and surprising results. When you put promotional signs in your office that say "Ask about our email-only specials," you will be surprised how many clients will give you their email addresses just because they do not want to be left out when there is a special available.

Newspaper

Newspaper advertising is a proven marketing method. In most cities, there are literally hundreds of ads for plastic surgery, spas, and medical skin care in weekend papers. When planning a newspaper advertisement, you should consider several questions: (1) Is your ad special or is it just one in the maze of many? (2) Are you participating in "advertorials"? (3) What is the competition doing?

   Although an effective method, advertising in newspapers can be an expensive tactic to acquire new patients. The question that must be answered when it comes to newspaper advertising (as with all tactics) is the cost to acquire. In other words how much money must be spent to get *one* new patient to walk through the door? Taken one step further, how many appointments will it take for the patient to spend enough money to cover the cost of the newspaper ad and begin to produce a profit for your clinic? Add into the financial mix the cost of ad design and additional marketing needs, and you may find that newspaper ads are too expensive unless you can really attract a substantial number of new patients.

cost to acquire
the average cost per new customer of any one marketing strategy

Radio

Radio advertising is a viable option for smaller markets. In larger metropolitan areas like Los Angeles or New York, the reach of the radio station may be too great to merit radio advertising. In other words, a large percentage of potential clients are simply too far away to consider driving to your clinic rather than to one closer to their house. However, even in these situations, radio provides great name recognition and branding. The important question to ask is, What is the primary objective of radio advertising? If it is to attract new clients, the larger the size of the city, the greater the risk of yielding an unsatisfactory number of new clients. Having said that, in smaller communities radio may work well, especially if there is a "morning drive time slot" and/or a DJ who will give live endorsements or testimonials.

In-House Strategies

In-house strategies are among the most effective and low-cost means of attracting new patients and increasing revenue. By implementing techniques such as cross-selling, "powering the patient database," and referral programs, you can create a sophisticated, layered initiative to generate additional revenue as well as flex your know-how.

First, business owners should learn and implement cross-selling, which is a technique of using an active patient in one category and moving him or her into other categories. For example, a client who is only in the clinic for Botox or dermal fillers may be open to the opportunity of experiencing hair removal. In fact, the client may be getting hair removal services at another clinic or spa. Cross-sales can be made by offering a gift certificate followed by a discount on a package sale. Cross-selling can also happen subtly when you combine procedures in a package. For example, when a client buys a facial package, include a couple of hair removal treatments. Almost everyone can benefit from hair removal, so it is really a win-win proposition for everyone.

Powering the database utilizes your existing database to uncover potential candidates for hair removal services. This method requires investigative work on the part of staff, but it is well worth the effort and time. Because it can cost 10 times more money to gain a new client than to keep an old client,[4] you should get to work on those clients who have already used your clinic. Look through the database and gather the names of clients who have not been in for awhile. Evaluate the number of "lost clients" and create a cross-selling campaign to entice them into the clinic again.

Use of a referral program will do a great job to collect new clients. Most clinics experience at least a 30 percent referral rate. In other words, each month 30 percent of your new clients come from the referral of satisfied clients. Do you reward those clients who send you business? If not, you might want to create a referral program for established clients. It is the easiest new patient you will get, and he or she is "pre-sold" because a

powering the patient database
in-house marketing strategy that involves innovative and detailed use of information already contained in a business database in order to increase traffic

referral programs
in-house marketing strategy that rewards an existing client for referring a new one

cross-selling
a term that describes the process of selling related, peripheral items to a customer

friend recommended your clinic as the best. The referral incentives could be gift certificates or cash rewards. That way everybody wins!

Literature

Having literature available describing the procedures you offer is an essential part of the in-house marketing campaign. Original literature specific to your practice can be informational, educational, and identifiable. If you do not print original literature, then be sure to have informational brochures that are supplied by the manufacturer of your equipment. If the manufacturer does not supply literature or brochures, vendors can often create "boilerplate" information that will work just fine. The important thing is that the literature is accurate and available.

Included in the literature category should be "posttreatment" instructions. Even if these are printed on your copy machine, you can still customize and enhance the presentation. However, the content is what is most important, and function should take obvious precedence over format. Written posttreatment instructions are important to ensure patients follow your instructions and that there are not any misunderstandings or unrealistic expectations.

Selling Hair Removal Treatments   So with all these marketing and advertising ideas in mind, how do you really sell hair removal treatments? It is more than the individual advantages of your device, or the personal style of each technician. As with any procedure or product, knowledge is the key to success (see Table 12–4): How much do you really know about the product or service you are selling? Assuming you are completely competent at the hair removal procedure, what you need is an organized plan to communicate the features and benefits to the client. The features describe how the program works, and the benefits list what it will do for the client. Organize your information by discussing the features first and concluding with the benefits.

> The best and worst forms of advertising are word of mouth or experienced based. These types of advertisements are reliable, affordable, achievable, and manageable. Try to make each client satisfied enough to want to tell at least one other person. Just think of the profound effect this would have on your business success. Conversely, making one client extremely disappointed in the services he or she received could have a detrimental impact on your business.

Table 12–4 Organizing Knowledge to Sell Your Treatment
What is hair removal?
What makes your treatment unique?
What are the features of your device?
Why do you prefer these features?
What home-care programs are associated with treatment?
What are the benefits of your hair removal program?

Well placed informational brochures throughout the clinic or spa inform and advertise.

Business Risks

In our litigious society, merely owning a business makes you susceptible to risk, let alone having a staff and equipment. Each year, the business owner should evaluate the potential risks that could damage the earning power of the company. Among the potentially harmful business risks are new government regulations, technology changes, decreased borrowing power of small businesses, and possible litigation. Make sure you have thought through potential problems and know what your plans are in response to a problem in the event your business faces a crisis.

Federal Government Regulations   Government regulations are a very real risk for the medical spa and luxury spa sector. For example, restrictions are put on who can perform hair removal and under what circumstances. The clinic director must be aware of the changes in government regulations.

State Government Regulations   Both the technician and the clinic should be aware of licensing regulations for hair removal. Each state is different, and the rules change often due to technology upgrades and physician input. Before beginning a laser hair removal business, be sure to check about licensure and the scope of practice in your particular state.

Technology Changes   Technology is advancing every day. Improvements in hand pieces, crystal management, and filters make new devices more attractive to technicians. Clients are more sophisticated than ever before, and, subsequently, their demands for the newest technology may drive decisions.

Liability Issues for the Clinic   Another important issue to investigate is malpractice insurance. Are new procedures covered by the insurance of the spa or the physician (if a medical spa)? Or will individuals need their own policies? Ask questions about training requirements because sometimes insurance carriers require additional training for employees providing hair removal. If the insurance is not provided by the physician or the spa, but by the technician individually, it is absolutely critical that copies of the policy be available to the spa director, the physician, and the medical spa, and that the technician understands that if there is a lapse in the policy that he or she will be suspended from providing services until the policy is renewed.

Just as the technician needs insurance, so does the clinic. A conversation with your insurance agent will direct you to the best approach and insurance company.

Indicators and Goals

Company history speaks not only to information such as, "this is where we came from and this is what we look like now," but also speaks to indicators and goals. While indicators and goals can sometimes sound financial in nature, indicators and goals really speak to history and the ability to exceed against the historical goals.

Setting goals for both the clinic and the technician is appropriate. Goals should reflect the number of patient calls, the number of patients scheduled, the number of patients treated, the referral patterns, and other important clinic indicators. Goals should translate directly to the revenue goal for the clinic.

The goals you establish should be attainable; otherwise, everyone gets discouraged. Failure is very harmful to employee morale and is something you do not want in your clinic. If hair removal services are being brought into an already established practice, the goals can be a little more aggressive because the client base is already established. If, on the other hand, your clinic is just starting, conservative numbers are in order. The goals should be established for the first six months, and evaluated monthly. This way you can determine how successful the process is, and, if needed, you can add more advertising or marketing to stimulate the number of visits or clients.

Set your goals and let the front desk and technician know these goals. Some managers like goal setting to be a collaborative process. This works only if you, as the manager, stretch your employees to accept goals that seem a bit out of reach. Because employees are a bit more conservative than managers, do not be surprised if your goals are a little higher than your employees'. Your goals might initially be broken down by: (a) how many clients are scheduled, and (b) how many clients are treated. Once you have these numbers, you can extrapolate the revenue. For example, if the goal is 50 clients and the price of the hair removal procedure is $210.00, your revenue treatment goal is $10,500.00 per month. In addition to the treatment goal, you should also calculate the product goal. For example, does every ticket need a product sale of at least $25.00? We know this will not happen, but the average product sales on hair removal tickets may come out to $25.00 and that is what you are looking to accomplish, a focus on additional sales.

Indicators track the progress of business goals. Daily or, at the longest interval, weekly review of each technician's hot-sheets will provide you with goal progress reports.

Without a weekly or daily hot-sheet, you do not have the opportunity for improvement. A hot-sheet for hair removal might include: number of

indicators
key values used to measure performance, over time, as it relates to an organization's goal progress

hot-sheets
daily or weekly progress reports that measure and provide daily insight into a business's or employee's performance

Initially you may find a daily review of indicators is not necessary. In that event, a weekly sheet will do. But only maintain weekly reviews for one week or else it becomes too easy to forget about the growth process. Unless daily reviews are conducted, at the end of the month you may be disappointed by the indicators, and by that point, nothing can be done to improve the numbers for the month.

Indicator Sheet

Hair Removal

	Week One	Week Two	Week Three	Week Four	Actual	Goal
Number of new clients booked						
Number of clients seen						
Number of clients rebooked (after treatment)						
Number of packages sold						
Revenue per ticket						
Service revenue per ticket						
Product revenue per ticket						

clients scheduled, number of clients seen, number of clients rebooked, average ticket revenue, and the breakdown between product and service revenue. You also might be interested in the referral pattern. The indicator hot-sheet should be the tool to evaluate, redirect, and grow the business. Over time it will be the comparative you use to measure your progress. Indicator sheets are simple in form. They need only the information you are looking for and should not be cumbersome.

Business Record Keeping　Record keeping is a broad category that includes business records and patient treatment records. We will discuss business record keeping in this section.

The records that should be kept for a business can be extensive, but with the computers and programs available today, it is much easier than it used to be. An organized business should include many different *sets* of information. Each set of information should be filed and organized monthly. Included in the financial information should be the following: tickets (i.e., cash, credit card), inventory, purchases, accounts payable (AP), and accounts receivable (AR). Other records that should be organized and on hand include: insurance records (health and liability), lease contracts, rent contracts, human resources records, marketing files, and patient database.

It is important to keep financial information organized and up-to-date. Financial data are the history of the company's performance and a road map to the future. Each year a notebook should be dedicated to your financial reports, and this should be divided into the 12 months with a 13th tab for a "year-end" report.

accounts payable
all accounting responsibilities associated with the recording and payment of all vendor related business expenditures

accounts receivable
all accounting responsibilities associated with the recording and allocation of all payments received by the business

All tickets should be kept with a notation whether the payment was cash or credit card. Refunds should be documented on a ticket and processed accordingly. It is wise to not allow cash refunds but offer store credit or product replacement. If a cash return has to be given, it should not be in cash from the register but refunded to a credit card or in the form of a check written and approved by the manager. The manager should approve all returns. Hopefully, you have a computer program that does the return for you. If so, a detailed printout should be made at the end of the month and placed in the notebook. The owner or bookkeeper should routinely go through the register tickets to look for irregularities and refunds. This protects the business from in-house theft.

Inventory should be done monthly. The worksheets to do the inventory and the computer printout should be filed in your notebook.

Purchases are the acquisitions of products, supplies, and other purchases you made throughout the month. A record of purchases (usually through a purchase order system) should be placed in your monthly notebook.

Accounts payable and accounts receivable reports should be placed monthly into the notebook. It is unusual to have account receivables, but if you do have house accounts, they should be very small.

Other records should be filed away in an accessible place and updated as required. Additional information that is accumulated should be placed into these files. These files do not change each year, but stay with the "timeless" files and always at hand.

Reading Income Statements

The income statement is a very important document. It is one of the documents a bank will ask to see when you are getting a loan or lease. You should review your income statement on a monthly basis. Review the *indicator hot-sheets* in tandem with income statements and then file them into the monthly notebook.

Learning to read an income statement is easy. Start at the top, look at the revenue or income line, which tells you how much money the business has made. It includes all the package treatments redeemed, but should not include the revenue from packages sold; that revenue goes onto the balance sheet in a category called deferred revenue. The revenue line should be broken into different types of revenue: facials, peels, hair removal, etc., so you know how much money you collected in each category.

The next line is cost of goods sold (COGS), which includes direct costs. Like the revenue, the COGS items should be broken into categories that correspond with the revenue categories.

purchase order system
a structured process a business undergoes in order to acquire materials needed for operation

income statement
the financial statement that summarizes the revenues generated and the expenses incurred by an entity during a period of time

balance sheet
document that states a business's assets and liabilities on a given date

deferred revenue
money that the organization has received, but has not yet earned as of the closing date on the balance sheet. The amount is carried as a liability until the organization provides the goods or services for which the money was received.

cost of goods sold
(COGS) directs costs of materials used in the products a business makes or sells

> The revenue on the income statement does not match the cash to the bank. Revenue on the income statement will reflect all treatments including redeemed package visits, which do not have cash attached because the package is generally prepaid.

The next line should be gross margin, which is the amount of money the business made before overhead costs. General costs should include: personnel, marketing, rent, telephone, and a general category. Finally, the income statement will include an item called income before taxes, which is the amount of money the business made before paying the government. A good computer system will allow you to look at all income statement categories with a percentage attached. This is an important feature because it helps understand the ratios at which the company is performing.

Understanding the Balance Sheet

The balance sheet is the partner document to the income statement. Banks require balance sheets because it tells them about the value of the business: your assets and your liabilities. The first category on the balance sheet is usually the assets, which includes equipment you own, cash in the bank, and other assets. The next category is the liabilities, which lists the company's debt. The balance sheet is a detailed snapshot of the company and helps anyone valuing the business clarity on its status.

Whether you are an independent technician renting a booth in a spa or a director of a multisite business, reviewing the income statement monthly and the indicator hot-sheet daily will help avoid some of this frustration of knowing where the money is being spent. When reviewing these documents, be sure to evaluate them against your budgeted estimates. Budgeting is a discipline that can help ensure that money goes to the categories you want and does not ooze into other places. But sometimes, despite your best efforts, it seems that you cannot direct the flow of cash. This usually means that you have a flawed budget or that costs are out of control. If this is happening, you may need a professional accountant to review your records and help locate problem areas. Keeping money where it belongs requires discipline and daily evaluation.

Conclusion

Starting a new business or adding to your existing business can be exhilarating and full of challenges. One thing that is always certain is that it is never as easy as it first appears. Those who are successful follow the intricate steps of business development, analysis, and the daily monitoring of progress. Hair removal is a worthwhile procedure, one that will improve the client's skin, and provides an expansion of the menu offerings. A well thought out and careful plan for implementing hair removal services will make a business competitive and successful.

▶ ▷ ▷ TOP 10 TIPS TO TAKE TO THE CLINIC

1. Hair removal packages are financially important to clinics and individual technicians.
2. A development plan can help a new and established business stay on target.
3. Direct costs are those associated with the procedure.
4. Indirect costs are also called overhead expenses.
5. Learning how to price procedures is important for the potential success of a business.
6. Banks like to review a business's balance sheet because it shows the value of the company.
7. Hot-sheets are the easiest way to track the success of a business.
8. Profit and loss statements are the monthly documents that show a company's performance.
9. Know how to cross-sell procedures.
10. Use your current patient database to help launch new procedures.

CHAPTER QUESTIONS

1. What is a balance sheet?
2. Why is it important?
3. Why should a hot-sheet be used?
4. What is the profit and loss statement?
5. How does a business development plan come together?
6. Why does a company need to understand direct costs?

CHAPTER REFERENCES

1. Cosmetic Surgery Times. (2001, August). *How to Buy a Hair Removal System Without Getting Skinned*. Available at http://www. cosmeticsurgerytimes.com
2. Brown, L., MD. (2003, March). *The Cosmetic Clinic: The Role of Hair Removal in Skin Care*. Available at http://www.skinandaging.com
3. Canada Business Service Centre. (2004, February 15). *Setting the Right Price*. Available at http://www.cbsc.org

4. Keller, K. L., Sternthal, B., & Tybout, A. (2002). Three Questions You Need to Ask About Your Brand. *Harvard Business Review*, 80(9).

BIBLIOGRAPHY

American Management Association. (2004, February 15). *A Baker's Dozen Pricing Strategies*. Available at http://www.amanet.org

Beer, K., MD. (2003, September). *The Cosmetic Clinic: Six Secrets to Success*. Available at http://www.skinandaging.com

Bennis, W. G., & Thomas, R. J. (2002). The Crucibles of Leadership. *Harvard Business Review*, 80(9).

Canada Business Service Centre. (2004, February 15). *Setting the Right Price*. Available at http://www.cbsc.org

Cosmetic Surgery Times. (2001, August). *How to Buy a Hair Removal System Without Getting Skinned*. Available at http://www.cosmeticsurgerytimes.com

Entrepreneur.com. (2001, October 2). *Avoid these "Destroy your business" Pitfalls*.

FaceForum. (2004, March 10). *Hair Removal Costs: How Much Does Hair Removal Cost?* Available at http://www.faceforum.com

Gail, S. (2003, July 1). *Mirror, Mirror on the Wall, Are Men So Vain After All?* Available at http://www.cosmeticsurgerytimes.com

Grima, D. (2004, February 15). *Keeping Tabs on Your Competition*. Available at http://www.santuccibrown.com

Intermediainc.com Weekend Reading. (2001, July 27). Acquire Consumers for Show, Retain Customers for the Dough.

Keller, K. L., Sternthal, B., & Tybout, A. (2002). Three Questions You Need to Ask About Your Brand. *Harvard Business Review*, 80(9).

Khurana, R. (2002). The Curse of the Superstar CEO. *Harvard Business Review*, 80(9).

MarketingTeacher.com. (2004, February 13). *Pricing Strategies Lesson*. Available at http://www.marketingteacher.com

Matarasso, S. L., Glogau, R. G., & Markley, A. C. (1994, June). Wood's Lamp for Superficial Chemical Peels. *Journal of American Academic Dermatology*, 30(6), 988–992.

Millenium Research Group. (2002, July). *US Hair Removal Market 2002*. Available at http://www.mindbranch.com

Nemko, M. (2000, March). *Perfecting Your Pricing Strategies*. Available at http://www.entrepreneur.com

Obagi. (2004, March 10). *Selecting a Hair Removal Device*. Available at http://www.obagi-me.com

Parisian Peel Medical Hair Removal. (2004, March 10). *Hair Removal Skin Renewal Market Study Confirms Growth, Cites "Second Generation Technology."* Available at http://www.parisianpeel.com

Parisian Peel Medical Hair Removal. (2000, October 10). *Aesthetic Buyers Guide: Hair Removal Market Study Defines Industrey Leaders and Market Size.* Available at http://www.parisianpeel.com

Smith-Isroelit, B. (2004, January 21). *Spa Finder's 2004 Trends and Predictions.* Available at http://www.spatrade.com

Spatrade. (2004, February 5). *Spas Leading Outlets for Professional Skin Care Brands.* Available at http://www.spatrade.com

Troy, B. (2003, October 1). *Patient Experience Makes Your Bottom Line.* Available at http://www.cosmeticsurgerytimes.com

Tutor2u.com. (2004, February 13). *Pricing.* Available at http://www.tutor2u.net

Urbany, J. (2003, Fall). *Getting the Price Right: What Gets in the Way.* Available at http://www.nd.edu

Glossary

A

absorption the uptake of one substance into another

accounts payable all accounting responsibilities associated with the recording and payment of all vendor related business expenditures

accounts receivable all accounting responsibilities associated with the recording and allocation of all payments received by the business

Accutane® An oral prescription medication used to treat acne

Achard-Thiers syndrome a disorder mainly affecting postmenopausal women, marked by diabetes mellitus and hirsutism, deep masculine voice, facial hypertrichosis, and obesity

acid mantle the bacteria-killing layer made of sweat and lipids

acne vulgaris the "common acne" characterized by blackheads and pimples; found most commonly in teenagers and young adults

acromegaly chronic condition affecting middle aged individuals characterized by bone enlargement and thickening of soft tissues

active medium the part of a laser that absorbs and stores energy

Addison's disease condition in which the adrenal glands fail to produce enough hormones

adenohypophysis the anterior part of the pituitary gland

adipose tissue connective tissue in animal bodies that contains fat

adrenal cortex outer portion of the adrenal gland

adrenal glands hormone producing glands situated above each kidney

adrenal medulla central portion of the adrenal gland

adrenogenital syndrome condition characterized by excessive androgen production; the stimulation of male characteristics

alternating current electric current that regularly reverses direction

ampere basic unit of electric current that measures the current's force

amplification the creation of a new photon of light, resulting from a chain reaction involving the collision of other photons

anagen the growth phase in the hair cycle in which a new hair is synthesized

303

anaphoresis process whereby ions are negatively charged

androgens hormones that promote the production of male characteristics

anions negatively charged ions

annual business plan growth plan that outlines business objectives, marketing plans, and budgets for the period of one fiscal year

anode pole pole used to positively charge ions

antidiuretic affects the volume of urine excreted

apocrine glands in the axillae and groin that secrete sweat and substances that, when contaminated with bacteria, produce body odor

appendages any anatomical structures associated with a larger structure; for the skin, its appendages include hair, glands, and pores

argon a chemical element in the form of an inert gas used in the creation of early lasers

arrector pili an appendage that is attached to the dermal papilla and to the hair shaft

arteries carry oxygenated blood away from the heart

avascular lacking in blood vessels and, thus, having a poor blood supply

axillae underarm

azulene an oil that is part of the chamomile essential oil, produced specifically by distillation

B

balance sheet document that states a business's assets and liabilities on a given date

blend method method of electrolysis that combines thermolysis and galvanic electrolysis

blending waxing technique that transitions wanted hair into unwanted hair, preventing a line from occurring

bloodborne pathogens infectious substances present in the blood that can cause infection or disease. HIV and HCV are bloodborne pathogens.

body dysmorphic disorder psychosocial disease that causes individuals to be inappropriately concerned with their appearance. Those affected with BDD are contraindicated for most aesthetic procedures.

C

candelilla wax a type of vegetable wax derived from the candelilla plant

career plan action taken on by an aesthetician to set goals and actions taken to ensure their realization

carnauba wax the hardest and most widely used vegetable wax; derived from the leaves of the carnauba palm tree

catagen the transition stage of the hair's growth cycle; the period between the growth and resting phases

cataphoresis the process whereby ions are positively charged

cathode pole pole used to negatively charge ions

cations positively charged ions

ceramides a class of lipids that do not contain glycerol

cholesterol an alcohol distributed in animal tissues and synthesized in the liver. A precursor to certain hormones and, in some individuals, coronary artery disease.

chromophores the elements that laser light is attracted to; blood, hair color

circuit route around which an electrical current can flow, beginning and ending at the same point

circuit breaker an automatic switch used in electricity to prevent the flow of electricity in an overload of electricity

clinic protocols any set of rules or guidelines established by a clinic for safe practice. These guidelines will vary by location, yet are expected to be observed by clinicians working within the individual clinic.

club hair hair that has lost its root structure and that, when shed from the follicle, exhibits a round shape

coherent light light waves that travel in parallel and in the same direction

collagen fiber made of protein that gives the skin its form and strength

collagenous of collagen fibers

collimated light refers to a very thin beam of laser light, in which all rays run parallel

conductor a substance that allows electricity to pass through it

connective tissue fibrous tissue that binds, protects, cushions, and supports the various parts of the body

constriction the process of narrowing

consultation initial visit with a professional during which the client and the professional both investigate whether a specific treatment or service is warranted or achievable

contaminated the act of making an item or compound nonsterile or impure

Continuing Education Units (CEU) any certified training or event which is intended to build or add skills

converter a device used to change alternating current to direct current

cornified hardening or thickening of the skin

corpus luteum endocrine secreting progesterone

cortex the middle layer of the hair; a fibrous protein core formed by elongated cells containing melanin

corticosteroids hormonal substances that regulate biochemical reactions to occur at prescribed optimal rates

cortisone a hormone secreted by the adrenal gland used to treat rheumatoid arthritis and allergies

cosmeceuticals those products that do more than decorate or camouflage but less than a drug would do

cost of goods sold (COGS) directs costs of materials used in the products a business makes or sells

cost to acquire the average cost per new customer of any one marketing strategy

cretinism congenital condition characterized by decreased mental and physical activity caused by reduced thyroid secretions

cross-selling a term that describes the process of selling related, peripheral items to a customer

cryogen a substance used to produce extremely low temperatures

Cushing's syndrome a disease that is caused by a high amount of adrenocortical hormone; the condition is characterized by excessive pituitary gland secretions

cuticle the outermost layer of hair consisting of one overlapping layer of transparent, scale-like cells

D

database an electronic compilation of extensive categorical information relevant to business processes such as marketing or inventory

deferred revenue money that the organization has received, but has not yet earned as of the closing date on the balance sheet. The amount is carried as a liability until the organization provides the goods or services for which the money was received.

dermal-epidermal junction where the dermis and the epidermis meet

dermal papilla small, cone-shaped indentation at the base of the hair follicle that fits into the hair bulb; also called the hair papilla

dermal scattering the change that occurs between the laser's spot size at the surface of the skin and the spot size deeper in the tissue

dermis underlying or inner layer of the skin

desmosomes small hair-like structures in the spiny layer of the epidermis

desquamation the act of exfoliating dead skin cells

diabetes insipidus type of diabetes characterized by excessive urine output

diabetes mellitus type of diabetes characterized by poor production or utilization of insulin

diathermy a treatment accomplished by passing high-frequency electric currents to generate heat; as it pertains to electrolysis, used synonymously with thermolysis

differentiate to make something stand out or be unique compared to something that would otherwise be similar

Differin® A topical prescription medication used to treat acne

dilation the process of widening or expanding

diopter unit of measurement relating to the power of a lens

direct costs costs that are directly and exclusively attributable to a specific product or service

direct current electric current that flows constantly in one direction

E

eccrine glands throughout the skin that excrete mainly water and salt

economy pricing the low pricing of a product or service as a means to entice costumers to buy

edema a condition of excessive fluid retention; swelling

effleurage a rhythmic, gentle stroking of the skin, often just using the fingertips, which does not attempt to move the muscle underneath

eflornithine chemical substance in the commercial cream Vaniqa™; blocks or inhibits hair growth

elastin connective tissue proteins

electrologist someone skilled in the use of electricity to remove moles, warts, or hair roots; synonymous with electrolysist

electrology the general study of electricity and its properties

electrolysis the use of an electric current to remove moles, warts, or hair roots

electrolysist someone skilled in the use of electricity to remove moles, warts, or hair roots: synonymous with electrologist

electrons stable, negatively charged elementary particles that orbit the nucleus of an atom

eleidin a substance in the stratum lucidum

endocrine system network of glands and organs that produce hormones

endocrinologist one who studies hormones and glands

energy fluence the energy level of a laser; measured in joules

energy source the device in a laser that supplies energy to the active medium

enzymes proteins that act as biochemical catalysts

epidermis the thin, outermost layer of the skin

epilepsy medical disorder involving episodes of abnormal electrical discharge in the brain characterized by seizures, convulsions, and loss of consciousness

epinephrine hormone that produces the fight or flight response

estrogen female hormone

ethyl alcohol a colorless liquid with a fruity smell produced by fermentation; often used as a solvent; synonymous with ethanol

excited states the conditions of a physical system in which the energy level is higher than the lowest possible level

excretion the act of discharging waste matter from tissues or organs

exocrine secreting externally through a gland

exogen fourth stage of hair, currently being studied

external root sheath the inner side of the follicular canal, which is made of horny epidermal tissue

F

fatlah Egyptian word for threading

fatty acids one of many molecules that are long chains of lipid-carboxylic acid found in fats and oils

fiber optics a delivery system for lasers; the light runs through small glass cables inside a handpiece

filaggrin synthesizes lipids (fats) that are thought to serve as "intercellular cement"; important component of NMF

Fitzpatrick Skin Typing method of skin typing that considers skin's complexion, hair color, eye color, ethnicity, and the individual's reaction to unprotected sun exposure

fixed price a price that remains the same, usually for a set time period

follicular canal the depression in the skin that houses the entire pilosebaceous unit

fuse an electrical safety device that contains a piece of metal that will melt if the current running through it exceeds a certain level

G

galvanic electrolysis a modality of electrolysis using direct current with positive and negative poles that causes the production of caustic lye in the hair follicle, which in turn causes the hair's destruction

glabella the area between the eyebrows that causes a frown

glucagons hormones that have the ability to increase blood glucose levels

glucocorticoids hormones that are involved in metabolism

glycerol ester a refined rosin product that can be mixed with honey to produce a wax-like substance

glycosaminoglycans (GAGs) polysaccharide chains, most prominent in the dermis, that bind with water, smoothing and softening the surface from below

goiter an enlargement of the thyroid gland

gonadotropic pertaining to the gonads

grand mal a serious form of epilepsy in which there is loss of consciousness and severe convulsions

ground state the condition of a physical system in which the energy is at its lowest possible level

ground substance consists mainly of glycosaminoglycans (hyaluronic acid, chondroitin sulfate, and dermatan sulfate); involved in maintenance and repair of dermis

H

hair follicle bulb the bulbous base of the hair follicle that houses the dermal papilla

hair matrix the germinating center of the hair follicle where mitotic activity occurs

hard wax depilatory wax used without a strip

hemophilia recessive genetic disorder occurring almost exclusively in men and boys in which the blood clots much more slowly than normal, resulting in extensive bleeding from even minor injuries

hirsutism condition characterized by abnormal hair growth

histamine a normal substance found in the body that is released from injured cells

hood when the upper eyelid falls over the upper eye lashes

hormones biochemical regulating agents of the body

hot-sheets daily or weekly progress reports that measure and provide daily insight into a business's or employee's performance

hydrochloric acid a colorless acid that is highly acidic

hydroquinone a white, crystalline compound used in skin bleaching

hyperpigment overstimulation of tyrosine in the melanocytes

hyperpigmentation overproduction and over deposits of melanin

hypertrichosis condition characterized by excessive hair

hypodermis layer of subcutaneous fat and connective tissue lying beneath the epidermis

hypopigmentation a lack of melanin product

hypothalamus part of the brain responsible for the release of hormones

hypothyroidism condition characterized by excessive release of thyroid hormones

I

image business type of business in which the way the public views the company is based largely upon how things look, or how they are perceived, more than actual performance

impressions lasting opinions or judgments of something

income statement the financial statement that summarizes the revenues generated and the expenses incurred by an entity during a period of time

indicators key values used to measure performance, over time, as it relates to an organization's goal progress

indirect costs costs necessary for the functioning of the organization as a whole, but that cannot be directly assigned to one service or product

in phase a property of light characterized by waves traveling in parallel and in the same direction

insulator a material or device that prevents or reduces the passage of electricity

integumentary system the skin and its accessory organs, such as the sebaceous and sweat glands, sensory receptors, hair, and nails

internal root sheath the innermost layer of the hair follicle, closest to the hair

interstitial fluid the fluid between cells

inventory an itemized list of merchandise or supplies on hand

ionization a process in which an atom or a molecule loses or gains electrons, acquiring an electrical charge

iontophoresis a method by which drugs or solutions are introduced into the body via electrical current

islets of Langerhans clusters of cells in the pancreas that are responsible for the production of insulin

isopropyl alcohol a colorless, flammable alcohol often used as a solvent

J

joules units of energy or work

K

keratin a protein found in the skin that helps guard against invasion

keratinization the process of living cells moving upward and changing to dead cells

keratinocytes any cell in the skin, hair, or nails that produces keratin

keratohyalin granules substance in cytoplasm cells of the stratum granulosum

khite Arabic word for threading

L

lactogenic hormone a hormone that induces the secretion of milk; prolactin

lamellar granules control lipids that produce NMF

Langerhans' cells cells found in the epidermis that warn against the invasion of microorganisms and respond to that invasion

lanugo soft, downy hair present on fetuses in utero, and infants at birth

leukocytes white blood cells or corpuscles

Leydig cells produces testosterone

lipids fat or fat-like substances, descriptive not chemical

luteinizing hormone hormone that stimulates the corpus luteum

lymph a fluid found in the lymphatic vessels

lymphocytes cells produced in the lymph nodes, spleen, and thymus gland that produce antibodies capable of attacking infection

M

malpighian a skin layer made of the stratum mucosum and the stratum germinativum

marketing strategies planned use of marketing elements and media pathways to create a strategy to introduce new clients or reactivate former clients

marketplace any environment where two or more people buy or sell a product or service

mast cells large tissue cells present in the skin that produce histamine and other acute symptoms of allergic reactions

medulla the innermost layer of hair; composed of round cells; often absent in fine hair

Meissner's corpuscles nerve endings in the skin that are sensitive to touch

melanin grains of pigment that give hair and skin its color

melanocytes melanin-forming cells

melatonin hormone responsible for color changes

melting points temperature at which wax begins to liquefy

Merkel cell usually close to nerve endings and may be involved in sensory perception

metabolism the ongoing conversion of food into energy and the distribution of required biochemicals throughout the body

metastable in an apparent state of equilibrium, but likely to change to a more truly stable state if conditions change

milliampere meter a device that measures electric current in units of 1/1000 of an ampere

milliamperes units of electric current, one of which equals 1/1000 of an ampere

mineralocorticoids hormones responsible for fluid balance; steroids that promote the reabsorption of salt and the excretion of potassium in the kidneys

mission statement written statement of a business's individual philosophy

mitosis the process by which a cell divides into two daughter cells

monochromatic light of one wavelength, which therefore appears as one color

muslin strips thin, plain-weave cotton cloth strips used for removing wax from the skin

myxedema condition characterized by hypofunctioning of the thyroid gland

N

nanometers each is one billionth of a meter

natural moisturizing factor (NMF) compound found only in the top layer of skin that gives cells their ability to bind with water

neurohypophysis hormone secreting part of the pituitary gland

Nikolski sign a condition on the skin characterized by blistering or epidermal separation, caused by lateral pressure on the skin

norepinephrine important neurotransmitter

O

Occupational Safety and Health Administration (OSHA) federal agency responsible for defining and regulating safety in the workplace

ohm a unit that measures the amount of resistance, indicating whether a higher voltage is required to push a current through a conductor

Ohm's law the law of physics that states that electric current is directly proportional to the voltage applied to a conductor and inversely proportional to that conductor's

optical cavity the part of the laser that contains the active medium

overhead costs indirect costs

oxytocin hormone that stimulates contractions of the womb during childbirth

P

Pacinian's corpuscles found in the subcutaneous tissue; sensory nerve endings

papillae cone-shaped, finger-like projections that protrude into the epidermis

papillary dermis the most superficial layer of the dermis

parahormone a chemical substance that has a stimulating effect, but does not originate from the endocrine system

parathyroid glands tiny masses of glands found on the back of the thyroid

Pellon strips a soft-woven, paper-like strip used for removing wax from the skin

penetration pricing pricing strategy in which the price is set low, to allow for introduction into an existing market

perception process by which individuals use their senses to make decisions or gather information

petit mal a form of epilepsy marked by episodes of brief loss of consciousness without convulsions or falling

pheromones chemicals produced by humans and other animals that, when secreted, influence other members of the same species

phlebitis inflammation of the wall of a vein

phoresis process in which chemical solutions can be forced into unbroken skin using galvanic current

photodynamic therapy a chemical reaction activated by light; this reaction selectively destroys tissue

photon cascade excited, parallel photons of light of the same energy, wavelength, and in phase

photons miniscule units of electromagnetic radiation or light

pilosebaceous unit hair follicle and accompanying sebaceous glands and arrector pili muscle

pineal gland secretes melonin

pituitary gland growth inducing gland found at the base of the brain; a major endocrine organ

point effect the concentration of high frequency current at the tip of the probe

polychromatic consisting of light of multiple wavelengths, appearing as different colors

polycystic ovary syndrome a disease that may constitute the following symptoms typically in childbearing women: high levels of androgens, an irregular or no menstrual cycle, possible small ovarian cysts

postinflammatory hyperpigmentation dyschromia associated with injury to the skin

powering the patient database in-house marketing strategy that involves innovative and detailed use of information already contained in a business database in order to increase traffic

premium pricing pricing strategy in which the price is set high to compensate for a high quality product, usually with a high production cost as well

pricing strategies process by which a business determines the best way to price its product or service in order to entice customers while allowing for profit

product bundling pricing pricing strategy in which one or more products or services are offered at a discount

professional ethics set of guidelines that should set a framework for professional behavior and responsibilities

progesterone female sex hormone

progressive improvement plan administrative document that is intended to record a problem and the actions that will be taken to improve the problem in order to prevent its reoccurrence

prostaglandins substances that resemble hormones

pseudofolliculitis barbae form of folliculitis, commonly seen as a result of shaving or waxing

psoriasis skin disease marked by red scaly patches

pulse duration the duration of an individual pulse of laser light; usually measured in milliseconds; also see "pulse width"

pulse width see "pulse duration"

pumping the process whereby the energy source supplies energy to the active medium

purchase order system a structured process a business undergoes in order to acquire materials needed for operation

R

rectifier an electronic device that converts alternating current (see preceding) to direct current

referral programs in-house marketing strategy that rewards an existing client for referring a new one

reflexology system of massage in which certain body parts are massaged in specific areas in order to favorably influence other body functions

resonator another term for "optical cavity"

reticula a protein fiber

reticular dermis a deep layer of the dermis; composed of dense bundles of collagen fibers; contains vessels, glands, nerve endings, and follicles

Retin-A® A topical medication originally used to treat acne; now also used to treat lines, wrinkles, and discolorations of the skin

rheostat a resistor designed to allow variation in resistance without breaking the electrical circuit

rosin a hard, translucent resin derived from the sap, stumps, and other parts of pine trees

S

Safety Bill of Rights original name for OSHA manual

safety manual OSHA document that outlines the hazardous materials and equipment specific to each location and the safety protocols for each

sebaceous glands oil glands of the skin connected to hair follicles

secretion the process of producing and discharging substances from glands

selective photothermolysis the selective targeting of an area using a specific wavelength to absorb light into that target area sufficient to damage the tissue of the target while allowing the surrounding area to remain relatively untouched

seminiferous producing semen

septum the part of the nose that divides the two nostrils

singlet state a state of higher energy of atoms arrived at upon excitation

skin condition fundamental skin classification in which an individual's skin is grouped according to the degree of moisture retention and/or its reaction to products or environment

skin typing a more detailed skin classification that gives indications as to how a certain skin type will react to various treatment conditions

splattering the appearance of tiny black spots, which are singed hairs, in hair follicles; caused by laser treatments

spontaneous emission the process whereby an excited atom, after holding extra energy for a fraction of a second, releases its energy as another photon, then falls back to its grounded state

spot size the width of a laser beam

standard pricing policy business document that outlines the specific price range of a given product or service, preferred pricing strategy, and circumstances during which each might change

Stein-Leventhal syndrome disease characterized by hyperandrogenism and chronic anovulation in women

steroid dependent dermatoses a condition in which the long-term overuse of topical steroid creams causes the skin to require continued usage to keep the offending condition away

steroids a group of chemicals that include hormones

stimulated emission the process whereby a newly created photon of light (generated through amplification) acquires energy equal to the photons that created it and travels in the same direction

stratified epithelium layers of tissue that lack blood vessels; acts as a surface barrier

stratum basale single cell layer that is the deepest layer of the epidermis

stratum corneum superficial sublayer of the epidermis; varies in thickness over the body

stratum germinativum the lower level of the epidermis where cell division occurs

stratum granulosum the granular layer of skin found at the bottom of the horny zone

stratum lucidum the layer between the stratum corneum and the stratum granulosum in the palms of the hands and the soles of the feet

stratum mucosum single-cell layer of the epidermis; found above the stratum germinativum

stratum spinosum the superior layer of the stratum germinativum; named for its shape and spiny, thorn-like protrusions; also known as the "prickle cell layer"

strip method technique of hair removal using a strip over the sugar or wax for removal

subcutis a layer of subcutaneous tissue

sudoriferous glands the skin's sweat glands

sugar wax a hair-removal product that is made primarily of sugar; technique sensitive

T

technique sensitive a procedure that is performed differently from aesthetician to aesthetician based on his or her experience and knowledge

telogen the resting phase of the hair follicle in its growth cycle

terminal hair hair found on the scalp, arms, legs, axillae, and pubic area (postpuberty)

thermal relaxation time the amount of time it takes a substance (e.g., dermal tissue), after heating, to return to its normal temperature

thermal storage coefficient the measure of heat stored in a chromophore

thermolysis the breakdown of a substance by heat; as it pertains to electrolysis, used synonymously with diathermy

thioglycolate a salt used in the solutions for hair permanents

threading method of hair removal using strands of thread

throcalcitonin thyroid hormone that reduces blood calcium levels, also called calcitonin

thrombosis formation or presence of one or more blood clots that may partially or completely block an artery, for example, flowing to the heart or brain or a vein

thymosin hormones responsible for the production of T cells

thymus organ responsible for the production of T cells

thyrotropic hormone hormone that stimulates the thyroid gland

thyroxine main thyroid hormone responsible for metabolism and growth

transepidermal water loss (TEWL) the process by which our bodies constantly lose water via evaporation

transformer a device that transfers electrical energy from one alternating circuit to another with a change in voltage, current, phase, or impedance

tubules very small tubes

tyrosine an amino acid present in melanocytes

U

Universal Precautions preventative actions taken to prevent the transmission of infectious diseases; involves the use of protective procedures and equipment, such as gloves and masks

unrealistic expectations belief that a certain outcome is possible, regardless of merit or circumstance

urticaria pigmentosa hives that pigment; Dariers sign

V

vasopressin hormone that is responsible for blood pressure

veins carry unoxygenated blood to the lungs

vellus fine, short hair with no pigment, found mainly on women's faces; also referred to as "peach fuzz"

volt the force needed to send 1 ampere of electric current through 1 ohm of resistance

watt the unit of power produced by a current of 1 ampere acting across a potential difference of 1 volt

wavelength the distance between two consecutive peaks or troughs in a wave

Y

yearly business objectives part of the annual business plan that identifies the goals a business would like to attain during a given fiscal year

Index

NOTES

NOTES

NOTES

NOTES

NOTES

NOTES

NOTES

NOTES

NOTES

NOTES

NOTES

NOTES